Diseases of the Gastrointestinal Tract and Associated Infections

Guest Editor

GUY D. ESLICK, PhD, MMedSc(Clin Epi), MMedStat

INFECTIOUS DISEASE CLINICS OF NORTH AMERICA

www.id.theclinics.com

Consulting Editor

ROBERT C. MOELLERING Jr, MD

December 2010 • Volume 24 • Number 4

SAUNDERS an imprint of ELSEVIER, Inc.

W.B. SAUNDERS COMPANY
A Division of Elsevier Inc.
1600 John F. Kennedy Blvd., Suite 1800, Philadelphia, PA 19103-2899.
http://www.theclinics.com
INFECTIOUS DISEASE CLINICS OF NORTH AMERICA Volume 24, Number 4
December 2010 ISSN 0891–5520, ISBN-13: 978-1-4377-2461-5

Editor: Barbara Cohen-Kligerman
Developmental Editor: Donald Mumford

Infectious Disease Clinics of North America (ISSN 0891–5520) is published in March, June, September, and December by Elsevier Inc., 360 Park Avenue South, New York, NY 10010-1710. Periodicals postage paid at New York, NY and additional mailing offices. Subscription prices are $251.00 per year for US individuals, $435.00 per year for US institutions, $124.00 per year for US students, $297.00 per year for Canadian individuals, $538.00 per year for Canadian institutions, $355.00 per year for international individuals, $538.00 per year for international institutions, and $171.00 per year for Canadian and international students. To receive student rate, orders must be accompained by name of affiliated institution, date of term, and the *signature* of program/residency coordinator on institution letterhead. Orders will be billed at individual rate until proof of status is received. Foreign air speed delivery is included in all *Clinics* subscription prices. All prices are subject to change without notice. **POSTMASTER**: Send address changes to *Infectious Disease Clinics of North America,* Elsevier Health Sciences Division, Subcription Customer Service, 3251 Riverport Lane, Maryland Heights, MO 63043. **Customer Service: 1-800-654-2452 (US). From outside of the US and Canada, call 1-314-447-8871. Fax: 1-314-447-8029. E-mail: JournalsCustomerService-usa@elsevier.com (print support) or JournalsOnlineSupport-usa@elsevier.com (online support).**

Infectious Disease Clinics of North America is also published in Spanish by Editorial Inter-Médica, Junin 917, 1er A 1113, Buenos Aires, Argentina.

Reprints. For copies of 100 or more, of articles in this publication, please contact the Commercial Reprints Department, Elsevier Inc., 360 Park Avenue South, New York, New York 10010-1710. Tel. (212) 633-3812, Fax: (212) 462-1935, E-mail: reprints@elsevier.com.

Infectious Disease Clinics of North America is covered in *MEDLINE/PubMed (Index Medicus), Current Contents/Clinical Medicine, Science Citation Alert, SCISEARCH,* and *Research Alert.*

Printed and bound by CPI Group (UK) Ltd, Croydon, CR0 4YY
Transferred to Digital Print 2011

Contributors

CONSULTING EDITOR

ROBERT C. MOELLERING JR, MD
Shields Warren-Mallinckrodt Professor of Medical Research, Harvard Medical School; Department of Medicine, Beth Israel Deaconess Medical Center, Boston, Massachusetts

GUEST EDITOR

GUY D. ESLICK, PhD, MMedSc(Clin Epi), MMedStat
The Whiteley-Martin Research Centre, Discipline of Surgery, The University of Sydney, Sydney Medical School, Sydney, Australia

AUTHORS

AHMED ABU-SHANAB, MB BCh, MSc, MRCP
Research Fellow, Alimentary Pharmabiotic Centre, University College Cork, Cork, Ireland

PREMYSL BERCIK, MD
Associate Professor, Department of Medicine, Farncombe Family Digestive Health Research Institute, Faculty of Health Sciences, McMaster University, Hamilton, Ontario, Canada

CAROLINA M. BOLINO, MD
Department of Medicine, Farncombe Family Digestive Health Research Institute, Faculty of Health Sciences, McMaster University, Hamilton, Ontario, Canada

CHIARA BRACONI, MD, PhD
Department of Internal Medicine, The Ohio State University Medical Center, Columbus, Ohio

MARKUS W. BÜCHLER, MD
Chairman, Department of General Surgery, University of Heidelberg, Heidelberg, Germany

ILSEUNG CHO, MD, MS
Division of Gastroenterology, Department of Medicine, New York University School of Medicine, New York, New York

PELAYO CORREA, MD
Professor of Medicine, Division of Gastroenterology, Vanderbilt University School of Medicine, Nashville, Tennessee

MEIRA EPPLEIN, PhD
Assistant Professor, Division of Epidemiology, Vanderbilt University School of Medicine, Nashville, Tennessee

GUY D. ESLICK, PhD, MMedSc(Clin Epi), MMedStat
The Whiteley-Martin Research Centre, Discipline of Surgery, The University of Sydney, Sydney Medical School, Sydney, Australia

SUBRATA GHOSH, MD, FRCP(C), FRCP(E)
Head and Professor of Medicine, Division of Gastroenterology, University of Calgary, Calgary, Alberta, Canada

NAZIA HASAN, MD, MPH
Department of Medicine, New York University School of Medicine, New York, New York

KABIR JULKA, MD
Senior Fellow, Division of Gastroenterology, University of Washington, Seattle, Washington

CYNTHIA W. KO, MD, MS
Associate Professor, Division of Gastroenterology, University of Washington, Seattle, Washington

LAURA W. LAMPS, MD
Professor and Vice-Chair; Director, Diagnostic Laboratories, Department of Pathology, University of Arkansas for Medical Sciences, Little Rock, Arkansas

REMO PANACCIONE, MD, FRCP(C)
Associate Professor of Medicine and Director, Inflammatory Bowel Disease Clinic, Division of Gastroenterology, University of Calgary, Calgary, Alberta, Canada

TUSHAR PATEL, MBChB
Professor of Medicine, Department of Internal Medicine, The Ohio State University Medical Center, Columbus, Ohio

M. BLANCA PIAZUELO, MD
Research Instructor, Division of Gastroenterology, Vanderbilt University School of Medicine, Nashville, Tennessee

ARI POLLACK, BA
Department of Medicine, Columbia University School of Medicine, New York, New York

EAMONN M.M. QUIGLEY, MD, FRCP, FACP, FACG, FRCPI
Professor of Medicine and Human Physiology, Alimentary Pharmabiotic Centre, University College Cork, Cork, Ireland

KEVIN RIOUX, MD, PhD, FRCP(C)
Assistant Professor, Division of Gastroenterology, Department of Microbiology and Infectious Diseases, Faculty of Medicine, University of Calgary, Calgary, Alberta, Canada

LEWIS R. ROBERTS, MBChB, PhD
Associate Professor of Medicine, Miles and Shirley Fiterman Center for Digestive Diseases, Division of Gastroenterology and Hepatology, College of Medicine, Mayo Clinic, Rochester, Minnesota

LUTZ SCHNEIDER, MD
Department of General Surgery, University of Heidelberg, Heidelberg, Germany

RACHEL VANDERPLOEG, BSc
Gastrointestinal Research Group, Faculty of Medicine, University of Calgary, Calgary, Alberta, Canada

JENS WERNER, MD
Head, Division of Pancreatic Surgery, Department of General Surgery, University of Heidelberg, Heidelberg, Germany

JU DONG YANG, MD
Research Fellow, Miles and Shirley Fiterman Center for Digestive Diseases, Division of Gastroenterology and Hepatology, College of Medicine, Mayo Clinic, Rochester, Minnesota

Contents

commonly thought to contribute to acute illness in patients. Acute calculous cholecystitis caused by an impacted gallstone is often complicated by secondary bacterial infection and is a major cause of morbidity and even mortality in patients. A wide variety of organisms can be associated with acute acalculous cholecystitis, a less common but potentially more severe form of acute cholecystitis. This review focuses on infections and their role in the above-mentioned processes involving the gallbladder.

Epidemiology and Management of Hepatocellular Carcinoma 899

Ju Dong Yang and Lewis R. Roberts

Hepatocellular carcinoma (HCC) is a major world health problem because of the high incidence and case fatality rate. In most patients, the diagnosis of HCC is made at an advanced stage, which limits the application of curative treatments. Most HCCs develop in patients with underlying chronic liver disease. Chronic viral hepatitis B and C are the major causes of liver cirrhosis and HCC. Recent improvements in treatment of viral hepatitis and in methods for surveillance and therapy for HCC have contributed to better survival of patients with HCC. This article reviews the epidemiology, cause, prevention, clinical manifestations, surveillance, diagnosis, and treatment approach for HCC.

Acute Pancreatitis with an Emphasis on Infection 921

Lutz Schneider, Markus W. Büchler, and Jens Werner

Acute pancreatitis is an inflammatory disease that is mild and self-limiting in about 80% of cases. However, severe necrotizing disease still has a mortality of up to 30%. Differentiated multimodal treatment concepts are needed for these patients, including a multidisciplinary team (intensivists, gastroenterologists, interventional radiologists, and surgeons). The primary therapy is supportive. Patients with infected pancreatic necrosis who are septic undergo interventional or surgical treatment, ideally not before the fourth week after onset of symptoms. This article reviews the pathophysiologic mechanisms of acute pancreatitis and describes clinical pathways for diagnosis and management based on the current literature and guidelines.

Small Intestinal Bacterial Overgrowth 943

Eamonn M.M. Quigley and Ahmed Abu-Shanab

Despite the current increase in interest in the role of the microbiota in health and disease and the recognition, for over 50 years, that an excess of colonic-type flora in the small intestine could lead to a malabsorption syndrome, small intestinal overgrowth remains poorly defined. This lack of clarity owes much to the difficulties that arise in attempting to arrive at consensus with regard to the diagnosis of this condition: there is currently no gold standard and the commonly available methodologies (the culture of jejunal aspirates and a variety of breath tests) suffer from considerable variations in their performance and interpretation, leading to variations in the prevalence of overgrowth in a variety of clinical contexts.

Treatment is similarly supported by a scant evidence base and the most commonly used antibiotic regimens owe more to custom than clinical trials.

Pathogenic Factors Involved in the Development of Irritable Bowel Syndrome: Focus on a Microbial Role 961

Carolina M. Bolino and Premysl Bercik

Irritable bowel syndrome (IBS) is a symptom complex characterized by recurrent abdominal pain or discomfort, and accompanied by abnormal bowel habits, in the absence of any discernible organic abnormality. Its origin remains unclear, partly because multiple pathophysiologic mechanisms are likely to be involved. A significant proportion of patients develop IBS symptoms after an episode of gastrointestinal infection. In addition to gastrointestinal pathogens, recent evidence suggests that patients with IBS have abnormal composition and higher temporal instability of their intestinal microbiota. Because the intestinal microbiota is an important determinant of normal gut function and immunity, this instability may constitute an additional mechanism that leads to symptom generation and IBS. More importantly, a role for altered microbiota composition in IBS raises the possibility of therapeutic interventions through selective antibiotic or probiotic administration. The new concept of functional bowel diseases incorporates the bidirectional communication between the gut and the central nervous system (gut–brain axis), which may explain the multiple facets of IBS by linking emotional and cognitive centers of the brain with peripheral functioning of the gastrointestinal tract and vice versa.

Influences of Intestinal Bacteria in Human Inflammatory Bowel Disease 977

Rachel Vanderploeg, Remo Panaccione, Subrata Ghosh, and Kevin Rioux

Microbes that reside in the human intestinal tract and interact with immune and epithelial cells are strongly implicated as causative or predisposing agents of inflammatory bowel disease (IBD). Recent studies using metagenomic approaches have revealed differences in the fecal and mucosa-associated microbiota of patients with IBD, but it remains unclear whether this is a cause or consequence of chronic intestinal inflammation. A few microbes have been singled out as candidate pathogens in IBD and remain the subject of ongoing study. Complex imbalances in gut bacterial community structure and/or deficiencies in their functional capabilities may be a greater issue in IBD development. A more complete understanding of host-microbiota interactions in IBD is hampered by several remaining but surmountable methodological and technical challenges.

Infectious Causes of Appendicitis 995

Laura W. Lamps

The pathologic spectrum of the inflamed appendix encompasses a wide range of infectious entities, some with specific histologic findings, and others with nonspecific findings that may require an extensive diagnostic evaluation. The appendix is exclusively involved in some of these disorders, and in others may be involved through extension from other areas of the gastrointestinal tract. This review discusses the pathologic features of bacterial, viral, fungal, and parasitic infections affecting the appendix, including adenovirus; cytomegalovirus; *Yersinia*, *Actinomyces*, *Mycobacterium*, or *Histoplasma* species; *Enterobius vermicularis;* schistosomiasis; and *Strongyloides stercoralis*. Pertinent ancillary diagnostic techniques and the clinical context and significance of the various infections are also discussed.

Infectious Causes of Colorectal Cancer **1019**

Nazia Hasan, Ari Pollack, and Ilseung Cho

Colorectal cancer is a major cause of cancer-related morbidity and mortality in the United States and many other regions of the world. Our understanding of the pathogenesis of colorectal cancer, from the precursor adenomatous polyp to adenocarcinoma, has evolved rapidly. Colorectal carcinogenesis is a sequential process characterized by the accumulation of multiple genetic and molecular alterations in colonic epithelial cells. However, the development of colorectal cancer involves more then just a genetic predisposition. External or environmental factors presumably play a significant role, and inflammatory bowel diseases, obesity, alcohol consumption, and a diet high in fat and low in fiber have all been implicated as risk factors for the development of either colonic adenomas or carcinomas. We are becoming increasingly aware of microbes as causes of malignancies. This article reviews the various microbes that have been associated with the development of colorectal carcinomas.

Future Perspectives on Infections Associated with Gastrointestinal Tract Diseases **1041**

Guy D. Eslick

There are a vast number of infectious agents that are associated with gastrointestinal (GI) tract diseases. The epidemiology of GI diseases is changing, with a greater number of conditions increasing in incidence. Challenges exist with establishing cause-and-effect relationships because of the ubiquitous nature of these organisms and the milieu in which they exist. Advances in technology should provide novel methods for identifying and diagnosing these organisms and the relationship they have with a specific digestive disease.

Index **1059**

FORTHCOMING ISSUES

March 2011

Infection Prevention and Control in the Hospital

Keith S. Kaye, MD, MPH, *Guest Editor*

June 2011

Global Health, Global Health Education, and Infectious Disease: the New Millennium, Part I

Anvar Velji, MD,
Guest Editor

September 2011

Global Health, Global Health Education, and Infectious Disease: the New Millennium, Part II

Anvar Velji, MD,
Guest Editor

RECENT ISSUES

September 2010

Emerging Respiratory Infections in the 21st Century

Alimuddin Zumla, FRCP, PhD(Lond), FRCPath, Wing-Wai Yew, MBBS, FRCP (Edinb), FCCP, and David SC Hui, MD(UNSW), FRACP, FRCP,
Guest Editors

June 2010

Infections in Transplant and Oncology Patients

Kieren A. Marr, MD, and
Aruna K. Subramanian, MD,
Guest Editors

March 2010

The Atypical Pneumonias

Burke A. Cunha, MD, MACP,
Guest Editor

ISSUES OF RELATED INTEREST

Clinics in Liver Disease August 2010 (Vol. 14, No. 3)
Chronic Hepatitis B: An Update
Naoky C.S. Tsai, MD, *Guest Editor*
Available at: http://www.liver.theclinics.com/

Foot and Ankle Clinics September 2010 (Vol. 15, No. 3)
Infection, Ischemia, and Amputation
Michael S. Pinzur, MD, *Guest Editor*
Available at: http://www.foot.theclinics.com/

Preface

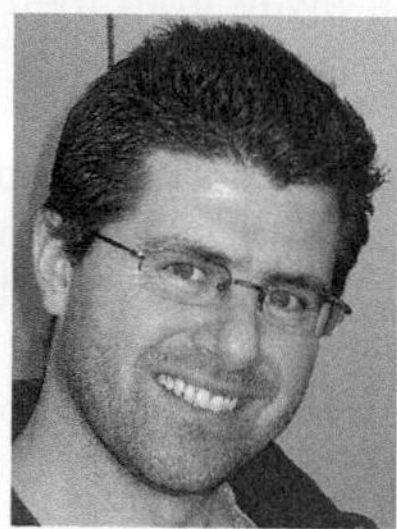

Guy D. Eslick, PhD,
MMedSc(Clin Epi), MMedStat
Guest Editor

"It was the best of times, it was the worst of times" and so it goes with infections associated with gastrointestinal disease. While advances are being made in some areas such as diagnostic technology (eg, molecular techniques), major limitations remain in controlling and preventing infections associated with gastrointestinal diseases. The prime example is infective diarrhea, which has been and unfortunately remains a major cause of morbidity and mortality among children, especially those under the age of 5 years and particularly in developing countries around the world.

However, with the emergence and identification of new infectious agents, interest in clinical infectious diseases and microbiology has been reignited and takes a prominent place in medicine today. Advances in technology have also allowed for great strides in the understanding of the pathophysiology, classification, and immunology of these pathogens. The most obvious example would be the most prevalent infection worldwide, namely *Helicobacter pylori*, which infects an estimated 3 billion people, a staggering number of individuals. In fact, there are gastrointestinal organisms (*Giardia, Cyclospora, Cryptosporidium* species) that were not considered significant pathogens in the 1970s but are now infections that must be reported to the Centers for Disease Control. Moreover, other controversial organisms such as *Blastocystis hominis* are the most frequently identified parasites in North America annually.

The microbiological spectrum of "bugs"—including bacteria, viruses, protozoa, and fungi—plays various roles in the development of gastrointestinal diseases, and there is an increasing interest in the role these organisms play in the development of gastrointestinal cancers. This issue of *Infectious Disease Clinics of North America* covers a broad range of gastrointestinal diseases and cancers, including esophageal cancer, gastric cancer, cholangiocarcinoma, gallbladder disease, hepatocellular carcinoma, acute pancreatitis, small intestinal bacterial overgrowth, irritable bowel syndrome, inflammatory bowel disease, appendicitis, and colorectal cancer.

I would like to thank the senior editor of *Infectious Disease Clinics of North America*, Barbara Cohen-Kligerman, for her support, assistance, and patience in putting this

Infect Dis Clin N Am 24 (2010) xiii–xiv
doi:10.1016/j.idc.2010.08.003

issue into publication. I would also like to sincerely thank Dr Robert Moellering for inviting me to develop this issue. In addition, special thanks to my family, Enid, Marielle, and Isaac, for their love and support as I spend time away from them to complete this work.

In developing this *Infectious Disease Clinics of North America* issue I have selected eminent leaders in their respective areas to write what I believe is an outstanding collection of articles on a diverse range of topics that should be of interest to all who engage in the diagnosis and treatment of infections associated with gastrointestinal diseases and cancers. It is hoped that these articles will provide insight for researchers and physicians in an exciting area of medicine that will continue to be dynamic for eons.

Guy D. Eslick, PhD, MMedSc(Clin Epi), MMedStat
The Whiteley-Martin Research Centre
Discipline of Surgery, Nepean Hospital
The University of Sydney, Level 5
South Block, PO Box 63, Penrith
New South Wales 2751, Australia

E-mail address:
eslickg@med.usyd.edu.au

Dedication

A teacher affects eternity; he can never tell where his influence stops.
~Henry Adams

I would like to dedicate this issue of the *Infectious Diseases Clinics of North America* to my friend and first mentor, Dr Harold M. Lukse, MBBS, FRCPA (**Fig. 1**). I first met Harry when I was 15 years old while I was undertaking a high school work experience program where I was fortunate enough to spend two weeks in the local hospital pathology laboratory. Two weeks turned into 10 years. All aspects of pathology intrigued me, but I was particularly interested in clinical microbiology and histopathology.

Harry was always keen to pass on his encyclopedic knowledge during the afternoon "cut-ups" of the surgical specimens. He is an excellent educator with a wonderful sense of humor. When I commenced my undergraduate studies, he was always supportive, and during one of my subjects in clinical microbiology I had to write a dissertation on an organism and related pathology. Harry suggested that I look at "this new bug that has been found in the human stomach and is supposed to cause peptic ulcer disease." For me, it was the beginning of a life-long interest in *Helicobacter pylori*, not to mention the impact this had on directing my career into gastrointestinal disease research.

I will never forget the multitudes of discussions we had. Whether it was in the lab while Harry dissected specimens or in the tea-room doing crossword puzzles or

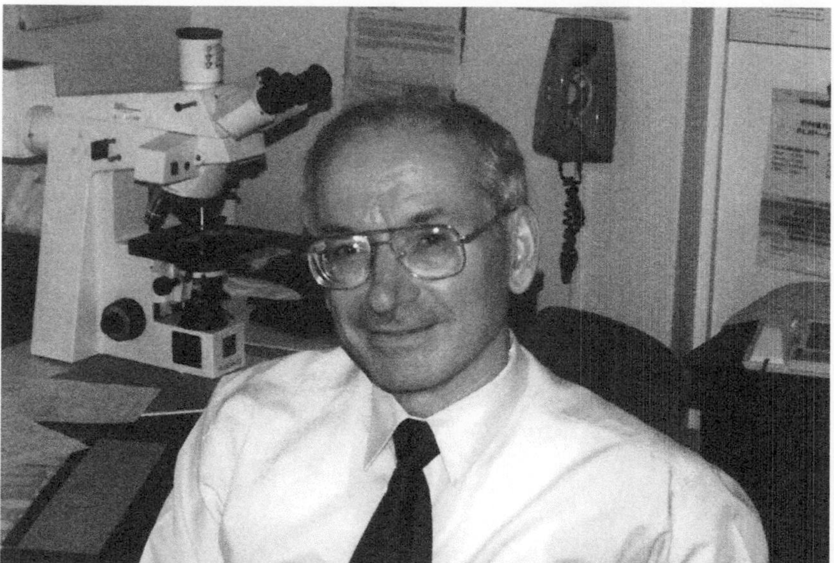

Fig. 1. Harold M. Lukse, MBBS, FRCPA.

Infect Dis Clin N Am 24 (2010) xv–xvi
doi:10.1016/j.idc.2010.08.004
0891-5520/10/$ – see front matter

reading the newspaper, it was always fun and educational. Harry would often call me over to the microscope and highlight cells and discuss the processes associated with that particular pathology and how the microscopic related to the macroscopic. I found it all so extremely fascinating.

For me, the two "H's" (Harry/*Helicobacter*) seem to go hand-in-hand, and one man's willingness to take an interest in the education of another has changed my life and provided me with a career of doing what I love most. Almost 25 years have passed since those initial days, I don't get to see Harry that often these days, but he is never far from my thoughts. I feel blessed to have known him and every time I visit the home of my childhood I try and catch-up with Harry. These days Harry is still making sure the margins are clear for those with cancer, and providing accurate diagnosis in difficult cases that require his outstanding diagnostic acumen. He still works long hours (including weekends) and gets few holidays. Harry is very dedicated to his work, and many thousands of patients who have never met Harry are in his debt. I know I am.

Guy D. Eslick

Infectious Causes of Esophageal Cancer

Guy D. Eslick, PhD, MMedSc(Clin Epi), MMedStat

KEYWORDS

• Esophageal cancer • Infectious agents • Bacteria • Viruses

The gastrointestinal environment provides a dynamic habitat via peristalsis, transport of food, host cells, and an enormous array of microorganisms.[1] It is estimated that a quadrillion (10^{15}) bacteria inhabit the gastrointestinal tract, with approximately 1000 different bacterial species from 11 different bacterial divisions.[2] These organisms consist of resident and transient groups that constantly interact with the gastrointestinal system from the mouth to the anus (**Fig. 1**). The types of organisms include opportunistic, facultative, and strict pathogens whose appearance will depend greatly on the surrounding normal commensal population of organisms and how these organisms interact in each gastrointestinal environment.

More recently, with the discovery of *Helicobacter pylori* in the human stomach and the subsequent discovery of many other *Helicobacter* species that occur not only in humans but also in a wide variety of animals, the idea that bacteria can live in such an environment that was previously thought to be sterile provides opportunities for future discovery that may not have been thought of or missed because of a lack of technology.

Infections of the esophagus are important in healthy and immunocompromised individuals (**Table 1**). Inflammation and invasion are required to be defined as an infection, rather than just colonization by organisms alone. Patients may have nonspecific complaints or may present with dysphagia or odynophagia. Chest pain or discomfort, heartburn, and nausea may also be present in these individuals. Types of pathology include ulcer, plaques, fistula, and mass, which can be found in various locations within the esophageal wall (**Fig. 2**).

THE ESOPHAGUS

The human esophagus is about 25 cm long and 2.5 cm in diameter and is 4 mm in thickness. It is the link between the mouth and the stomach and as such must be considered a potential haven of numerous organisms that make their way from the oral cavity via peristalsis (both primary and secondary) to the stomach.

Conflict of Interest: None.

The Whiteley-Martin Research Centre, Discipline of Surgery, Nepean Hospital, The University of Sydney, Level 5, South Block, PO Box 63, Penrith, New South Wales 2751, Australia
E-mail address: eslickg@med.usyd.edu.au

Infect Dis Clin N Am 24 (2010) 845–852
doi:10.1016/j.idc.2010.08.001 **id.theclinics.com**

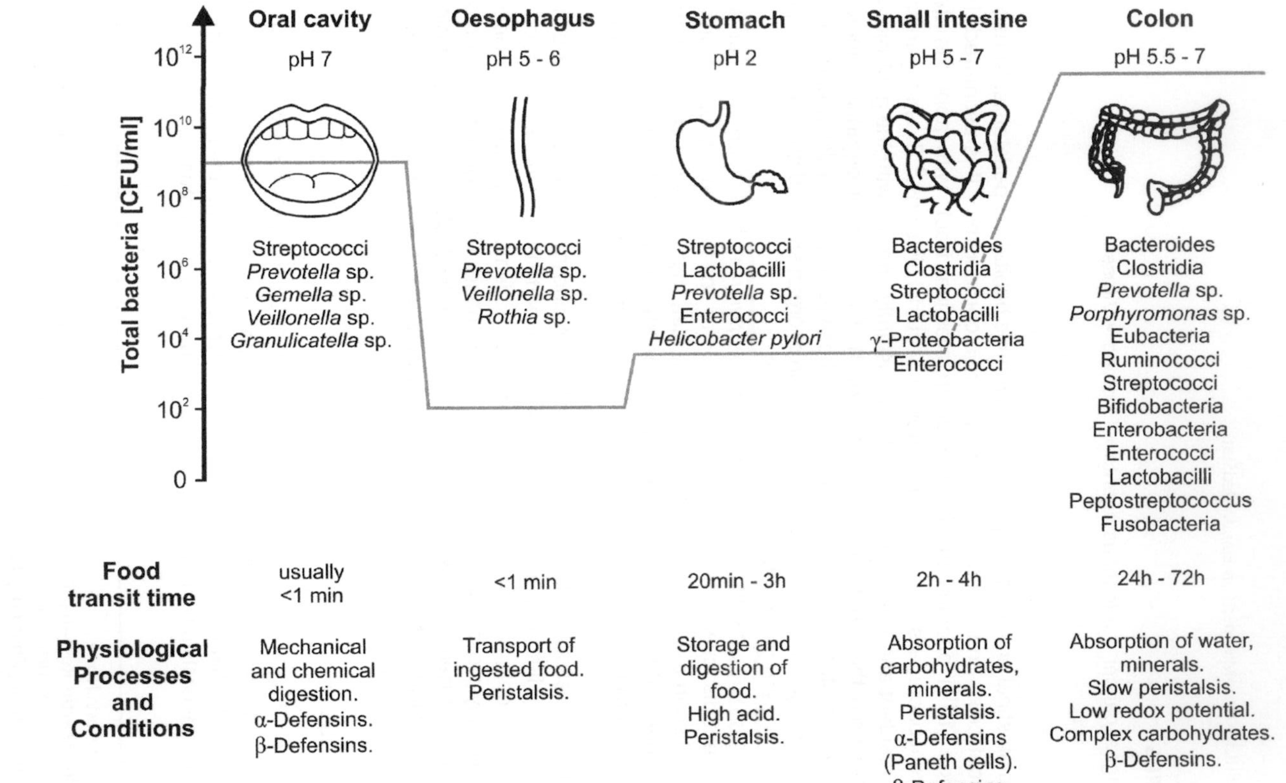

Fig. 1. Microbiota of the gastrointestinal system. (*From* Manson JM, Rauch M, Gilmore MS. The commensal microbiology of the gastrointestinal tract. In: Huffnagle GB, Mairi N, editors. GI microbiota and regulation of the immune system. New York: Springer; 2008. p. 19; with permission.)

Table 1
Esophageal infections in humans

Healthy	Immunocompromised
Common Candida species	Common *Candida* species Cytomegalovirus (CMV) Herpes Simplex virus (HSV) Human Immunodeficiency virus (HIV)
Uncommon Herpes Simplex virus (HSV) Epstein-Barr virus (EBV)	Uncommon Oral flora *Aspergillus* species Varicella zoster virus (VZV)
Rare Varicella zoster virus (VZV) *Mycobacterium tuberculosis* *Histoplasma*	

ORAL FLORA

There are a myriad of organisms that reside in the mouth, nasopharynx, and oropharynx that make their way down the esophagus into the stomach and the intestinal system.[3] The oral flora include *Streptococcus*, *Neisseria*, *Veillonella*, *Fusobacterium*, *Bacteroides*, *Lactobacillus*, *Staphylococcus*, Enterobacteriaceae, and yeasts.

ORGANISM TRANSFER

Organisms can also be introduced into the esophagus through the process of swallowing food and liquids.[4]

POTENTIAL INFECTIOUS AGENTS

Bacteria

There are several studies that have aimed to determine the microbiological flora (bacteria) of the esophagus (**Boxes 1–3**).[5–8] These studies have been conducted on

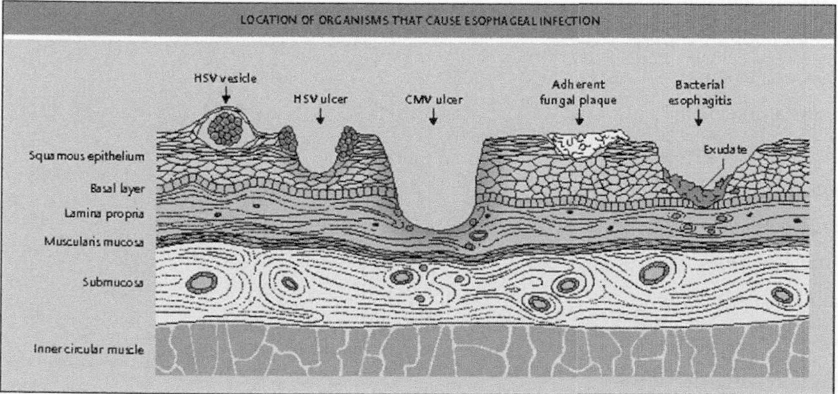

Fig. 2. Location of organisms causing infections of the esophagus. (*From* Weinstein WM, Hawkey CJ, Bosch J. Clinical gastroenterology and hepatology. New York: Elsevier; 2005; with permission.)

Box 1
Microbiological flora found in the healthy esophagus

Streptococcus

Neisseria

Veillonella

Fusobacterium

Bacteroides

Lactobacillus

Staphylococcus

Prevotella

Enterobacteriaceae

Yeast

Box 2
Microbiological flora found in patients with esophageal cancer

α-Hemolytic *Streptococcus*

β-Hemolytic *Streptococcus*

Bacteroides fragilis

Bacteroides melaninogenicus

Bacteroides spp

Clostridium spp

Coagulase-negative *Staphylococcus*

Corynebacterium spp

Escherichia coli

Fusobacterium spp

Haemophilus influenzae

Lactobacillus spp

Neisseria catarrhalis

Non-hemolytic *Streptococcus*

Peptococcus

Pneumococcus

Proteus mirabilis

Staphylococcus albus

Staphylococcus aureus

Streptococcus pyogenes

Streptococcus viridans

Yeast

Box 3
Organisms that cause pathology of the esophagus

Candida albicans

Cytomegalovirus (CMV)

Epstein-Barr virus (EBV)

Fusarium spp

Herpes simplex virus (HSV)

Histoplasma capsulatum

Mycobacterium avium

Mycobacterium tuberculosis

Cryptosporidium

Varicella zoster virus (VZV)

various types of patients, including those who are healthy and those with esophagitis, Barrett esophagus, and esophageal carcinoma. Recently, a study found that nitrate-reducing *Campylobacter* species (*C concisus*, *C rectus*) were clinically important among patients with Barrett esophagus and may promote the development of adenocarcinoma.[8]

Helicobacter pylori

The relationship between *H pylori* and esophageal cancer is an interesting one, with most data from meta-analyses suggesting that there is an inverse relationship, where the presence of *H pylori* is protective against esophageal squamous cell carcinoma.[9–11] The most recent meta-analysis found 19 studies of case-control or nested case-control design. For esophageal adenocarcinoma, the pooled estimate is 0.56 (95% confidence interval [CI]: 0.46–0.68). There was little heterogeneity among studies (I^2 = 15%). Further research is required.

Streptococcus anginosus

There have been several studies conducted looking at the relationship between *Streptococcus anginosus* and esophageal cancer.[12,13] Most of these studies do not provide substantial evidence to support the investigators' claims that *S anginosus* is associated with esophageal cancer. One study found that *S anginosus* occurred in 44% of esophageal cancer tissue samples.[12] There are now several *Streptococcus* species being assessed to determine what role if any they might play in the development of esophageal cancer. Future studies must be better designed and not rely on purely laboratory-based designs.

Treponema denticola

This is a periodontopathic spirochete that causes matrix destruction of the gingival and periodontitis. A study of esophageal carcinoma tissue, normal tissue, and saliva were obtained from patients and underwent molecular analysis including polymerase chain reaction (PCR) and Northern blot analysis.[14] Almost half (45%) of the organisms found in the esophageal cancer samples were from *T denticola*. It was suggested by the authors that this organism has a preference for infecting the normal mucosa of the esophagus and esophageal cancer tissue.

Viruses

JC virus

Currently, there is only one study looking at human polyomavirus JC virus (JCV) and esophageal cancer development.[15] Molecular DNA of 70 esophageal biopsy specimens from individuals with various types of esophageal disorders (achalasia, reflux esophagitis, Barrett esophagus, adenocarcinoma, squamous call carcinoma) and healthy controls was analyzed.

JCV DNA was isolated from 85% of normal esophageal tissues, and 100% of esophageal carcinomas. Among carcinoma samples, immunohistochemistry revealed JCV T antigen in 53%, agnoprotein in 42%, p53 tumor suppressor in 58%, and β-catenin in 21%. JCV DNA was found in normal, benign, and malignant esophageal tissue samples; however, it was active only in carcinoma cells where viral expression of proteins occurred. The investigators suggest that these data provide evidence that infection with JCV may play a role in the subsequent development of esophageal carcinoma. Further research is required.

Epstein-Barr virus

There are a handful of studies assessing EBV in relation to esophageal cancer. There were 2 early studies from 1999 and then a German group published 2 studies in 2002 and 2005.[16–19] Lam[16] conducted a study in Hong Kong on 40 sporadic mesenchymal tumors of the esophagus that underwent immunohistochemical study for EBV (mRNA probes: EBER, BamHI W). None of the tumors were positive for either of the two EBV markers. Another early study, conducted in northern China on 51 esophageal squamous cell carcinoma specimens that also used the EBV BamHI W fragment, found no link using in situ hybridization and PCR.[17]

A study of 72 squamous cell carcinoma and 40 adenocarcinoma specimens from Russia were assessed for EBV using PCR.[18] One-third of esophageal squamous cell carcinoma and adenocarcinomas had EBV DNA in the nuclei of tumor-infiltrating lymphocytes, suggesting that EBV plays no role in the development of esophageal cancer. In another earlier study from this group, just over one-third of esophageal squamous cell carcinomas (35%) and adenocarcinomas (36%) were positive for EBV DNA from 37 specimens.[19] The investigators also assessed human papillomavirus (HPV) among these samples but none of them were positive for HPV.

Herpes simplex virus

No studies currently exist assessing the role of HSV in the development of esophageal cancer.

Human papillomavirus

This is currently the most studied organism in relation to not only infection of the esophagus but also its potential relationship with the development of esophageal cancer. High incidences of HPV positivity have been reported among esophageal squamous cell carcinoma in high-risk areas such as China, Korea, South Africa, and Alaska. But HPV is rarely identified in esophageal squamous cell carcinoma in Japan, the United States, the United Kingdom, the Netherlands, and low-risk areas of China. There is obvious geographic variation, which may help explain the differences in rates of HPV seen around the world in esophageal cancers. Variation also exists by HPV type, with the following types associated with esophageal squamous cell carcinoma: 5, 6, 9, 11, 16, 18, 20, 20, 21, 24, 25, 27, 31, 32, 33, 39, 45, 52, 53, 58, 67, and 87.[20] The major HPV type linked with esophageal cancer is HPV 16. There has been a substantial amount of research into HPV 16, including potential mechanisms.[21] The strength of an association for HPV 16 and esophageal squamous cell carcinoma is relatively high, with studies reporting an odds ratio as high as 6.3 (95% CI: 1.6–23.7).[22]

Fungi

Several mycotoxins have been linked to esophageal cancer, however the data are circumstantial, with greater research required in this area.[23–25]

Parasites

Currently, no parasites have been identified in the esophagus, nor have any been linked with esophageal cancers. However, in animals, dogs do get a rare esophageal cancer that can occur following infection by the esophageal parasite *Spirocerca lupi*.

SUMMARY

The causes of esophageal cancer in many cases remains unknown. The potential for an infectious agent as a cause still remains. There are several types of bacteria and viruses associated with esophageal cancer. Many of these studies require replication in various geographic locations. The availability of modern molecular techniques will provide greater advances in future studies.

REFERENCES

1. Manson JM, Rauch M, Gilmore MS. The commensal microbiology of the gastrointestinal tract. In: Huffnagle GB, Mairi N, editors. GI microbiota and regulation of the immune system. New York: Springer; 2008. p. 18.
2. Ouwehand AC, Vaughan EE, editors. Gastrointestinal microbiology. New York: Taylor Francis; 2006. p. 28–9.
3. Sjostedt S. The upper gastrointestinal microbiota in relation to gastric diseases and gastric surgery. Acta Chir Scand Suppl 1989;551:1–57.
4. Dantas RO, Oliveira RB, Aprile LR, et al. Saliva transport to the distal esophagus. Scand J Gastroenterol 2005;40:1010–6.
5. Pei Z, Yang L, Peek RM, et al. Bacterial biota in reflux esophagitis and Barrett's esophagus. World J Gastroenterol 2005;11:7277–83.
6. Pei Z, Bini EJ, Yang L, et al. Bacterial biota in the human distal esophagus. Proc Natl Acad Sci U S A 2004;101:4250–5.
7. Gagliardi D, Makihara S, Corsi PR, et al. Microbial flora of the normal esophagus. Dis Esophagus 1998;11:248–50.
8. Macfarlane S, Furrie E, Macfarlane GT, et al. Microbial colonization of the upper gastrointestinal tract in patients with Barrett's esophagus. Clin Infect Dis 2007;45:29–38.
9. Islami F, Kamangar F. *Helicobacter pylori* and esophageal cancer risk: a meta-analysis. Cancer Prev Res (Phila Pa) 2008;1:329–38.
10. Rokkas T, Pistiolas D, Sechopoulos P, et al. Relationship between *Helicobacter pylori* infection and esophageal neoplasia: a meta-analysis. Clin Gastroenterol Hepatol 2007;5:1413–7.
11. de Martel C, Llosa AE, Farr SM, et al. *Helicobacter pylori* infection and the risk of development of esophageal adenocarcinoma. J Infect Dis 2005;191:761–7.
12. Narikiyo ME, Yokoyama M, Yano A, et al. Predominant presence of *Streptococcus anginosus* in the saliva of alcoholics. Oral Microbiol Immunol 2005;20:362–5.
13. Morita E, Narikiyo ME, Yano A, et al. Different frequencies of *Streptococcus anginosus* infection in oral cancer and esophageal cancer. Cancer Sci 2003;94:492–6.

14. Narikiyo ME, Tanabe C, Yamada Y, et al. Frequent and preferential infection of *Treponema denticola, Streptococcus mitis*, and *Streptococcus anginosus* in esophageal cancers. Cancer Sci 2004;95:569–74.
15. Del Valle L, White MK, Enam S, et al. Detection of JC virus DNA sequences and expression of viral T antigen and agnoprotein in esophageal carcinoma. Cancer 2005;103:516–27.
16. Lam KY. Oesophageal mesenchymal tumours: clinicopathological features and absence of Epstein-Barr virus. J Clin Pathol 1999;52:758–60.
17. Wang J, Noffsinger A, Stemmermann G, et al. Esophageal squamous cell carcinoma arising in patients from a high-risk area of North China lack an association with Epstein-Barr virus. Cancer Epidemiol Biomarkers Prev 1999;8:1111–4.
18. Awerkiew S, zur Hausen A, Baldus SE, et al. Presence of Epstein-Barr virus in esophageal cancer is restricted to tumor infiltrating lymphocytes. Med Microbiol Immunol 2005;194:187–91.
19. Awerkiew S, Bollschweiler E, Metzger R, et al. Esophageal cancer in Germany is associated with Epstein-Barr virus but not with papillomavirus. Med Microbiol Immunol 2003;192:137–40.
20. Syrjanen KS. HPV infections and oesophageal cancer. J Clin Pathol 2002;55:721–8.
21. Zhou Y, Pan Y, Zhang S, et al. Increased phosphorylation of p70 S6 kinase is associated with HPV 16 infection in cervical cancer and esophageal cancer. Br J Cancer 2007;97:218–22.
22. Han C, Qiao G, Hubbert NL, et al. Serologic association between human papillomavirus type 16 infection and esophageal cancer in Shaanxi Province, China. J Natl Cancer Inst 1996;88:1467–71.
23. Marasas WF, van Rensburg SJ, Mirocha CJ. Incidence of *Fusarium* species and the mycotoxins, deoxynivalenol and zearalenone, in corn produced in esophageal cancer areas in Transkei. J Agric Food Chem 1979;27:1108–12.
24. Shephard GS, Marasas WF, Leggott NL, et al. Natural occurrence of fumonisins in corn from Iran. J Agric Food Chem 2000;48:1860–4.
25. Chu FS, Li GY. Simultaneous occurrence of fumonisin B1 and other mycotoxins in moldy corn collected from the people's republic of China in regions with high incidences of esophageal cancer. Appl Environ Microbiol 1994;60:847–52.

Gastric Cancer: An Infectious Disease

M. Blanca Piazuelo, MD[a,*], Meira Epplein, PhD[b], Pelayo Correa, MD[a]

KEYWORDS

• Gastric cancer • Gastric adenocarcinoma • *Helicobacter pylori*
• Epidemiology

Although viral and parasitic agents have been implicated in human cancers, gastric cancer is currently the only malignant neoplasia recognized as causally associated in humans with a bacterium. In 1994, the International Agency for Research on Cancer (IARC) concluded that "there is sufficient evidence in humans for the carcinogenicity of infection with *Helicobacter pylori*."[1] At that time, they concluded that "there is inadequate evidence in experimental animals for the carcinogenicity of infection with *Helicobacter pylori*." Since then, experimental evidence of carcinogenicity has been documented, especially using the Mongolian gerbil model.[2] In 2009, the evidence was reevaluated and confirmed by the IARC.[3] *H pylori* is associated with causation of gastric adenocarcinoma and gastric mucosa–associated lymphoid tissue lymphoma.[3] Because gastric adenocarcinomas account for more than 90% of all gastric malignancies,[4] this review focuses on adenocarcinomas.

Although gastric cancer rates have been decreasing in many countries, this disease is the second most common cause of death from cancer worldwide and ranks fourth worldwide in cancer incidence (**Table 1**).[5] Approximately 1 million new cases were estimated in 2007.[6] There are marked differences in gastric cancer rates among populations worldwide. The highest incidences are in Japan, Korea, China, eastern Europe, and the Andean portions of Latin America. Lower rates are seen in Africa, Oceania, North America, and Brazil (**Fig. 1**). Despite the low overall rates in gastric cancer incidence and mortality in the United States, there are some ethnic groups at increased risk, including African Americans, Native Americans, and immigrants from east Asia and Latin America.[7–9] In addition, although overall incidence of gastric cancer has been steadily declining in the United States, a recent observational study based on data from the National Cancer Institute's Surveillance, Epidemiology, and

This work was supported by the grant P01-CA28842 from the National Cancer Institute.
[a] Division of Gastroenterology, Vanderbilt University School of Medicine, 2215 Garland Avenue, 1030 MRB IV, Nashville, TN 37232, USA
[b] Division of Epidemiology, Vanderbilt University School of Medicine, 2525 West End Avenue Suite 600, Nashville, TN 37203, USA
* Corresponding author.
E-mail address: maria.b.piazuelo@vanderbilt.edu

Infect Dis Clin N Am 24 (2010) 853–869
doi:10.1016/j.idc.2010.07.010
id.theclinics.com
0891-5520/10/$ – see front matter

Table 1
New cases and deaths by cancer site worldwide, 2002

	New Cases	Deaths
Lung	1,352,132	1,178,918
Breast	1,151,298	410,712
Colon and rectum	1,023,152	528,978
Stomach	933,937	700,349
Liver	626,162	598,321
Prostate	679,023	221,002
Cervix uteri	493,243	273,505
Esophagus	462,117	385,892
Bladder	356,557	145,009
Non-Hodgkin lymphoma	300,571	171,820
Leukemia	300,522	222,506
Pancreas	232,306	227,023
All sites but skin	10,862,496	6,723,887

Data from Parkin DM, Bray F, Ferlay J, et al. Global cancer statistics, 2002. CA Cancer J Clin 2005;55(2):74–108.

End Results Program identified increasing rates of noncardia cancer in white US residents aged 25 to 39 years in the past 3 decades.[10] The causes of this phenomenon are unclear.

AGENT-HOST-ENVIRONMENT INTERACTIONS

Infection with *H pylori* is the strongest known risk factor for gastric cancer[1,11–13]; however, only a small minority of people infected with *H pylori* develop gastric

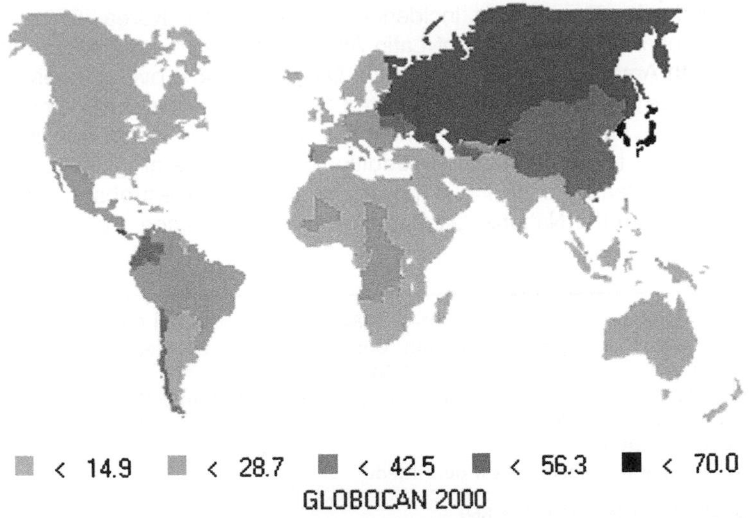

Fig. 1. Incidence of stomach cancer in men worldwide (age-standardized rates). (*Courtesy of* GLOBOCAN, 2000; http://www-dep.iarc.fr/; with permission.)

cancer or gastric precancerous lesions. The epidemiologic triangle, a conceptual model that posits that the outcome depends on the complex interplay of the agent with environmental and host factors,[14] can be applied to better understand the cause of gastric cancer. Factors specific to the host, such as genetic background, diet, and smoking behavior, as well as factors related to the environment, including neighborhood socioeconomic status, parasites endemic to the region, and possibly even climate, play key roles in whether gastric cancer develops in a particular individual. There is clearly a strong environmental component that affects cancer risk. Migrant populations from high-risk areas of the world show a decrease in risk in the second generation when they move to a lower-risk area.[15] Some of these factors work on both the individual and societal level, and can be viewed as factors associated with host, environment, or both, depending on the specific characteristic. A change in this precarious balance of agent, host, and environment, such as infection with a more virulent strain of *H pylori* or increased salt intake, can affect the speed of the cascade of events that lead to the development of gastric cancer.

THE INFECTIOUS AGENT

H pylori

H pylori is a gram-negative microaerophilic spiral bacterium that localizes mostly extracellularly within the gastric lumen (**Fig. 2**). Identified and cultured for the first time in 1982 by Marshall and Warren,[16] *H pylori* is present in more than 50% of the human population[17] and is highly adapted to colonize the human stomach. It possesses a potent urease that allows it to live in the acid microenvironment of the gastric lumen by hydrolyzing the urea that filters into the lumen, resulting in an ammonium cloud that protects the bacterium from the acid pH. In the same reaction, carbon dioxide is produced and immediately eliminated with the exhaled air. Oral administration of ^{13}C-urea is used as a diagnostic test because $^{13}CO_2$ is exhaled if the infection is present. Other factors that contribute to the persistence of the bacterium in the stomach are certain characteristics of the lipopolysaccharide that reduce the intensity

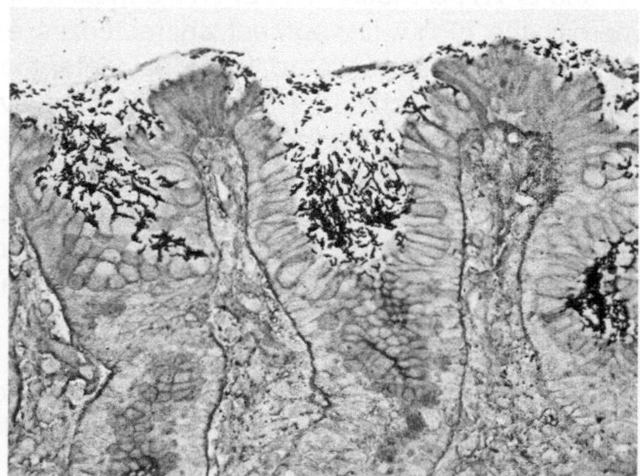

Fig. 2. Gastric mucosa colonized by abundant *H pylori* organisms (modified Steiner silver stain, ×400).

of the host immune response and the expression of adhesins that confer intimate adherence to the gastric epithelium.[18,19]

H pylori has been part of the native human flora since time immemorial. Both species migrated out of Africa some 60,000 years ago and have traveled together since then to other continents. Molecular microbiological studies have shown that the genome of the bacteria evolves frequently, mostly from recombination. Achtman and colleagues,[20] using the multilocus sequence typing (MLST) of 7 housekeeping genes, identified bacterial strains that originate in specific populations of Africa (hpAfrica), Europe (hpEurope), and Asia (hpEAsia).[20–22] The original Amerindian strains in the Americas, after being exposed to European strains, supposedly then acquired the *cag* pathogenicity island (*cag* PAI), a recognized virulence factor.[23–26] It is not clear whether the Amerindian strains were totally replaced by European strains or whether they acquired some of their genes by recombination.[26] Preliminary results from an ongoing study in Colombia show that *H pylori* isolates from the high–gastric-cancer-risk populations of the Andes Mountains, of mestizo extraction (mixed Amerindian and European ancestry), display European genotypes by MLST, presumably indicating the exposure of Amerindian strains to European strains. In contrast, inhabitants of the low–gastric-cancer-risk area on the Pacific coast, of mixed African and European extraction, display heterogeneity of their *H pylori* strains: some harbor West African genotypes and some harbor European genotypes (data not published). These findings suggest that the ancestry of the bacterial strains may be linked to cancer risk.

Despite the widespread dissemination of *H pylori* infection, it is estimated that only a minute fraction of infected patients ever develop gastric adenocarcinoma. However, it is also estimated that 77% of noncardia gastric cancer is attributable to *H pylori* infection.[17] Several components of the *H pylori* genome are linked to carcinogenicity. *cag* PAI, a major determinant of virulence, is a cluster of genes present in about 60% of *H pylori* isolates from Western countries and in almost all of the isolates from east Asian countries.[27] One gene (*cagA*) in the *H pylori cag* PAI encodes an effector protein (CagA) and others encode proteins for a type IV secretion apparatus that translocates CagA into gastric epithelial cells.[23,24] Infection with *cagA*-positive *H pylori* strains has been associated with increased risk for development of peptic ulcer,[24,28] gastric precancerous lesions, and gastric adenocarcinoma.[29–31] *cagA*-positive strains are more prevalent in high–cancer-risk than in low-risk populations: approximately 90% in the Andes Mountains and 70% in the Pacific coast of Colombia.[32] The CagA protein is polymorphic, as shown by the sequences flanking the so-called EPIYA motifs. Most strains have EPIYA-A and EPIYA-B motifs. The EPIYA-C motif is characteristic of the Western strains, whereas the EPIYA-D segment characterizes east Asian strains. These motifs become tyrosine phosphorylated when they enter the epithelial cells of the host, presumably starting the chain of events that may eventually result in neoplastic transformation.[27] Another virulence factor is a protein known as VacA, a multifunctional cytotoxin that causes intracellular vacuoles and forms membrane channels in epithelial cells.[33] The *vacA* gene is present in all *H pylori* strains, and comprises several variable loci (designed s, i, and m). The combination of different alleles determines the production of cytotoxin and is associated with the pathogenicity of the bacterium.[18,33]

Both types of peptic ulcers (gastric and duodenal) are causally linked to *H pylori* infection, but gastric peptic ulcer is associated with a high risk of gastric cancer, whereas duodenal ulcer is associated with a low risk compared with the general population.[13,34] Patients with gastric ulcers typically have multifocal atrophic gastritis. Patients with duodenal ulcers have antrum-predominant gastritis but none of the atrophic changes.

Epstein-Barr Virus

Increasing evidence indicates the possibility of a role of Epstein-Barr virus (EBV) in the cause of some gastric cancers. Multiple studies around the world have found the presence of the EBV in 5% to 16% of gastric adenocarcinomas. A recent meta-analysis including 70 articles estimated that the overall EBV positivity was 8.7% among gastric cancer cases and that EBV-associated adenocarcinomas are more frequent in men than in women, in gastric cardia or corpus than in antrum, and in tumors of post-surgical gastric stump/remnants.[35] In addition, a strong association (>90%) was confirmed between EBV and the uncommon histologic-type lymphoepitheliomalike gastric carcinoma.[35] Several observations support the causal involvement of EBV in some gastric cancers, including the uniform presence of clonal EBV in all malignant cells of EBV-positive tumors but not in surrounding normal epithelial cells.[36] However, the precise role of EBV in gastric carcinogenesis is still unclear.

THE ENVIRONMENT

Diet

In 2007, an expert panel from the World Cancer Research Fund released a report declaring that high intakes of vegetables and fruit probably decrease risk of gastric cancer, and that high intakes of salt and salty food probably increase risk of gastric cancer.[37] Most of the evidence for these associations comes from case-control studies; cohort studies have been more inconsistent and have primarily found weaker, nonsignificant associations. The mechanism for the inverse association of gastric cancer risk with high vegetable and fruit intake has been hypothesized to be related to the presence of antioxidants, which protect against oxidative damage. The positive association with salt has been more clearly delineated, because salt acts directly on the stomach lining, destroying the mucosal barrier and causing gastritis, increasing epithelial proliferation.[38] A synergistic interaction between diet and *H pylori* infection with risk of gastric cancer has been proposed,[39] and studies on this topic have generally suggested a stronger effect among individuals who are *H pylori* positive.[40,41]

Smoking

Tobacco smoking is the risk factor associated with the largest number of cancer cases worldwide, and the causal link with stomach cancer is recognized.[42] A recent meta-analysis of 32 studies, including 18 cohort studies, found significant positive associations of smoking with risk of both cardia and noncardia gastric cancer among most studies, overall increasing risk by 62% for male current smokers (95% confidence interval [CI] 1.50–1.75) and 20% for female current smokers (95% CI 1.01–1.43).[43] Tobacco smoke contains multiple well-known chemical carcinogens.[44] Although the mechanisms by which smoking increases the risk of gastric cancer are not completely understood, it is possible that tobacco smoke carcinogens affect gastric cancer risk directly through contact with the stomach mucosa or indirectly through the blood flow.[45]

Nonsteroidal Antiinflammatory Drugs

Observational studies have consistently found a protective effect of regular use of nonsteroidal antiinflammatory drugs (NSAIDs), particularly aspirin, on risk of gastric cancer. Specifically, a 2009 meta-analysis found that regular NSAID users had an 18% to 20% reduced risk of gastric cardia adenocarcinoma and a 32% to 36% reduced risk of distal gastric adenocarcinoma.[46] NSAIDs are considered to be chemopreventive agents because they suppress the production of cyclooxygenase enzymes, which are involved in prostaglandin biosynthesis.[47] Although clinical trials of NSAIDs and risk of colorectal adenoma among high-risk populations have mostly met with success,[48] there has been only 1 clinical trial with gastric cancer or a gastric cancer precursor. In this randomized trial of the COX-2 inhibitor rofecoxib, the drug did not reduce risk of gastric intestinal metaplasia after a 2-year period.[49] However, it is possible that the duration of drug use was not long enough, and/or that intervention with NSAIDs may be effective at a later stage of the carcinogenesis process. A recent international consensus statement on aspirin and cancer prevention concluded that future research should focus on high-risk individuals and aim to resolve the questions of optimal dose, age to begin therapy, and treatment duration.[50]

Socioeconomic Status

Lower socioeconomic status, whether measured by education or income, has been consistently associated with an at least twofold greater risk of gastric cancer.[51] This gradient has been observed within both high-risk countries (such as Japan) and low-risk countries (including the United States).[52] The factors creating this association are most likely characteristics related to low socioeconomic status that increase likelihood of transmission and reinfection with *H pylori*, such as household crowding, large family size, poor household sanitation, and less-frequent use of antibiotics. Low socioeconomic status could be an indicator of a diet lower in fresh fruits and vegetables. The high gastric cancer risk seen in a few countries with overall high socioeconomic status, such as Japan and South Korea, is not completely understood, but it is possibly caused by the prevalence of highly virulent strains of *H pylori* in these countries.[53]

The African Enigma

H pylori infects more than half of the world's population, with variable rates of prevalence across countries and among ethnic groups.[17] However, discordance between the high prevalence of *H pylori* infection and the low rates of gastric cancer has been observed in some areas, especially in the African continent. This phenomenon has been called the African enigma.[54] Studies carried out in different regions of Africa have shown that most populations are infected with *H pylori*, with 61% to 80% showing evidence of antibodies to *H pylori*, and that acquisition of the infection occurs at an early age.[54,55] In sub-Saharan Africa, despite overall high *H pylori* infection prevalence, gastric cancer incidences are low.[55] A similar pattern has been found in other geographic regions. In Colombia, our group has identified a high-risk area for gastric cancer in the Andes Mountains and a low-risk area on the Pacific coast.[56] The 2 populations have similar prevalence of *H pylori* infection in the adult population (74% and 80%)[32] and a common pattern of early age at infection.[57] In Costa Rica, marked regional heterogeneity in cancer incidence has been observed in spite of no significant variation in *H pylori* infection prevalence.[58] In both Colombia and Costa Rica, greater prevalence of more virulent strains has been observed in the high-risk areas.[32,59,60] However, it is unlikely that these differences are large enough to completely explain the differences in gastric cancer risk.

The lack of correlation between gastric cancer incidence and *H pylori* infection prevalence indicates that other factors, such as environmental factors, host genetic background, and coinfections, may modulate the outcome of the infection. One important factor is diet. High-risk populations tend to have excessive salt intake, whereas low-risk communities on the coastal regions of Colombia more frequently consume fish and seafood and fruits. Another factor is the type of immune response of the host to the *H pylori* infection. Intestinal parasites, especially helminths, are more frequent in tropical climates and they tend to modulate the immune response toward a Th2 anti-inflammatory type.[61,62] In Colombia, we observed that children in the low-risk area (on the coast) were more than twice as likely to be infected with helminths, and both adults and children had serum immunoglobulin E levels several times higher than those in the high-risk area (mountains).[62] In addition, significantly greater eosinophilic infiltration of the gastric mucosa was observed in infected adult subjects in the low-risk area compared with subjects in the high-risk area.[63] In an animal model, supporting this hypothesis, concurrent helminth infection considerably reduced *Helicobacter*-associated gastric inflammatory cytokines and chemokines associated with a Th1 response and gastric atrophy.[64] Similar evidence from a Chinese population indicates that a concurrent helminth infection modifies the immune response to *H pylori* and reduces the probability of developing gastric corpus atrophy.[65] These results suggest that early acquisition of the parasite induces an antiinflammatory Th2 immune response against the *H pylori* infection. This antiinflammatory response may aid in ameliorating the chronic damage to the gastric mucosa, subsequently decreasing the risk of gastric cancer.

THE HOST

Host Genetics in H pylori–induced Gastric Cancer

The association between chronic inflammation and cancer is well established, and gastric adenocarcinoma is usually accompanied by an evident inflammatory infiltrate. The long-standing inflammatory response against *H pylori* in the gastric mucosa may cause sustained tissue injury leading to the development of distal gastric cancer. Host genetic factors may influence the nature and intensity of the immune response to *H pylori*. Polymorphisms in cytokine genes have been associated with risk for gastric cancer. Biologically, the genetic polymorphisms are believed to modulate risk by increasing expression of proinflammatory factors that enhance and prolong the inflammatory response in gastric mucosa. El-Omar and colleagues[66,67] were the first to show that polymorphisms in *IL1B* and *IL1RN* genes (*IL1B* encoding interleukin [IL]-1β and *IL1RN* encoding its naturally occurring receptor antagonist) were associated with increased risk for hypochlorhydria and gastric cancer in subjects with *H pylori* infection. IL-1β is a proinflammatory cytokine and a potent inhibitor of gastric acid secretion. It has been hypothesized that a profound acid secretion suppression promotes proliferation and dissemination of *H pylori* from the antrum to the corpus, leading to a severe and more extensive gastritis that favors the development of atrophy and subsequently adenocarcinoma.[68] A meta-analysis concluded that *IL1B-511 T* and *IL1RN*2* polymorphisms are associated with gastric cancer in white people but not in Asian people, and that the association of *IL1B-511 T* in white people was stronger when intestinal type and noncardia gastric cancer cases were examined.[69] Polymorphisms in other cytokine genes have also been associated with cancer risk, including tumor necrosis factor α[70–72] and IL-10.[70] Studies combining host susceptibility with bacterial virulence factors have shown that gastric cancer risk is highest among those with both host and bacterial high-risk genotypes.[73,74] An increasing amount of evidence shows the possible role of multiple other polymorphisms in genes mainly related to processes involved in carcinogenesis and/or cell defense and repair.[75]

PATHOLOGY

Gastric adenocarcinomas are classified anatomically as proximal (cardia) and distal (noncardia). Distal adenocarcinomas are commonly associated with *H pylori* infection, but the association of this infection with cardia adenocarcinomas is less well defined. Gastric cardia adenocarcinomas are associated with gastroesophageal reflux disease.[76] For reasons that are unclear, the incidence of gastric cardia adenocarcinoma has been increasing during the last decades in conjunction with an increase in esophageal adenocarcinoma, especially among white men.[76–79] In the United States, gastric cardia adenocarcinomas have lower overall 5-year survival rates than distal adenocarcinomas (14% vs 26%).[76] In addition to the problem of distinguishing gastric cardia from noncardia adenocarcinomas, there is the difficulty in separating true cardia tumors from adenocarcinomas of the distal esophagus, frequently involving the gastroesophageal junction (GEJ). Thus, according to the Siewert and Stein classification, 3 types of carcinomas develop around the GEJ: (1) adenocarcinomas of the distal esophagus; (2) true cardia carcinomas, extending 1 cm above and 2 cm below the anatomic GEJ; and (3) subcardiac gastric cancers, tumors located more than 2 cm below the anatomic GEJ that may infiltrate the GEJ from below.[80]

Carcinoma of the stomach may be detected either in an early stage or in an advanced stage. Early gastric cancer is defined as an adenocarcinoma confined to the gastric mucosa or submucosa regardless of lymph node metastasis.[81] Most patients with early gastric cancer are asymptomatic. Among symptomatic patients, dyspepsia and epigastric pain are the most common symptoms. The macroscopic appearance of advanced carcinomas may be polypoid, fungating, ulcerated, or infiltrative (Borrmann classification), with occasional combinations of types. Histologically, there are several classifications for gastric adenocarcinomas. The most widely used in the United States is the Lauren classification, which recognizes 2 main types: intestinal and diffuse (**Fig. 3**).[82] Intestinal-type tumors predominate in geographic areas with a high incidence of gastric cancer, whereas diffuse-type tumors are found more uniformly throughout the world.

The Precancerous Process

Intestinal-type adenocarcinomas develop through a series of sequential lesions in the gastric mucosa (**Fig. 4**). This multistep precancerous process was described in 1975[83,84] based on observations in Colombian populations with high risk of gastric cancer,[56,85,86] and before the identification of *H pylori* infection as a carcinogen. The process starts when *H pylori* colonizes the gastric mucosa, initially in the antropyloric region, avoiding the lower pH in the acid-producing areas (fundus and corpus) of the stomach. The immune response induced by the bacterium may vary in severity, but usually causes a nonatrophic chronic gastritis that may last decades unless treatment eradicates the bacterium. In time, the infection may spread proximally to the oxyntic mucosa, mainly in patients taking proton pump inhibitors. Prolonged and severe infection may eventually result in loss of glandular tissue (multifocal atrophic gastritis) and sometimes in gastric ulcers. The atrophic changes usually start in the incisura angularis and may extend to the antrum and the corpus mucosa, as the foci become progressively larger and coalesce. In some patients with multifocal atrophic gastritis, the lost glands are then replaced by glandular structures with intestinal phenotype, displaying characteristics of small intestine (complete intestinal metaplasia) or colonic epithelium (incomplete intestinal metaplasia). The complete type displays absorptive enterocytes with brush border, well-developed goblet cells, and Paneth cells. In incomplete intestinal metaplasia, there are goblet cells of variable size, absence of brush border, and sometimes presence of sulfomucins. There is evidence that intestinal metaplasia of the incomplete type is associated with increased risk of gastric cancer.[87,88] A small proportion of patients with intestinal metaplasia eventually

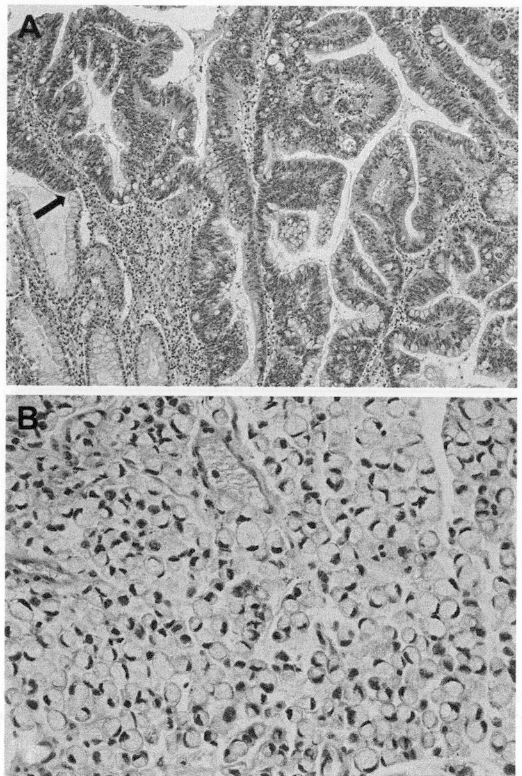

Fig. 3. Gastric adenocarcinoma. (*A*) Intestinal type, showing tumor cells cohesively arranged to form irregular glandular structures. On the left lower corner there are a few glands with intestinal metaplasia. An arrow shows the transition zone between intestinal metaplasia and adenocarcinoma (×100). (*B*) Diffuse type, with tumor cells that show lack of cohesiveness infiltrating diffusely. In this subtype, the signet-ring adenocarcinoma, the nuclei are pushed to the periphery by the abundant mucinous cytoplasmic content (×400).

progress to dysplasia (synonyms: intraepithelial neoplasia, noninvasive neoplasia, adenoma), which is classified as low grade or high grade. Some patients with dysplasia develop adenocarcinoma, defined as invasion of the lamina propria or beyond. *H pylori* tends to disappear as intestinal metaplasia develops. Therefore, previous or current *H pylori* infection may be underestimated in patients with intestinal metaplasia or more advanced lesions.

Intestinal-type Adenocarcinoma

Besides *H pylori* infection, other environmental factors, including diet and smoking, are recognized risk factors for intestinal-type adenocarcinoma. More recently (as described earlier), the etiopathogenic role of host genetic factors is increasingly recognized in this type of carcinoma. Most cases of intestinal-type adenocarcinomas are diagnosed between the ages of 50 and 70 years, and the incidence rate is approximately double in men compared with women. Microscopically, intestinal-type adenocarcinomas are formed by tumor cells arranged cohesively in irregular tubular or papillary structures infiltrating the stroma. Epithelium with intestinal metaplasia is frequently seen in neighboring mucosa (see **Fig. 3**A). Based on architectural and

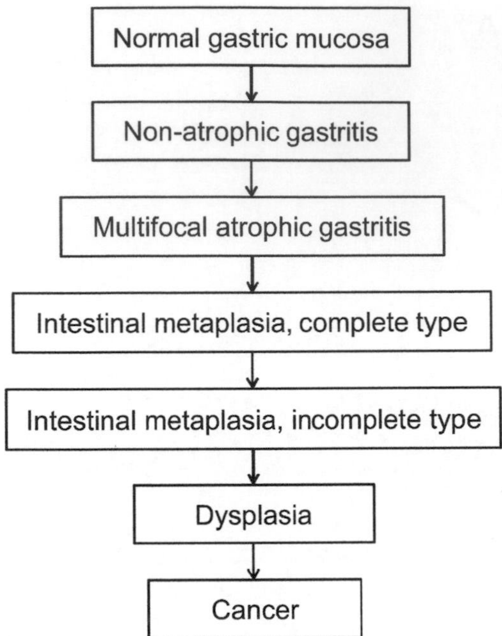

Fig. 4. Sequential steps in the gastric precancerous process. (*Adapted from* Correa P. Human gastric carcinogenesis: a multistep and multifactorial process–First American Cancer Society Award Lecture on Cancer Epidemiology and Prevention. Cancer Res 1992;52(24):6735–40; with permission.)

cellular characteristics, the tumors have variable degrees of differentiation. In the better-differentiated adenocarcinomas, most of the cells are columnar and contain cytoplasmic mucin. Poorly differentiated adenocarcinomas have a predominantly solid pattern.

Diffuse-type Adenocarcinoma

Diffuse-type adenocarcinoma is more frequent in populations at low risk for gastric cancer and in younger people, and environmental factors have been believed to play a less important role than genetic factors. Because atrophic changes are not severe in diffuse-type gastric cancer, it was previously considered to have little relation to *H pylori* infection. However, epidemiologic and histopathologic studies[30,89] have shown that the development of diffuse-type cancer is also related to *H pylori* infection. Gross alterations include thickening and rigidity of the gastric wall, a condition known as linitis plastica. Microscopically, the tumoral cells of the diffuse type are usually round and small, and are arranged as single cells with minimal, or an absence of, intercellular cohesion (see **Fig. 3**B).

Hereditary diffuse gastric cancer is an autosomal dominant disorder that accounts for less than 1% of all cases of gastric cancer. Mutations in the E-cadherin gene (*CDH1*) are germline defects associated with this syndrome.[90–92] *CDH1* encodes E-cadherin, a cell-to-cell adhesion molecule that plays a fundamental role in the maintenance of the normal architecture of epithelial tissues. Diffuse gastric cancer is the most important cause of cancer mortality in these families.[93] In addition to mutation, epigenetic inactivation of E-cadherin by promoter hypermethylation has frequently been reported in sporadic diffuse gastric cancer.[94,95]

CANCER CONTROL

The high mortality from gastric cancer is believed to be primarily caused by late-stage diagnoses. In the United States, two-thirds of gastric cancer cases are diagnosed when the tumor has invaded the muscularis propria, and the overall 5-year survival rate is about 25%.[96] Early gastric cancer is generally small and asymptomatic, and surgery or endoscopic resection can offer the chance of a cure. In Japan, a country with one of the highest incidences of gastric cancer, more than 50% of cases are diagnosed at an early stage because of a massive screening program. The 5-year survival rate in this group is more than 90%.[97] A recent review article by gastric cancer experts from the Asia Pacific Working Group on Gastric Cancer recommended multistage screening using serum-pepsinogen testing (to determine the presence and extension of atrophic gastritis) and *H pylori* serology to identify patients at high risk, who should then go on to endoscopic surveillance.[98] *H pylori* eradication has also been proposed as a method of gastric cancer prevention. In studies of precancerous gastric lesions, *H pylori* eradication generally reduced the rate of progression.[99] Although individual randomized, controlled trials of *H pylori* eradication on gastric cancer risk have generally found non–statistically significant suggestions of protection, a recent meta-analysis of these trials found that, when considering these trials together (and thus increasing the power to observe an association), *H pylori* eradication treatment does significantly reduce risk of gastric cancer.[100] In addition, a recent retrospective cohort study in Taiwan concluded that, for patients with peptic ulcers, early *H pylori* eradication (defined as within 1 year of hospitalization for the ulcer) decreased the risk of gastric cancer.[101] However, large-scale *H pylori* eradication strategies face challenges such as the development of antibiotic resistant strains. In the United States, because of the low incidence of gastric cancer, endoscopic surveillance is recommended only in patients with low-grade dysplasia. Patients with high-grade dysplasia need to undergo endoscopic or surgical resection.[102] However, surveillance of patients with gastric intestinal metaplasia should be considered in the presence of risk factors for gastric cancer such as family history of gastric cancer, ethnicity, and extensive or incomplete-type intestinal metaplasia.[88,103,104]

An *H pylori* vaccine has been in development for years, but there has been little success and currently an efficacious human vaccine does not exist. Both *H pylori* strategies of eradication and vaccine development have also been criticized because of the potential unexpected effects of *H pylori* eradication, including increased risk of esophageal adenocarcinoma, gastroesophageal reflux–related diseases, and possibly allergic and autoimmune diseases.[105–108]

SUMMARY

The role of infectious agents and chronic inflammation in carcinogenesis is being increasingly recognized. It has been estimated that about 18% of cancers are directly linked to infections, particularly gastric adenocarcinoma (*H pylori*), cervical carcinoma (human papilloma viruses), and hepatocarcinoma (hepatitis B and C viruses).[17] Multiple clinical trials of COX-2 inhibitors and antiinflammatory agents have shown a beneficial effect on the development of diverse tumors, such as those of the colon, prostate, and breast.[50] However, their mechanism of action is not completely understood and may differ among the infectious agents and tumor types.

REFERENCES

1. IARC Monographs on the evaluation of carcinogenic risks to humans. Schistosomes, liver flukes and *Helicobacter pylori*. Lyon (France): International Agency for Research on Cancer; 1994. p. 177–240.
2. Honda S, Fujioka T, Tokieda M, et al. Development of *Helicobacter pylori*-induced gastric carcinoma in Mongolian gerbils. Cancer Res 1998;58(19):4255–9.
3. Bouvard V, Baan R, Straif K, et al. A review of human carcinogens–Part B: Biological agents. Lancet Oncol 2009;10(4):321–2.
4. Coleman MP, Esteve J, Damiecki P, et al. Trends in cancer incidence and mortality. Lyon (France): International Agency for Research on Cancer; 1993.
5. Parkin DM, Bray F, Ferlay J, et al. Global cancer statistics, 2002. CA Cancer J Clin 2005;55(2):74–108.
6. Thun MJ, DeLancey JO, Center MM, et al. The global burden of cancer: priorities for prevention. Carcinogenesis 2010;31(1):100–10.
7. Espey DK, Wu XC, Swan J, et al. Annual report to the nation on the status of cancer, 1975–2004, featuring cancer in American Indians and Alaska Natives. Cancer 2007;110(10):2119–52.
8. Wu X, Chen VW, Andrews PA, et al. Incidence of esophageal and gastric cancers among hispanics, non-hispanic whites and non-hispanic blacks in the United States: subsite and histology differences. Cancer Causes Control 2007;18(6):585–93.
9. Wu X, Chen VW, Ruiz B, et al. Incidence of esophageal and gastric carcinomas among American Asians/Pacific Islanders, whites, and blacks: subsite and histology differences. Cancer 2006;106(3):683–92.
10. Anderson WF, Camargo MC, Fraumeni JF Jr, et al. Age-specific trends in incidence of noncardia gastric cancer in US adults. JAMA 2010;303(17):1723–8.
11. Helicobacter and Cancer Collaborative Group. Gastric cancer and *Helicobacter pylori*: a combined analysis of 12 case control studies nested within prospective cohorts. Gut 2001;49(3):347–53.
12. Kamangar F, Dawsey SM, Blaser MJ, et al. Opposing risks of gastric cardia and noncardia gastric adenocarcinomas associated with *Helicobacter pylori* seropositivity. J Natl Cancer Inst 2006;98(20):1445–52.
13. Uemura N, Okamoto S, Yamamoto S, et al. *Helicobacter pylori* infection and the development of gastric cancer. N Engl J Med 2001;345(11):784–9.
14. Leavell HR, Clark EG. Preventive medicine for the doctor in his community; an epidemiologic approach. New York: McGraw-Hill; 1965.
15. Haenszel W, Kurihara M. Studies of Japanese migrants. I. Mortality from cancer and other diseases among Japanese in the United States. J Natl Cancer Inst 1968;40(1):43–68.
16. Marshall BJ, Warren JR. Unidentified curved bacilli in the stomach of patients with gastritis and peptic ulceration. Lancet 1984;1(8390):1311–5.
17. Parkin DM. The global health burden of infection-associated cancers in the year 2002. Int J Cancer 2006;118(12):3030–44.
18. Cover TL, Blaser MJ. *Helicobacter pylori* in health and disease. Gastroenterology 2009;136(6):1863–73.
19. Peek RM Jr, Crabtree JE. *Helicobacter* infection and gastric neoplasia. J Pathol 2006;208(2):233–48.
20. Achtman M, Azuma T, Berg DE, et al. Recombination and clonal groupings within *Helicobacter pylori* from different geographical regions. Mol Microbiol 1999;32(3):459–70.

21. Falush D, Wirth T, Linz B, et al. Traces of human migrations in *Helicobacter pylori* populations. Science 2003;299(5612):1582–5.
22. Linz B, Balloux F, Moodley Y, et al. An African origin for the intimate association between humans and *Helicobacter pylori*. Nature 2007;445(7130):915–8.
23. Censini S, Lange C, Xiang Z, et al. Cag, a pathogenicity island of *Helicobacter pylori*, encodes type I-specific and disease-associated virulence factors. Proc Natl Acad Sci USA 1996;93(25):14648–53.
24. Covacci A, Censini S, Bugnoli M, et al. Molecular characterization of the 128-kDa immunodominant antigen of *Helicobacter pylori* associated with cytotoxicity and duodenal ulcer. Proc Natl Acad Sci USA 1993;90(12): 5791–5.
25. Devi SM, Ahmed I, Khan AA, et al. Genomes of *Helicobacter pylori* from native Peruvians suggest admixture of ancestral and modern lineages and reveal a western type cag-pathogenicity island. BMC Genomics 2006;7:191.
26. Dominguez-Bello MG, Perez ME, Bortolini MC, et al. Amerindian *Helicobacter pylori* strains go extinct, as European strains expand their host range. PLoS One 2008;3(10):e3307.
27. Hatakeyama M. *Helicobacter pylori* and gastric carcinogenesis. J Gastroenterol 2009;44(4):239–48.
28. Tham KT, Peek RM Jr, Atherton JC, et al. *Helicobacter pylori* genotypes, host factors, and gastric mucosal histopathology in peptic ulcer disease. Hum Pathol 2001;32(3):264–73.
29. Blaser MJ, Perez-Perez GI, Kleanthous H, et al. Infection with *Helicobacter pylori* strains possessing *cagA* is associated with an increased risk of developing adenocarcinoma of the stomach. Cancer Res 1995;55(10): 2111–5.
30. Parsonnet J, Friedman GD, Orentreich N, et al. Risk for gastric cancer in people with CagA positive or CagA negative *Helicobacter pylori* infection. Gut 1997; 40(3):297–301.
31. Plummer M, van Doorn LJ, Franceschi S, et al. *Helicobacter pylori* cytotoxin-associated genotype and gastric precancerous lesions. J Natl Cancer Inst 2007;99(17):1328–34.
32. Bravo LE, van Doom LJ, Realpe JL, et al. Virulence-associated genotypes of *Helicobacter pylori*: do they explain the African enigma? Am J Gastroenterol 2002;97(11):2839–42.
33. Cover TL, Blanke SR. *Helicobacter pylori* VacA, a paradigm for toxin multifunctionality. Nat Rev Microbiol 2005;3(4):320–32.
34. Hansson LE, Nyren O, Hsing AW, et al. The risk of stomach cancer in patients with gastric or duodenal ulcer disease. N Engl J Med 1996;335(4):242–9.
35. Murphy G, Pfeiffer R, Camargo MC, et al. Meta-analysis shows that prevalence of Epstein-Barr virus-positive gastric cancer differs based on sex and anatomic location. Gastroenterology 2009;137(3):824–33.
36. Akiba S, Koriyama C, Herrera-Goepfert R, et al. Epstein-Barr virus associated gastric carcinoma: epidemiological and clinicopathological features. Cancer Sci 2008;99(2):195–201.
37. World Cancer Research Fund/American Institute for Cancer Research. Food, nutrition, physical activity, and the prevention of cancer: a global perspective. Washington, DC: AICR; 2007.
38. Fox JG, Dangler CA, Taylor NS, et al. High-salt diet induces gastric epithelial hyperplasia and parietal cell loss, and enhances *Helicobacter pylori* colonization in C57BL/6 mice. Cancer Res 1999;59(19):4823–8.

39. Yamaguchi N, Kakizoe T. Synergistic interaction between *Helicobacter pylori* gastritis and diet in gastric cancer. Lancet Oncol 2001;2(2):88–94.
40. Epplein M, Nomura AM, Hankin JH, et al. Association of *Helicobacter pylori* infection and diet on the risk of gastric cancer: a case-control study in Hawaii. Cancer Causes Control 2008;19(8):869–77.
41. Gonzalez CA, Pera G, Agudo A, et al. Fruit and vegetable intake and the risk of stomach and oesophagus adenocarcinoma in the European Prospective Investigation into Cancer and Nutrition (EPIC-EURGAST). Int J Cancer 2006;118(10):2559–66.
42. Secretan B, Straif K, Baan R, et al. A review of human carcinogens–Part E: tobacco, areca nut, alcohol, coal smoke, and salted fish. Lancet Oncol 2009;10(11):1033–4.
43. Ladeiras-Lopes R, Pereira AK, Nogueira A, et al. Smoking and gastric cancer: systematic review and meta-analysis of cohort studies. Cancer Causes Control 2008;19(7):689–701.
44. IARC Monographs on the evaluation of carcinogenic risks to humans. Tobacco smoke and involuntary smoking. Lyon (France): International Agency for Research on Cancer; 2004. p. 59–94.
45. Gonzalez CA, Pera G, Agudo A, et al. Smoking and the risk of gastric cancer in the European Prospective Investigation Into Cancer and Nutrition (EPIC). Int J Cancer 2003;107(4):629–34.
46. Abnet CC, Freedman ND, Kamangar F, et al. Non-steroidal anti-inflammatory drugs and risk of gastric and oesophageal adenocarcinomas: results from a cohort study and a meta-analysis. Br J Cancer 2009;100(3):551–7.
47. Thun MJ, Henley SJ, Patrono C. Nonsteroidal anti-inflammatory drugs as anticancer agents: mechanistic, pharmacologic, and clinical issues. J Natl Cancer Inst 2002;94(4):252–66.
48. Baron JA. Aspirin and NSAIDs for the prevention of colorectal cancer. Recent Results Cancer Res 2009;181:223–9.
49. Leung WK, Ng EK, Chan FK, et al. Effects of long-term rofecoxib on gastric intestinal metaplasia: results of a randomized controlled trial. Clin Cancer Res 2006;12(15):4766–72.
50. Cuzick J, Otto F, Baron JA, et al. Aspirin and non-steroidal anti-inflammatory drugs for cancer prevention: an international consensus statement. Lancet Oncol 2009;10(5):501–7.
51. Nyren O, Adami H-O. Stomach cancer. In: Adami H-O, Hunter D, Trichopoulos D, editors. Textbook of cancer epidemiology. New York: Oxford University Press; 2002. p. 162–87.
52. Nomura A. Stomach cancer. In: Schottenfeld D, Fraumeni J, editors. Cancer epidemiology and prevention. 2nd edition. New York: Oxford University Press; 1996. p. 707–24.
53. Nguyen LT, Uchida T, Murakami K, et al. *Helicobacter pylori* virulence and the diversity of gastric cancer in Asia. J Med Microbiol 2008;57(Pt 12):1445–53.
54. Holcombe C. *Helicobacter pylori*: the African enigma. Gut 1992;33(4):429–31.
55. Segal I, Ally R, Mitchell H. Gastric cancer in sub-Saharan Africa. Eur J Cancer Prev 2001;10(6):479–82.
56. Correa P, Cuello C, Duque E, et al. Gastric cancer in Colombia. III. Natural history of precursor lesions. J Natl Cancer Inst 1976;57(5):1027–35.
57. Camargo MC, Yepez MC, Ceron C, et al. Age at acquisition of *Helicobacter pylori* infection: comparison of two areas with contrasting risk of gastric cancer. Helicobacter 2004;9(3):262–70.

58. Tsuji S. The "Costa Rican enigma" of *Helicobacter pylori* CagA and gastric cancer. J Gastroenterol 2006;41(7):716–7.
59. Con SA, Valerin AL, Takeuchi H, et al. *Helicobacter pylori* CagA status associated with gastric cancer incidence rate variability in Costa Rican regions. J Gastroenterol 2006;41(7):632–7.
60. Sicinschi LA, Correa P, Peek RM Jr, et al. *Helicobacter pylori* genotyping and sequencing using paraffin-embedded biopsies from residents of Colombian areas with contrasting gastric cancer risks. Helicobacter 2008;13(2):135–45.
61. Mitchell HM, Ally R, Wadee A, et al. Major differences in the IgG subclass response to *Helicobacter pylori* in the first and third worlds. Scand J Gastroenterol 2002;37(5):517–22.
62. Whary MT, Sundina N, Bravo LE, et al. Intestinal helminthiasis in Colombian children promotes a Th2 response to *Helicobacter pylori*: possible implications for gastric carcinogenesis. Cancer Epidemiol Biomarkers Prev 2005;14(6):1464–9.
63. Piazuelo MB, Camargo MC, Mera RM, et al. Eosinophils and mast cells in chronic gastritis: possible implications in carcinogenesis. Hum Pathol 2008; 39(9):1360–9.
64. Fox JG, Beck P, Dangler CA, et al. Concurrent enteric helminth infection modulates inflammation and gastric immune responses and reduces *Helicobacter*-induced gastric atrophy. Nat Med 2000;6(5):536–42.
65. Du Y, Agnew A, Ye XP, et al. *Helicobacter pylori* and *Schistosoma japonicum* co-infection in a Chinese population: helminth infection alters humoral responses to *H. pylori* and serum pepsinogen I/II ratio. Microbes Infect 2006;8(1):52–60.
66. El-Omar EM, Carrington M, Chow WH, et al. Interleukin-1 polymorphisms associated with increased risk of gastric cancer. Nature 2000;404(6776):398–402.
67. El-Omar EM, Carrington M, Chow WH, et al. The role of interleukin-1 polymorphisms in the pathogenesis of gastric cancer [erratum]. Nature 2001;412(6842):99.
68. El-Omar EM. The importance of interleukin 1beta in *Helicobacter pylori* associated disease. Gut 2001;48(6):743–7.
69. Camargo MC, Mera R, Correa P, et al. Interleukin-1beta and interleukin-1 receptor antagonist gene polymorphisms and gastric cancer: a meta-analysis. Cancer Epidemiol Biomarkers Prev 2006;15(9):1674–87.
70. El-Omar EM, Rabkin CS, Gammon MD, et al. Increased risk of noncardia gastric cancer associated with proinflammatory cytokine gene polymorphisms. Gastroenterology 2003;124(5):1193–201.
71. Gorouhi F, Islami F, Bahrami H, et al. Tumour-necrosis factor-A polymorphisms and gastric cancer risk: a meta-analysis. Br J Cancer 2008;98(8):1443–51.
72. Machado JC, Figueiredo C, Canedo P, et al. A proinflammatory genetic profile increases the risk for chronic atrophic gastritis and gastric carcinoma. Gastroenterology 2003;125(2):364–71.
73. Figueiredo C, Machado JC, Pharoah P, et al. *Helicobacter pylori* and interleukin 1 genotyping: an opportunity to identify high-risk individuals for gastric carcinoma. J Natl Cancer Inst 2002;94(22):1680–7.
74. Sicinschi LA, Lopez-Carrillo L, Camargo MC, et al. Gastric cancer risk in a Mexican population: role of *Helicobacter pylori* CagA positive infection and polymorphisms in interleukin-1 and -10 genes. Int J Cancer 2006;118(3): 649–57.
75. Correa P, Camargo MC, Piazuelo MB. Overview and pathology of gastric cancer. In: Wang TC, Fox JG, Giraud AS, editors. The biology of gastric cancers. New York: Springer; 2009. p. 1–24.

76. Brown LM, Devesa SS. Epidemiologic trends in esophageal and gastric cancer in the United States. Surg Oncol Clin N Am 2002;11(2):235–56.
77. Blot WJ, Devesa SS, Kneller RW, et al. Rising incidence of adenocarcinoma of the esophagus and gastric cardia. JAMA 1991;265(10):1287–9.
78. Devesa SS, Blot WJ, Fraumeni JF Jr. Changing patterns in the incidence of esophageal and gastric carcinoma in the United States. Cancer 1998;83(10): 2049–53.
79. Devesa SS, Fraumeni JF Jr. The rising incidence of gastric cardia cancer. J Natl Cancer Inst 1999;91(9):747–9.
80. Siewert JR, Stein HJ. Classification of adenocarcinoma of the oesophagogastric junction. Br J Surg 1998;85(11):1457–9.
81. Japanese Gastric Cancer Association. Japanese classification of gastric carcinoma - 2nd English edition. Gastric Cancer 1998;1(1):10–24.
82. Lauren P. The two histological main types of gastric carcinoma: diffuse and so called intestinal-type carcinoma. Acta Pathol Microbiol Scand 1965;64:31–49.
83. Correa P. Human gastric carcinogenesis: a multistep and multifactorial process–first American Cancer Society Award Lecture on Cancer Epidemiology and Prevention. Cancer Res 1992;52(24):6735–40.
84. Correa P, Haenszel W, Cuello C, et al. A model for gastric cancer epidemiology. Lancet 1975;2(7924):58–60.
85. Correa P, Bolanos O, Garcia F, et al. The cancer registry of Cali, Colombia. Epidemiologic studies of gastric cancer. Recent Results Cancer Res 1975;50: 155–69.
86. Correa P, Cuello C, Duque E. Carcinoma and intestinal metaplasia of the stomach in Colombian migrants. J Natl Cancer Inst 1970;44(2):297–306.
87. Filipe MI, Munoz N, Matko I, et al. Intestinal metaplasia types and the risk of gastric cancer: a cohort study in Slovenia. Int J Cancer 1994;57(3):324–9.
88. Tava F, Luinetti O, Ghigna MR, et al. Type or extension of intestinal metaplasia and immature/atypical "indefinite-for-dysplasia" lesions as predictors of gastric neoplasia. Hum Pathol 2006;37(11):1489–97.
89. Kikuchi S, Wada O, Nakajima T, et al. Serum anti-*Helicobacter pylori* antibody and gastric carcinoma among young adults. Research Group on Prevention of Gastric Carcinoma among Young Adults. Cancer 1995;75(12):2789–93.
90. Guilford P, Hopkins J, Harraway J, et al. E-cadherin germline mutations in familial gastric cancer. Nature 1998;392(6674):402–5.
91. Guilford PJ, Hopkins JB, Grady WM, et al. E-cadherin germline mutations define an inherited cancer syndrome dominated by diffuse gastric cancer. Hum Mutat 1999;14(3):249–55.
92. Lynch HT, Kaurah P, Wirtzfeld D, et al. Hereditary diffuse gastric cancer: diagnosis, genetic counseling, and prophylactic total gastrectomy. Cancer 2008; 112(12):2655–63.
93. Pharoah PD, Guilford P, Caldas C. Incidence of gastric cancer and breast cancer in CDH1 (E-cadherin) mutation carriers from hereditary diffuse gastric cancer families. Gastroenterology 2001;121(6):1348–53.
94. Machado JC, Oliveira C, Carvalho R, et al. E-cadherin gene (*CDH1*) promoter methylation as the second hit in sporadic diffuse gastric carcinoma. Oncogene 2001;20(12):1525–8.
95. Tamura G, Yin J, Wang S, et al. E-Cadherin gene promoter hypermethylation in primary human gastric carcinomas. J Natl Cancer Inst 2000;92(7):569–73.
96. Jemal A, Siegel R, Ward E, et al. Cancer statistics, 2009. CA Cancer J Clin 2009; 59(4):225–49.

97. Sano T, Katai H, Sasako M, et al. The management of early gastric cancer. Surg Oncol 2000;9(1):17–22.
98. Leung WK, Wu MS, Kakugawa Y, et al. Screening for gastric cancer in Asia: current evidence and practice. Lancet Oncol 2008;9(3):279–87.
99. Mera R, Fontham ET, Bravo LE, et al. Long term follow up of patients treated for *Helicobacter pylori* infection. Gut 2005;54(11):1536–40.
100. Fuccio L, Zagari RM, Eusebi LH, et al. Meta-analysis: can *Helicobacter pylori* eradication treatment reduce the risk for gastric cancer? Ann Intern Med 2009;151(2):121–8.
101. Wu CY, Kuo KN, Wu MS, et al. Early *Helicobacter pylori* eradication decreases risk of gastric cancer in patients with peptic ulcer disease. Gastroenterology 2009;137(5):1641–8.
102. Lauwers GY, Srivastava A. Gastric preneoplastic lesions and epithelial dysplasia. Gastroenterol Clin North Am 2007;36(4):813–29.
103. Correa P, Piazuelo MB, Wilson KT. Pathology of gastric intestinal metaplasia: Clinical implications. Am J Gastroenterol 2010;105(3):493–8.
104. de Vries AC, Haringsma J, de Vries RA, et al. The use of clinical, histologic, and serologic parameters to predict the intragastric extent of intestinal metaplasia: a recommendation for routine practice. Gastrointest Endosc 2009;70(1):18–25.
105. Blaser MJ, Falkow S. What are the consequences of the disappearing human microbiota? Nat Rev Microbiol 2009;7(12):887–94.
106. Chen Y, Blaser MJ. Inverse associations of *Helicobacter pylori* with asthma and allergy. Arch Intern Med 2007;167(8):821–7.
107. Islami F, Kamangar F. *Helicobacter pylori* and esophageal cancer risk: a meta-analysis. Cancer Prev Res (Phila Pa) 2008;1(5):329–38.
108. Peek RM Jr, Blaser MJ. *Helicobacter pylori* and gastrointestinal tract adenocarcinomas. Nat Rev Cancer 2002;2(1):28–37.

Cholangiocarcinoma: New Insights into Disease Pathogenesis and Biology

Chiara Braconi, MD, PhD, Tushar Patel, MBChB*

KEYWORDS

• Biliary tract cancers • Liver flukes • Liver cancers

OVERVIEW

Recent studies have shown an increased global incidence of cholangiocarcinomas, rare malignant tumors with morphologic features of biliary tract epithelia. This aggressive and poorly understood malignancy remains largely incurable. Biliary tract inflammation resulting from liver fluke infection or other causes is a well-defined risk factor for cholangiocarcinoma. Recent studies have explored the relationship between inflammatory mediators and biliary tract carcinogenesis and provided an insight into the molecular and genetic perturbations involved in the pathogenesis of cholangiocarcinoma.

CLASSIFICATION

Cholangiocarcinomas are classified into 2 major categories based on their anatomic location. Intrahepatic cholangiocarcinomas (ICCs) arise within the hepatic parenchyma and most often present as a mass lesion without major bile duct obstruction or jaundice. Ductal cholangiocarcinoma arises within the large bile ducts, namely common bile duct, common hepatic duct, and right or left hepatic duct up to the secondary bifurcation. Perihilar cholangiocarcinomas, or Klatskin tumors, are often considered separately but should be classified as ductal cholangiocarcinomas based on their location and presentation. These lesions can extend into the hepatic parenchyma and have also been classified as intrahepatic or extrahepatic. The lack of a consistent convention has led to inaccurate reporting of the epidemiology, natural history, and prognosis. Among the hilar lesions, the Bismuth classification has been widely used as a guide to surgical intervention. Intrahepatic and ductal cholangiocarcinomas can be further classified on the basis of the pathology. The staging system

Funding support: Supported in part by the National Institutes of Health, DK 06378.
Department of Internal Medicine, The Ohio State University Medical Center, 395 West 12th Avenue, Columbus, OH 43210, USA
* Corresponding author.
E-mail address: tushar.patel@osumc.edu

Infect Dis Clin N Am 24 (2010) 871–884
doi:10.1016/j.idc.2010.07.006 id.theclinics.com
0891-5520/10/$ – see front matter

used by the Liver Cancer Study Group of Japan classifies ICCs as mass forming, periductal infiltrating, intraductal, or mixed. Similarly, extrahepatic ductal cholangiocarcinoma can be further described as sclerosing, nodular, or papillary.[1] However, these clinical and pathologic classifications require modifications to incorporate hilar lesions. The TNM classification for biliary tract cancers has not been useful in clinical practice because the T category does not differentiate prognosis, for example, in T2 and T3 tumors.[2] In a recent study, the number of lesions and presence of vascular invasion were important prognostic factors, whereas tumor size was not.[2]

EPIDEMIOLOGY

The incidence of these cancers shows a marked variation worldwide. In regions where liver flukes are endemic, the rates of ICC are extremely high; for example, in the Khon Kaen region in Thailand, cholangiocarcinoma accounts for more than 85% of all cancers. In the United States, the incidence ranges from 3 to 8 per 100,000. In most other parts of the world, the incidence of ICC has increased during the last few decades, with an annual percentage change of about 9%.[3,4] However, observations during the past decade have indicated that the rate of increase may be leveling off. The grouping together of ICC and hepatocellular cancer in epidemiologic reports has confounded an analysis of the true incidence of these cancers in the United States. The incidence of ductal cholangiocarcinoma is less variable. The reported incidence of extrahepatic cholangiocarcinoma, for example, is twice as high in Manitoba, Canada, compared with that in the United Kingdom.[5]

There are racial and gender differences in the incidence of these cancers. The incidence of ICC is higher in men than in women,[6,7] whereas the incidence of extrahepatic cholangiocarcinoma is comparable between the 2 sexes.[6] The incidence is increased in African Americans (1.5-fold), American Indians and Hispanics (1.8-fold), and Asian Americans and Pacific Islanders (2.5-fold) compared with whites in the United States. Overall, the prevalence is greater in men, except in Hispanics, in whom the prevalence is greater in women.[7] The overall age-adjusted mortality rates for ICC in the United States are highest for the American Indian/Alaska Native and Asian/Pacific groups. However, the increase in mortality rates is similar for all racial groups, with an annual percentage change of greater than 3.5%, except for Asian/Pacific Islander women, for whom mortality rates have been slightly decreasing.[7] According to the American Cancer Society, in the United States, the estimated number of deaths caused by extrahepatic cholangiocarcinoma in 2008 were 3340 per year, with 62% of these occurring in men.[6]

RISK FACTORS

Several risk factors have been identified for cholangiocarcinoma (**Box 1**). Although the risk factors vary geographically, there is a strong association of cholangiocarcinoma with chronic biliary tract infection and inflammation. Well-characterized risk factors include liver fluke infestations, chronic viral hepatitis, hepatolithiasis, choledochal cysts, and primary sclerosing cholangitis (PSC).

Liver Fluke Infestation

Infestation with either *Clonorchis sinensis* or *Opisthorchis viverrini* leads to an increased risk of cholangiocarcinoma. Both these liver flukes are now considered as grade 1 carcinogens by the World Health Organization and International Agency for Research on Cancer.

C sinensis infection is endemic in south China, Japan, Korea, and Taiwan because of a long tradition of consuming raw fish or shellfish. Chronic infection with heavy parasite

Box 1
Risk factors for cholangiocarcinoma

- Liver fluke (*C sinensis, O viverrini*) infection
- Primary sclerosing cholangitis
- Choledochal cysts
- Viral hepatitis B and C infection
- Human immunodeficiency virus infection
- Cirrhosis
- Hepatolithiasis
- Toxins, including alcohol
- Lynch syndrome
- Diabetes
- Obesity

loads has been associated with various hepatobiliary diseases. *Clonorchis* dwells in the bile ducts and induces an inflammatory reaction that causes a malignant transformation of cholangiocytes. Patients affected by clonorchiasis have a higher risk for developing cholangiocarcinoma. In a recent analysis of more than 3000 Korean patients, the incidence of cholangiocarcinoma was 8.6%.[8] Since the introduction of praziquantel, the incidence of clonorchiasis has been reduced in the endemic areas. However, this condition has not been eradicated, and chronic infestation remains the main cause of cholangiocarcinoma in these areas. The detection of *C sinensis* is problematic because fecal examination for eggs has low sensitivity and, in the intradermal test, diluted antigens of *Clonorchis* can cross-react with other parasites such as *Paragonimus westermani*.[9] Thus, the diagnosis can be missed. Adult worms can remain in the peripheral intrahepatic bile ducts for 20 to 30 years, causing chronic persistent infection[10] and subsequently resulting in cholangiocarcinoma.

O viverrini is highly prevalent in Thailand and Laos. As with *C sinensis*, humans are infected by ingesting undercooked fish containing infective metacercariae. This infection is associated with several benign hepatobiliary diseases, including cholangitis, obstructive jaundice, hepatomegaly, and cholecystitis. The risk of cholangiocarcinoma depends on the intensity of the infection,[11] previous or current exposure to infection, and host genetic polymorphisms.[12] Less than 10% of people infected with *O viverrini* may develop cholangiocarcinoma.[13] However, other than for Thailand, cancer registration and statistics are not available for many other countries in the region. Thus, an accurate estimation of the risk of developing cholangiocarcinoma is difficult.[14] Conversely, in Thailand, more than 80% of cholangiocarcinomas test positive for the presence of *O viverrini* by real-time polymerase chain reaction (PCR).[15] Repeated infection with *O viverrini* induces oxidative DNA lesions, such as 8-oxo-7,8-dihydro-2′-deoxyguanosine (8-oxodG), in the bile duct epithelium, which are carcinogenic. The urinary level of 8-oxodG was found to be significantly higher in patients with cholangiocarcinoma than in *O viverrini*–infected patients and healthy subjects. Praziquantel is effective against *O viverrini* and can significantly decrease the urinary level of 8-oxodG. Thus, urinary 8-oxodG may be a useful biomarker to monitor infection and the efficacy of treatment, as well as for surveillance for tumors.[16] Repeated infections with *O viverrini* may accelerate DNA damage.[17] Thus, a preventive strategy to reduce infection, such as by decreasing the consumption of infected fish, may be more rational to reduce the incidence of cholangiocarcinoma than a strategy that is focused on treating established infections.

Primary Sclerosing Cholangitis

In the Western world, the incidence of liver fluke infestation is quite low, and PSC is the main risk factor for cholangiocarcinoma. PSC is a chronic idiopathic inflammatory disorder characterized by fibrosis and bile duct strictures. The risk of cholangiocarcinoma varies from 7% to 40%.[18,19] The duration of PSC does not correlate with the development of cholangiocarcinoma, and the estimated risk of cholangiocarcinoma at 10 years is similar to that at 20 years.[19] In a recent study, the median interval between the diagnosis of PSC and cholangiocarcinoma was 2.5 years, with all cases developing within 3 years. Thus, it is unclear whether or not cholangiocarcinoma occurs as a synchronous condition or as a consequence of PSC in these patients.[20]

Congenital Abnormalities of the Biliary Tract

Patients with choledochal cysts, congenital cystic dilations of the biliary tract, are at risk of malignancy. Similarly, patients with Caroli disease or congenital hepatic fibrosis, which are developmental abnormalities resulting in multiple intrahepatic cysts, are also at risk of developing cholangiocarcinoma.

Chronic Viral Hepatitis

Hepatitis C virus (HCV) infection has been recently described as a risk factor for cholangiocarcinoma. In a retrospective US cohort study, HCV infection was significantly associated with an increased risk of cholangiocarcinoma. Although the rate of infection remained low (4 per 100,000 person-years), the risk was more than doubled in the HCV-infected cohort than in the uninfected cohort. The risk for extrahepatic cholangiocarcinoma was not increased.[21] A prospective cohort study from Japan showed that 2.3% of 600 patients with HCV-related cirrhosis developed ICC during a mean follow-up of 7 years and had a significantly higher risk of developing cholangiocarcinoma than the general population.[22] Although growing evidence is supporting the carcinogenic effects of HCV proteins in hepatocellular carcinoma, the involvement of HCV in cholangiocarcinogenesis is less clear. The HCV core protein can alter cellular proliferation and apoptosis in hilar cholangiocarcinoma cells.[23] Because ICC and hepatocellular carcinoma may arise from the same progenitor cells, common mechanisms may account for the malignant transformation.[24]

Hepatitis B virus (HBV) infection is also a recognized risk factor. In China, where HBV infection is endemic, the main risk factors are HBV infection and hepatolithiasis. The prevalence of hepatitis B surface antigen (HBsAg) seropositivity and hepatolithiasis was increased from 9% to 48% and from 1% to 5%, respectively, in patients with ICC compared with controls.[25] In studies conducted in other regions such as Korea, Italy, and the United States, HBsAg seropositivity in patients with ICC ranged from 0.2% to 13%.[26–29] It is hoped that screening and vaccination strategies for HBV in regions of high endemicity may lead to a reduction of cholangiocarcinoma, similar to the dramatic effects of these strategies in reducing hepatocellular cancer.

Hepatolithiasis

The relationship between hepatolithiasis and cholangiocarcinoma has been long recognized.[30] In cholangiocarcinoma associated with hepatolithiasis, the stones are closely situated within or adjacent to the tumor foci. Carcinomatous cells spread along the luminal surface of the stone-containing bile ducts and invade the ductal walls. Features of chronic proliferative cholangitis are usually found within these bile ducts.[31]

A wide range of molecular alterations has been described in this setting, such as inactivation of p16, increased expression of cyclooxygenase (COX)-2 and prostaglandin E_2, overexpression of the proto-oncogene c-met, and lack of the tumor suppressor, caudal-related homeobox gene 2. These alterations have been noted in precursor lesions and in established cholangiocarcinoma.[32] Most primary hepatolithiasis involves calcium bilirubinate; cases of cholesterol hepatolithiasis have also been described, although rare.[33]

Alcohol and Toxins

Certain exposures may lead to increased risk of cholangiocarcinoma. Multiple case-control analyses have reported an association between cholangiocarcinoma and alcohol use.[34,35] Several cases of cholangiocarcinoma have been described after the iatrogenic exposure to thorium dioxide (Thorotrast), a radiocontrast agent used in the past.[36] Exposure to toxins may be linked to outbreaks of cholangiocarcinoma, which have been noted in Italy, West Virginia, and British Columbia, although convincing evidence for any likely culprits is lacking.

Cirrhosis and Other Causes

Cirrhosis has been previously associated with a higher incidence of cholangiocarcinoma in a large cohort study in Denmark.[37] The risk of cholangiocarcinoma might be mediated by HCV-induced liver cirrhosis. Analysis of the Surveillance, Epidemiology and End Results–Medicare database established the relationship between several risk factors in the US population. Cirrhosis and primary biliary cirrhosis were significantly more common among extrahepatic cholangiocarcinoma and ICC cases than in controls.[38] Alcoholic liver disease, type 2 diabetes, obesity, and human immunodeficiency virus infection are also significantly associated with cholangiocarcinoma.

SCREENING FOR CHOLANGIOCARCINOMA

The lifetime risk for cholangiocarcinoma varies according to the specific risk factors involved. These tumors are usually silent or associated with nonspecific symptoms, and diagnosis is frequently late (**Fig. 1**). Although early detection is needed to improve survival rates, there are no proven effective screening tests to date. Serum or stool tests for liver flukes and estimation of urinary levels of 8-oxodG might be promising

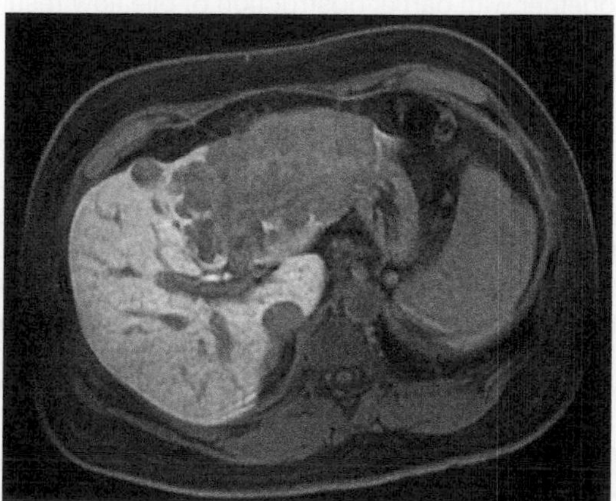

Fig. 1. Magnetic resonance image of the liver showing a multifocal, poorly differentiated ICC with vascular invasion.

strategies in endemic areas. Several tumor markers may support a diagnosis of cholangiocarcinoma, but none are sensitive enough to be used for screening purposes. The most commonly used markers are carbohydrate antigen 19-9 and carcinoembryonic antigen. However, the levels of these markers can be elevated in the presence of other malignancies as well as in benign conditions such as cholangitis and hepatolithiasis. Moreover, the value of screening for cholangiocarcinoma is debatable given the poor response to treatment.

PATHOGENESIS

Study of the pathogenesis of cholangiocarcinoma provides a paradigm for the study of the role of infection and chronic epithelial inflammation in malignancy. The pathogenic mechanisms involved in biliary fluke-associated cholangiocarcinoma are likely to be multifactorial. Biliary tract injury arises as a consequence of mechanical injury caused by the migration of the flukes, metabolic toxins, and immunopathologic processes.[39]

Metabolic products released by liver flukes may be directly toxic or may promote an immunologic response that results in proliferation of fibroblasts and overexpression of transforming growth factors (TGFs)[40] and metalloproteinases.[41] Evidence for fluke-induced host inflammatory response in mediating biliary damage is further provided by the expression of opisthorchis antigens in peripheral macrophages and epithelioid cells.[42] Subsequent cytokine-dependent activation of effector cells results in oxidative stress, which causes cytotoxicity and enhances mutagenesis. This oxidative stress results in DNA damage with malfunctioning of mismatch repair systems and aberrant regulation of cellular apoptosis. *N*-nitroso compounds are primary carcinogens leading to cholangiocarcinoma. Humans infected with *Opisthorchis* seem to have a higher endogenous nitrosation potential than uninfected people, as a result of the production of nitric oxide (NO) and the stimulation of NO synthase (NOS). Population-based variations in the expression of genes involved in the detoxification of carcinogens may also contribute to the higher incidence in endemic areas, such as Thailand, than in nonendemic areas.[43]

Biliary Constituents

Carcinogenesis of biliary epithelia is a multistep process that involves the transformation from hyperplasia to dysplasia and eventually to carcinoma. Chronic inflammation and cellular injury together with partial obstruction of bile flow result in bile stasis and chronic exposure of biliary cells to the carcinogenic action of bile components. The bile from patients with inflammatory biliary injuries contains increased levels of oxysterols, oxygenated derivatives of cholesterol. Oxysterols and bile acids, such as deoxycholic acid, may promote carcinogenesis by inducing the expression of COX-2, transactivating the epidermal growth factor receptor (EGFR), repressing E-cadherin, and blocking the degradation of the antiapoptotic myeloid cell leukemia protein 1 (Mcl-1).[44,45] In experimentally induced cholestasis, levels of reduced glutathione (GSH) and the enzymes indispensable for GSH synthesis are decreased in the bile. GSH participates in the detoxification of many molecules and in the defense against oxidative stress. Therefore, the alteration in GSH content may lead to DNA damage and deregulation of apoptosis in cells of patients with chronic biliary disorders.[46]

Genetic and Epigenetic Abnormalities

Neoplastic transformation of biliary epithelia is accompanied by several molecular and genetic alterations. Activation of autonomous growth signaling molecules, such as hepatocyte growth factor (HGF)/met, interleukin (IL)-6, c-erbB2, K-ras (20%–50%), BRAF, and COX-2, are responsible for abnormal cell proliferation and survival. Abnormalities of DNA mismatch repair, such as microsatellite instability, increase the risk of genetic damages. Immortalization of biliary cells is mediated by the modulation of telomerase activity.[47] Several tumor suppressor genes are inactivated in cholangiocarcinoma. For example, p53 is usually lost in cholangiocarcinoma cells (20%–70%) because of the loss of heterozygosity or inactivating mutations, and $p16^{Ink4A}$ is frequently silenced by promoter hypermethylation. Inactivation of p16, together with the lack of $p21^{WAF1/CIP1}$, $p27^{KIP1}$, and $p57^{KIP2}$ and increased levels of cyclin D1, is responsible for cell cycle dysregulation. Regulation of apoptosis is aberrant in cholangiocarcinoma cells because of the overexpression of antiapoptotic proteins, such as Bcl2, Bclxl, and Mcl-1. Specific mucin antigen expression profiles have been associated with predictive value. Invasion and metastasis are favored by the loss of E-cadherin and catenins. Cholangiocarcinoma growth may be facilitated by increased angiogenesis mediated by overexpression of vascular endothelial growth factor, COX-2, and TGF-β1.[48,49]

Cytokine-Mediated Signaling Pathways

Several cytokines or growth factors, such as IL-6, HGF, TGF-α, endothelial growth factor, c-erbB2, heterogeneous IgA, and leukocyte inhibitory factor, are known to have mitogenic or proliferative effects on biliary cells via an autocrine or a paracrine effect. Neoplastic transformation of biliary cells is associated with a constitutive production of IL-6, as demonstrated by positive cytoplasmic immunohisotchemical staining and overexpression of IL-6 messenger RNA and protein in cholangiocarcinoma cells.[50] This production is significantly enhanced by other inflammatory cytokines, such as tumor necrosis factor α and IL-1, as a result of the complex paracrine-autocrine stimulation that takes place in inflammatory-mediated carcinogenesis.[51] In addition, expression of IL-6 receptor on tumor cells makes the cells hypersensitive to the exogenous IL-6 from environmental sources, such as stromal and immune cells.[51,52] The response to IL-6 stimulation differs between normal and malignant cholangiocytes, with aberrant expression of p38 mitogen-activated protein kinase (MAPK) in the latter.[51,53–55] IL-6 signaling modulates gene expression and sustains mitogenic signals that promote cholangiocarcinoma cell growth and survival through different mechanisms.[55] Some of these effects are exerted through the modulation of microRNAs, small noncoding RNAs that regulate gene expression. In in vitro and animal models, IL-6 overexpression was shown to reduce the expression of miR-370, resulting in the enhancement of p38 MAPK activation.[56] In other disease models, IL-6 expression is regulated by microRNAs, suggesting that a circulatory loop might be responsible for the sustained expression of IL-6 in cholangiocarcinoma. IL-6 may also alter the methylation status of cholangiocarcinoma cells by increasing the expression of DNA methyltransferase 1, which results in methylation-mediated silencing of oncosuppressor genes and promotion of cellular proliferation and survival.[57] Furthermore, IL-6 mediates chemoresistance of cholangiocarcinoma cells by the p38- and STAT 3–dependent modulation of the antiapoptotic protein Mcl-1.[54,55] Together, these data suggest that IL-6 signaling plays a central role in colangiocarcinogenesis and provide the rationale for the evaluation of IL-6 targeting agents as sensitizers or cytotoxic agents useful in cholangiocarcinoma treatment.

Oxidative Injury and DNA Damage

Biliary injury of diverse causes results in the recruitment of inflammatory cells and release of proinflammatory cytokines, which increase the generation of NO by inducing NOS. NO may favor the possibility of oncogenic mutations, may inhibit apoptosis through the nitrosylation of caspase 9, and may cause bile ductular cholestasis by inhibiting ion transporters of the biliary cells.[58]

All this evidence confirms that the pathogenesis of cholangiocarcinoma is enhanced by inflammatory mediators that mediate oncogenic signaling. The relevance of inflammation in cholangiocarcinoma is also supported by recent findings that show that patients with a neutrophil to lymphocyte ratio greater than 5 have larger tumors with intrahepatic satellite lesions, microvascular invasion, and lymph node involvement; the ratio also predicts poorer overall and disease-free survival in patients undergoing radical surgery. This index may reflect a weaker lymphocyte-mediated immune response to the tumor and the enrichment of cytokines produced by circulating and intratumoral neutrophils that can enhance tumor cell growth.[59]

DIAGNOSIS

Clinical Presentation

A suspicion of cholangiocarcinoma may be raised in several different clinical scenarios (**Box 2**). ICCs usually present as a mass lesion within the liver and may be asymptomatic until they are quite advanced. Ductal cancers are more likely to be symptomatic because of biliary obstruction and often present with jaundice. Because of the tendency of these cancers to spread along the biliary tract, they may also be more extensive at the time of diagnosis.

Risk Factor Analysis

In regions where liver flukes are endemic, an assessment of liver fluke infection can be performed using stool studies to look for eggs. PCR-based techniques capable of amplifying DNA taken directly from eggs of species of flukes have a better sensitivity and specificity than the standard microscopic examination of stool samples.[60] Use of these or other similar noninvasive assays may be helpful for diagnosis as well as for epidemiologic surveys of the distribution of liver flukes and may enable individual or population-based targeted approaches. In patients with known ulcerative colitis, evaluation for serum markers of cholestasis, abdominal imaging, ultrasonography, or cholangiography may be useful to diagnose PSC.

Diagnostic Studies

A combination of tumor markers, imaging, and cytologic studies may be used to diagnose cholangiocarcinoma (**Table 1**). The diagnosis is difficult to make, especially in patients with underlying PSC who may have biliary strictures. For patients with ICC, biopsy may reveal adenocarcinoma, which may prompt evaluation and exclusion of potential other primary sites.

Box 2
Clinical scenarios in which a suspicion of cholangiocarcinoma should be raised

- Jaundice, systemic illness, and weight loss in patients with known risk factors, such as liver fluke infection, PSC, and hepatolithiasis
- Jaundice or systemic illness in patients from areas with liver fluke endemicity
- Bile duct stricture causing jaundice
- Intrahepatic liver mass

Table 1
Diagnostic tests for cholangiocarcinoma

Diagnostic Test	Sensitivity (%)
Tumor markers	
CA 19-9	80–90
CEA	30
Radiology	
Computed tomography	50–60
Magnetic resonance imaging	50–90
Intraductal ultrasonography	89–95
Endoscopy	
Cholangiography and sampling	45–75
Nuclear medicine	
Positron emission tomography	85 (18 in infiltrative CCA)
Cytologic analysis	
Routine cytology	16–68
Digital imaging analysis	44
Fluorescence in situ hybridization	43

Abbreviations: CA, carbohydrate antigen; CCA, cholangiocarcinoma; CEA, carcinoembryonic antigen.

TREATMENT

Surgery

Survival from cholangiocarcinoma is extremely poor, with an average 5-year survival rate of approximately 5%. Surgical resection or transplantation could be curative in selected patients who have no evidence of distant spread, vascular invasion, or extrahepatic spread with limited resectable disease. For patients with ductal carcinomas, exploration to assess resectability may be appropriate. For ICC, hepatic resection may be appropriate. Reported outcomes show a wide variation with 5 year survival ranging from ~10–40%. Although recent series suggest that outcomes have improved in recent years, variable classifications and differing patient populations make interpretation difficult. Liver transplantation is appropriate for very few individuals with localized, early-stage disease and is offered only at a handful of centers worldwide. Neither transplantation nor resection is appropriate for individuals with evidence of portal vein or hepatic artery invasion on preoperative imaging or endoscopic ultrasonography. There are no data on the benefit of using adjuvant therapy after a margin-negative resection.

Photodynamic Therapy

Photodynamic therapy involves the intravenous administration of a photosensitizer followed by endoscopic delivery of light at a specific wavelength, which causes tumor cell death because of oxidative injury. Use of this approach with stenting can improve survival compared with stenting alone. Photodynamic therapy should be considered for patients with locally advanced disease, but it is not widely available.

Medical

Cholangiocarcinoma is highly resistant to chemotherapy. However, systemic chemotherapy may be considered in patients with advanced cholangiocarcinoma, as there may be some benefit compared with best supportive care.[61] The literature is limited and consists of several small series involving multiple tumor types. Various chemotherapeutic agents, dosing regimens, and combinations have been tested with overall poor survival improvement. 5-Fluorouracil, gemcitabine, oxaliplatin, and docetaxel have shown the most activity as single agents.[62] A recent phase 3 trial evaluated the combination of gemcitabine and cisplatin and showed this combination to be superior to single-agent chemotherapy, with a higher response rate and a prolonged overall survival that reached 11.7 months in the combination arm. According to these data, gemcitabine and cisplatin should be considered as the standard therapy for locally advanced and metastatic cholangiocarcinomas.[63] Several new molecular targeted agents and biologic agents are being explored for the treatment of cholangiocarcinoma.

Palliative Therapy

In patients with biliary tract obstruction, decompression may be helpful. Cholestatic liver dysfunction and biliary cirrhosis may rapidly occur in patients with unrelieved obstruction. However, placement of stents in patients who are candidates for surgery may interfere with preoperative evaluation for resectability and intraoperative determination of tumor extent.

PREVENTION

In regions of high liver fluke endemicity, the optimal approach to chemoprevention involves appropriate public health measures and education to reduce the effect and incidence of liver fluke infestation. However, an estimated 40 million to 50 million people in Southeast Asia may have fluke infection and may be candidates for eradication efforts. Although reducing the consumption of uncooked fish may be an effective strategy, these cultural and traditional practices are deeply entrenched and difficult to change. Active surveillance for fluke infection and potential interventions for eradication using chemotherapy may reduce the development of cholangiocarcinoma, but such approaches have not been evaluated for their chemopreventive efficacy in reducing the incidence of cholangiocarcinoma.

In the West, chemopreventive strategies may be considered for patients with PSC, who have a higher frequency of cholangiocarcinoma and may be associated with inflammatory bowel disease or colorectal cancer. Ursodeoxycholic acid (UDCA) is a hydrophilic bile salt that may protect the biliary tree by stabilizing bile duct epithelium and hepatocyte cell membranes and increasing bile flow from the liver, thereby reducing intrahepatic bile stasis and exposure time to toxic bile salts.[64] UDCA also seems to exert a protective effect on colic mucosa by reducing fecal concentrations of deoxycholic acid.[65] UDCA has been evaluated as a potential chemopreventive measure for PSC, but there is no clear benefit of efficacy in reducing the rate of tumor formation.[20,66] Further evaluation in randomized trials is necessary.

Novel approaches to chemoprevention may be based on new insights from molecular pathogenesis. The EGFR gene, for example, is located on the short arm of chromosome 7. Patients with PSC who show trisomy 7 and/or EGFR expression in biliary tract epithelia may be appropriate to consider for chemoprevention with EGFR blockers, if they have a higher risk of cholangiocarcinoma. Overexpression of COX-2 has been reported in extrahepatic cholangiocarcinoma, and COX-2 inhibitors could be potentially useful chemopreventive agents in such patients.[67]

CHALLENGES IN CHOLANGIOCARCINOMA

Cholangiocarcinoma has a dismal prognosis and is almost always incurable because it is refractory to most currently used surgical or medical interventions. A major limitation in the management of cholangiocarcinoma has been that the disease and its nosology are poorly defined, which has limited the information that can be obtained from epidemiologic studies and has made it difficult to compare outcomes of different management strategies. Oncologic trials for biliary cancers, for example, have often included intrahepatic and extrahepatic malignancies. A clinically useful classification system that separates these 2 different diseases with different risk factors, pathogenetic mechanisms, and clinical behavior is needed. Risk factors for cholangiocarcinoma vary considerably, being primarily infectious in the East and noninfectious in the West. Thus, the clinical behavior and management of this tumor show regional variations despite shared pathogenetic mechanisms. Investigation on the role of inflammatory mediators and processes on cholangiocarcinoma pathogenesis is likely to be beneficial, given the common involvement of chronic biliary tract inflammation in cholangiocarcinoma. The epidemiologic trends are concerning, in that they show a global increase in incidence and mortality, but the disease has received little interest among research funding bodies and public health administrators, and it continues to be regarded as a rare disease of little importance in the West. There are many challenges in the current management and approach to cholangiocarcinoma, both from the perspective of the individual as well as from a public health perspective.

REFERENCES

1. Yamasaki S. Intrahepatic cholangiocarcinoma: macroscopic type and stage classification. J Hepatobiliary Pancreat Surg 2003;10(4):288–91.
2. Nathan H, Aloia TA, Vauthey JN, et al. A proposed staging system for intrahepatic cholangiocarcinoma. Ann Surg Oncol 2009;16(1):14–22.
3. Patel T. Increasing incidence and mortality of primary intrahepatic cholangiocarcinoma in the United States. Hepatology 2001;33(6):1353–7.
4. Patel T. Worldwide trends in mortality from biliary tract malignancies. BMC Cancer 2002;2:10.
5. El-Serag HB, Petersen NJ, Carter J, et al. Gastroesophageal reflux among different racial groups in the United States. Gastroenterology 2004;126(7):1692–9.
6. Jemal A, Siegel R, Ward E, et al. Cancer statistics, 2008. CA Cancer J Clin 2008; 58(2):71–96.
7. McLean L, Patel T. Racial and ethnic variations in the epidemiology of intrahepatic cholangiocarcinoma in the United States. Liver Int 2006;26(9):1047–53.
8. Kim HG, Han J, Kim MH, et al. Prevalence of clonorchiasis in patients with gastrointestinal disease: a Korean nationwide multicenter survey. World J Gastroenterol 2009;15(1):86–94.
9. Kim Si A. Clonorchis sinensis-specific antigen that detects active human clonorchiasis. Korean J Parasitol 1998;36(1):37–45.
10. Hou PC. The pathology of Clonorchis sinensis infestation of the liver. J Pathol Bacteriol 1955;70(1):53–64.
11. Haswell-Elkins MR, Satarug S, Tsuda M, et al. Liver fluke infection and cholangiocarcinoma: model of endogenous nitric oxide and extragastric nitrosation in human carcinogenesis. Mutat Res 1994;305(2):241–52.
12. Honjo S, Srivatanakul P, Sriplung H, et al. Genetic and environmental determinants of risk for cholangiocarcinoma via Opisthorchis viverrini in a densely infested area in Nakhon Phanom, Northeast Thailand. Int J Cancer 2005;117(5):854–60.
13. Sriamporn S, Pisani P, Pipitgool V, et al. Prevalence of Opisthorchis viverrini infection and incidence of cholangiocarcinoma in Khon Kaen, Northeast Thailand. Trop Med Int Health 2004;9(5):588–94.
14. Andrews RH, Sithithaworn P, Petney TN. Opisthorchis viverrini: an underestimated parasite in world health. Trends Parasitol 2008;24(11):497–501.

15. Suksumek N, Leelawat K, Leelawat S, et al. TaqMan real-time PCR assay for specific detection of Opisthorchis viverrini DNA in Thai patients with hepatocellular carcinoma and cholangiocarcinoma. Exp Parasitol 2008;119(2):217–24.
16. Thanan R, Murata M, Pinlaor S, et al. Urinary 8-oxo-7, 8-dihydro-2'-deoxyguanosine in patients with parasite infection and effect of antiparasitic drug in relation to cholangiocarcinogenesis. Cancer Epidemiol Biomarkers Prev 2008;17(3):518–24.
17. Pinlaor S, Ma N, Hiraku Y, et al. Repeated infection with Opisthorchis viverrini induces accumulation of 8-nitroguanine and 8-oxo-7, 8-dihydro-2'-deoxyguanine in the bile duct of hamsters via inducible nitric oxide synthase. Carcinogenesis 2004;25(8):1535–42.
18. Burak K, Angulo P, Pasha TM, et al. Incidence and risk factors for cholangiocarcinoma in primary sclerosing cholangitis. Am J Gastroenterol 2004;99(3):523–6.
19. Claessen MM, Lutgens MW, van Buuren HR, et al. More right-sided IBD-associated colorectal cancer in patients with primary sclerosing cholangitis. Inflamm Bowel Dis 2009;15(9):1331–6.
20. Kitiyakara T, Chapman RW. Chemoprevention and screening in primary sclerosing cholangitis. Postgrad Med J 2008;84(991):228–37.
21. El-Serag HB, Engels EA, Landgren O, et al. Risk of hepatobiliary and pancreatic cancers after hepatitis C virus infection: a population-based study of U.S. veterans. Hepatology 2009;49(1):116–23.
22. Kobayashi M, Ikeda K, Saitoh S, et al. Incidence of primary cholangiocellular carcinoma of the liver in Japanese patients with hepatitis C virus-related cirrhosis. Cancer 2000;88(11):2471–7.
23. Chen RF, Li ZH, Chen JS, et al. [Human normal biliary epithelial cells transformation and tumor development induced by hepatitis C virus core protein]. Zhonghua Wai Ke Za Zhi 2005;43(3):153–6 [in Chinese].
24. Roskams T. Different types of liver progenitor cells and their niches. J Hepatol 2006;45(1):1–4.
25. Zhou YM, Yin ZF, Yang JM, et al. Risk factors for intrahepatic cholangiocarcinoma: a case-control study in China. World J Gastroenterol 2008;14(4):632–5.
26. Lee TY, Lee SS, Jung SW, et al. Hepatitis B virus infection and intrahepatic cholangiocarcinoma in Korea: a case-control study. Am J Gastroenterol 2008;103(7):1716–20.
27. Shin HR, Lee CU, Park HJ, et al. Hepatitis B and C virus, Clonorchis sinensis for the risk of liver cancer: a case-control study in Pusan, Korea. Int J Epidemiol 1996;25(5):933–40.
28. Donato F, Gelatti U, Tagger A, et al. Intrahepatic cholangiocarcinoma and hepatitis C and B virus infection, alcohol intake, and hepatolithiasis: a case-control study in Italy. Cancer Causes Control 2001;12(10):959–64.
29. Shaib YH, El-Serag HB, Davila JA, et al. Risk factors of intrahepatic cholangiocarcinoma in the United States: a case-control study. Gastroenterology 2005;128(3):620–6.
30. Falchuk KR, Lesser PB, Galdabini JJ, et al. Cholangiocarcinoma as related to chronic intrahepatic cholangitis and hepatolithiasis. Case report and review of the literature. Am J Gastroenterol 1976;66(1):57–61.
31. Nakanuma Y, Terada T, Tanaka Y, et al. Are hepatolithiasis and cholangiocarcinoma aetiologically related? A morphological study of 12 cases of hepatolithiasis associated with cholangiocarcinoma. Virchows Arch A Pathol Anat Histopathol 1985;406(1):45–58.

32. Kuroki T, Tajima Y, Kanematsu T. Hepatolithiasis and intrahepatic cholangiocarcinoma: carcinogenesis based on molecular mechanisms. J Hepatobiliary Pancreat Surg 2005;12(6):463–6.
33. Kawakami H, Kuwatani M, Onodera M, et al. Primary cholesterol hepatolithiasis associated with cholangiocellular carcinoma: a case report and literature review. Intern Med 2007;46(15):1191–6.
34. Donato F, Tagger A, Gelatti U, et al. Alcohol and hepatocellular carcinoma: the effect of lifetime intake and hepatitis virus infections in men and women. Am J Epidemiol 2002;155(4):323–31.
35. Torbenson M, Yeh MM, Abraham SC. Bile duct dysplasia in the setting of chronic hepatitis C and alcohol cirrhosis. Am J Surg Pathol 2007;31(9):1410–3.
36. Zhu AX, Lauwers GY, Tanabe KK. Cholangiocarcinoma in association with thorotrast exposure. J Hepatobiliary Pancreat Surg 2004;11(6):430–3.
37. Sorensen HT, Friis S, Olsen JH, et al. Risk of liver and other types of cancer in patients with cirrhosis: a nationwide cohort study in Denmark. Hepatology 1998;28(4):921–5.
38. Welzel TM, Graubard BI, El-Serag HB, et al. Risk factors for intrahepatic and extrahepatic cholangiocarcinoma in the United States: a population-based case-control study. Clin Gastroenterol Hepatol 2007;5(10):1221–8.
39. Sripa B, Kaewkes S, Sithithaworn P, et al. Liver fluke induces cholangiocarcinoma. PLoS Med 2007;4(7):e201.
40. Thuwajit C, Thuwajit P, Uchida K, et al. Gene expression profiling defined pathways correlated with fibroblast cell proliferation induced by Opisthorchis viverrini excretory/secretory product. World J Gastroenterol 2006;12(22):3585–92.
41. Prakobwong S, Pinlaor S, Yongvanit P, et al. Time profiles of the expression of metalloproteinases, tissue inhibitors of metalloproteases, cytokines and collagens in hamsters infected with Opisthorchis viverrini with special reference to peribiliary fibrosis and liver injury. Int J Parasitol 2009;39(7):825–35.
42. Sripa B, Kaewkes S. Localisation of parasite antigens and inflammatory responses in experimental opisthorchiasis. Int J Parasitol 2000;30(6):735–40.
43. Jinawath N, Chamgramol Y, Furukawa Y, et al. Comparison of gene expression profiles between Opisthorchis viverrini and non-Opisthorchis viverrini associated human intrahepatic cholangiocarcinoma. Hepatology 2006;44(4):1025–38.
44. Yoon JH, Werneburg NW, Higuchi H, et al. Bile acids inhibit Mcl-1 protein turnover via an epidermal growth factor receptor/Raf-1-dependent mechanism. Cancer Res 2002;62(22):6500–5.
45. Fukase K, Ohtsuka H, Onogawa T, et al. Bile acids repress E-cadherin through the induction of Snail and increase cancer invasiveness in human hepatobiliary carcinoma. Cancer Sci 2008;99(9):1785–92.
46. Celli A, Que FG, Gores GJ, et al. Glutathione depletion is associated with decreased Bcl-2 expression and increased apoptosis in cholangiocytes. Am J Physiol 1998;275(4 Pt 1):G749–57.
47. Yamagiwa Y, Meng F, Patel T. Interleukin-6 decreases senescence and increases telomerase activity in malignant human cholangiocytes. Life Sci 2006;78(21):2494–502.
48. Sirica AE. Cholangiocarcinoma: molecular targeting strategies for chemoprevention and therapy. Hepatology 2005;41(1):5–15.
49. Okuda K, Nakanuma Y, Miyazaki M. Cholangiocarcinoma: recent progress. Part 2: molecular pathology and treatment. J Gastroenterol Hepatol 2002;17(10):1056–63.

50. Sugawara H, Yasoshima M, Katayanagi K, et al. Relationship between interleukin-6 and proliferation and differentiation in cholangiocarcinoma. Histopathology 1998;33(2):145–53.
51. Park J, Tadlock L, Gores GJ, et al. Inhibition of interleukin 6-mediated mitogen-activated protein kinase activation attenuates growth of a cholangiocarcinoma cell line. Hepatology 1999;30(5):1128–33.
52. Okada K, Shimizu Y, Nambu S, et al. Interleukin-6 functions as an autocrine growth factor in a colangiocarcinoma cell line. J Gastroenterol Hepatol 1994; 9(5):462–7.
53. Yokomuro S, Tsuji H, Lunz JG III, et al. Growth control of human biliary epithelial cells by interleukin 6, hepatocyte growth factor, transforming growth factor beta1, and activin A: comparison of a cholangiocarcinoma cell line with primary cultures of non-neoplastic biliary epithelial cells. Hepatology 2000;32(1):26–35.
54. Isomoto H, Kobayashi S, Werneburg NW, et al. Interleukin 6 upregulates myeloid cell leukemia-1 expression through a STAT3 pathway in cholangiocarcinoma cells. Hepatology 2005;42(6):1329–38.
55. Meng F, Yamagiwa Y, Ueno Y, et al. Over-expression of interleukin-6 enhances cell survival and transformed cell growth in human malignant cholangiocytes. J Hepatol 2006;44(6):1055–65.
56. Meng F, Wehbe-Janek H, Henson R, et al. Epigenetic regulation of microRNA-370 by interleukin-6 in malignant human cholangiocytes. Oncogene 2008;27(3):378–86.
57. Wehbe H, Henson R, Meng F, et al. Interleukin-6 contributes to growth in cholangiocarcinoma cells by aberrant promoter methylation and gene expression. Cancer Res 2006;66(21):10517–24.
58. Spirli C, Fabris L, Duner E, et al. Cytokine-stimulated nitric oxide production inhibits adenylyl cyclase and cAMP-dependent secretion in cholangiocytes. Gastroenterology 2003;124(3):737–53.
59. Gomez D, Morris-Stiff G, Toogood GJ, et al. Impact of systemic inflammation on outcome following resection for intrahepatic cholangiocarcinoma. J Surg Oncol 2008;97(6):513–8.
60. Traub RJ, Macaranas J, Mungthin M, et al. A new PCR-based approach indicates the range of Clonorchis sinensis now extends to Central Thailand. PLoS Negl Trop Dis 2009;3(1):e367.
61. Glimelius B, Hoffman K, Sjoden PO, et al. Chemotherapy improves survival and quality of life in advanced pancreatic and biliary cancer. Ann Oncol 1996;7(6): 593–600.
62. Hezel AF, Zhu AX. Systemic therapy for biliary tract cancers. Oncologist 2008; 13(4):415–23.
63. Valle J, Harpreet W, Palmer DH, et al. Cisplatin plus gemcitabine versus gemcitabine for biliary tract cancer. N Engl J Med 2010;362:1273–8.
64. Colombo C, Crosignani A, Assaisso M, et al. Ursodeoxycholic acid therapy in cystic fibrosis-associated liver disease: a dose-response study. Hepatology 1992;16(4):924–30.
65. Pardi DS, Loftus EV Jr, Kremers WK, et al. Ursodeoxycholic acid as a chemopreventive agent in patients with ulcerative colitis and primary sclerosing cholangitis. Gastroenterology 2003;124(4):889–93.
66. Forsmo HM, Horn A, Viste A, et al. Survival and an overview of decision-making in patients with cholangiocarcinoma. Hepatobiliary Pancreat Dis Int 2008;7(4): 412–7.
67. Wu GS, Wang JH, Liu ZR, et al. Expression of cyclooxygenase-1 and -2 in extrahepatic cholangiocarcinoma. Hepatobiliary Pancreat Dis Int 2002;1(3):429–33.

Infectious Diseases and the Gallbladder

Kabir Julka, MD, Cynthia W. Ko, MD, MS*

KEYWORDS

• Cholecystitis • Acute cholecystitis • Acalculous cholecystitis

The gallbladder is located on the undersurface of the right lobe of the liver. The gallbladder connects to the biliary tree via the cystic duct. The cystic duct joins with the common hepatic duct to form the common bile duct, which ultimately drains directly into the duodenum.

The gallbladder's main function is to store bile acids excreted from the liver in preparation for a meal. On stimulation by meals and hormones such as cholecystokinin, the gallbladder contracts and excretes bile acids into the cystic duct. From the cystic duct, bile travels down the common bile duct into the duodenum. The delivered bile acids are used to help digest lipids. At any given point, the gallbladder can store 30 to 50 mL of bile. Blood supply to the gallbladder is exclusively via the cystic artery, an end arterial branch of the right hepatic artery. There is no collateral circulation that supplies the gallbladder, rendering the gallbladder susceptible to ischemia if the cystic artery is damaged.[1]

Commonly, disorders of the gallbladder cause gastrointestinal illness. Gallstone disease is among the most common gastrointestinal reasons for hospitalization and has been estimated to incur a cost of approximately $6.5 billion annually.[2] It is estimated that more than 20 million Americans have gallstones and more than 700,000 cholecystectomies are performed each year in the United States alone.[3]

Gallstones are usually asymptomatic but can lead to other symptoms. Conditions related to gallstones can range from symptomatic cholecystitis to severe acute cholecystitis to fulminant sepsis. The biochemical composition of gallstones may vary, and infection may play a role in the formation of certain types of gallstones.

Complications of gallbladder disease can often be treated with cholecystectomy. Cholecystectomy is commonly performed for symptomatic cholelithiasis, but other complications can also require surgery. Acute cholecystitis is the most common complication of gallstone disease. The vast majority of acute cholecystitis are caused by a gallstone impacted in the cystic duct leading to gallbladder obstruction (calculous cholecystitis). Acute acalculous cholecystitis occurs in a minority of cases, often in patients who are critically ill from other causes. Secondary infections often complicate cholecystitis, both calculous and acalculous.

Division of Gastroenterology, University of Washington, Box 356424, Seattle, WA 98195, USA
* Corresponding author.
E-mail address: cwko@u.washington.edu

Infect Dis Clin N Am 24 (2010) 885–898
doi:10.1016/j.idc.2010.07.003 id.theclinics.com
0891-5520/10/$ – see front matter

This article focuses on infections and their role in the gallbladder. Ranging from a role in gallstone formation to a secondary complication of cholecystitis, infections can be frequently seen in the gallbladder. If an infection is part of a spectrum of cholecystitis, identifying and treating the infection can be crucial to a patient's care.

GALLSTONE PATHOGENESIS AND THE ROLE OF BACTERIA

Gallstones are typically asymptomatic in most patients. It has been estimated that only about one-third of patients with gallstones have clinical symptoms.[4] The 3 main types of gallstones are cholesterol stones, mixed stones, and pigment stones. In the Western world, the vast majority of gallstones are cholesterol stones. Gallstone prevalence increases with age and they are more prevalent in women across the age spectrum.[2] Certain ethnic groups, such as the Pima Indians of North America, are at much higher risk for developing gallstones, suggesting that genetic factors may play a role.[4]

Pigment stones are primarily composed of bilirubin. It is known that these gallstones, in particular, may be precipitated by a bacterial infection. In contrast to cholesterol gallstones, ethnicity does not seem to play a role in predisposition. The 2 types of pigment gallstones are black and brown. In the United States, black pigment stones are found in the gallbladder and are not associated with infections. Black pigment stones are associated with a range of conditions from chronic hemolysis to advancing age and cirrhosis.

Brown pigment stones, on the other hand, are strongly associated with infection.[5–8] As opposed to cholesterol stones and black pigment stones, brown pigment stones may be found within the bile ducts and the gallbladder. Brown pigment stones are more common in the Asian population.[9] *Escherichia coli* infection, in particular, is highly prevalent in patients with brown pigment stones, suggesting that bacterial infection plays a critical role in stone formation.[10–12]

In the liver, bilirubin, a hydrophobic molecule, is conjugated with glucuronic acid and is rendered water soluble before its secretion into bile. Bacteria within the biliary system produce β-glucuronidase, which deconjugates bilirubin to its water-insoluble form. Once this process occurs, calcium salts of unconjugated bilirubin, deconjugated bile acids, and saturated long-chain fatty acids can form a brown stone.[13,14] Molecular studies have demonstrated that bacterial DNA is present in most gallstones, including cholesterol stones, confirming a role for bacteria in stone formation.[15–17] Organisms implicated in the formation of brown pigment stones range from *E coli* to parasitic organisms, such as *Clonorchis sinensis, Opisthorchis viverrini*, and *Ascaris lumbricoides*.[3]

Bacterial activity alone is not thought to be sufficient to form pigment gallstones. Another process that likely contributes is gallbladder stasis. Stasis can facilitate bacterial infection and permit nonenzymatic deconjugation of bilirubin diglucuronide, which leads to the precipitation of bilirubin and subsequent formation of pigment stones.[18,19]

Cholesterol stones, which are the most common type of gallstones, have generally not been considered to have an infectious origin. This concept may change as the understanding of cholesterol stone formation increases. To form a cholesterol gallstone, 3 main factors are involved: supersaturation of cholesterol, nucleation of bile into cholesterol crystals, and gallbladder hypomotility (**Fig. 1**).[13]

Cholesterol is insoluble in water and requires bile salts and phospholipids to remain soluble in bile. At lower levels of cholesterol, bile salts and phospholipids solubilize cholesterol molecules in the form of mixed micelles. As the cholesterol concentration in bile increases, vesicles are formed instead of micelles. Vesicles are larger, have higher concentrations of cholesterol, and have no bile salts to help solubilize

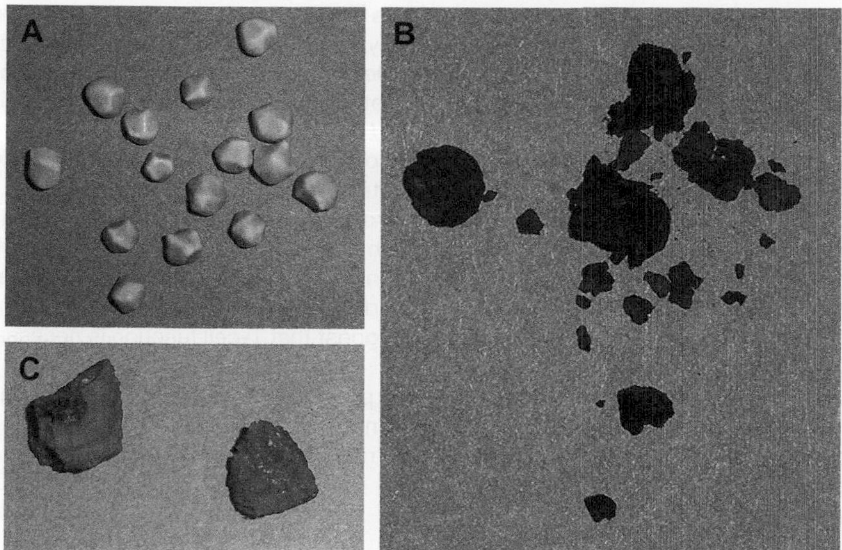

Fig. 1. (*A*) Cholesterol gallstones. (*B*) Black pigment gallstones. (*C*) Brown pigment gallstones. (*Courtesy of* Drs Sum Lee, University of Hong Kong and Geoffrey Haigh, University of Washington, USA.)

cholesterol. As such, vesicles are more prone to aggregate, with cholesterol precipitating into crystals.[13]

Cholesterol precipitation from a solution depends on several factors including the relative proportions of cholesterol, bile salts, and phospholipids in bile. Typically, the most important factor is excess secretion of cholesterol from the liver, which can occur from several causes including obesity, aging, and various drug effects.[20,21] Once bile is supersaturated with cholesterol, the excess cholesterol separates from micelles and forms vesicles of cholesterol that can aggregate into microscopic crystals, known as biliary sludge. These cholesterol crystals further aggregate to form macroscopic gallstones. Finally, gallbladder hypomotility plays a critical role in cholesterol gallstone formation. Patients with gallbladder hypomotility have been shown to have increased frequency of gallstones and biliary sludge, a potential precursor of gallstones.[13,22]

Despite the well-characterized risk factors for gallstone formation as described earlier, research has continued to look into other factors that may cause gallstones formation. Although biliary sludge is considered a risk factor to progress to gallstone formation, many patients do not ultimately progress to gallstones formation and may in fact have regression of sludge.[23] Similarly, genetically identical mice raised with the same diet but in different laboratory environments have different rates of gallstone formation. One of the areas of interest has been whether or not colonization with gastrointestinal microbes with subsequent immune response and inflammation could contribute to gallstone formation. Work on mouse models showed that mice infected with certain *Helicobacter* spp formed gallstones at a much higher rate than genetically identical mouse models that were kept free of infection. Mice without infection still developed gallstones, although at a much lower rate, suggesting that infection with *Helicobacter* spp accelerated gallstone formation.[24]

Numerous studies have demonstrated bacterial presence in bile, cholesterol stones, and within the gallbladder of patients with cholesterol gallstones. Bacteria have been found in up to 81% of gallstone cores.[25,26] *Helicobacter pylori* has received attention as a possible infectious agent that may cause gallstones. Numerous studies have found *H pylori* in gallstones and bile.[27–30] Despite these findings, the studies have come under some criticism regarding the methods, and the association remains unclear. A part of the debate is whether other *Helicobacter* spp rather than *H pylori* may be associated with gallstones.[22] It is also unclear whether bacterial infection occurred during initial gallstone formation or after the gallstones had formed.

The role of the immune system in cholesterol gallstone formation has also been examined by investigators. Genetically altered mice with only T cell–mediated immunity develop gallstones more frequently than nonmodified mice. Mice with only B cell–mediated immune responses have a decreased prevalence of gallstones compared with nonmodified mice. Results of this study suggest that T-cell function is necessary to form cholesterol gallstones in mice.[31]

Overall, there is significant research into the potential causative role of bacteria in the formation of cholesterol gallstones in humans. The data available are not conclusive, and more work is yet to be done in humans to determine the actual role of bacteria in forming cholesterol gallstones.

ACUTE CALCULOUS CHOLECYSTITIS

Overview and Pathogenesis

Acute cholecystitis is most frequently caused by gallstones. Although gallstones are frequently found in asymptomatic patients, acute cholecystitis is estimated to occur in 1% to 3% of patients with symptomatic gallstones.[32] The overwhelming majority of cases of acute cholecystitis are secondary to cystic duct obstruction by an impacted gallstone or biliary sludge (acute calculous cholecystitis). A cascade of events is triggered by prolonged cystic duct obstruction. With cystic duct obstruction, the intraluminal pressure within the gallbladder increases. Combined with bile that is supersaturated with cholesterol, an acute inflammatory response is triggered.[32–34]

Because the gallbladder mucosa gets damaged and distended by the obstruction, a prostaglandin-mediated response is stimulated, which mediates the inflammatory response of the body.[35,36] As inflammation progresses and the gallbladder distends, the wall thickens and becomes edematous and a pericholecystic inflammatory exudate develops. This exudate is initially sterile in most patients, but secondary bacterial infection can occur and complicate the process. Most patients with secondary bacterial infection from acute calculous cholecystitis are infected with species of the family Enterobacteriaceae or other anaerobic species.[37,38] Other organisms, such as gas-forming organisms, may complicate acute cholecystitis and lead to gas accumulation within the gallbladder wall, which is known as emphysematous cholecystitis. Patients with secondary bacterial infection can often develop sepsis and may have worse outcomes when compared with uncomplicated patients. Complications of acute cholecystitis are discussed later.

Diagnosis

Most commonly, the diagnosis of acute calculous cholecystitis can be made by abdominal ultrasonography or hepatobiliary scintigraphy (hepatobiliary iminodiacetic acid scan). Plain radiography has minimal utility in diagnosing cholelithiasis or cholecystitis (approximately 15%–20% gallstones may show up on radiography) but may show air within the gallbladder wall in emphysematous cholecystitis.[39] Other modalities that can be used include computed tomography (CT) and magnetic resonance imaging (MRI).

In the right clinical setting, ultrasonography has a positive predictive value between 92% and 95%. Without abnormal findings suspicious for acute cholecystitis, the negative predictive value of an abdominal ultrasonography is approximately 95%.[40] Suggestive findings on abdominal ultrasonography include thickened gallbladder wall, presence of pericholecystic fluid, and tenderness in the right upper quadrant with pressure from the ultrasonography probe (sonographic Murphy sign) (**Fig. 2**).[41]

Hepatobiliary scintigraphy is considered more accurate for diagnosing acute cholecystitis than abdominal ultrasonography but is clinically used less often with the widespread availability of ultrasonography.[42] After a 2- to 4-hour fast, an intravenous (IV) injection of a technetium Tc 99m-labeled iminodiacetic acid derivative is administered. This agent is taken up by the liver, excreted into the bile ducts, and then taken up into the gallbladder, from where it is later excreted into the common bile duct and small intestine. Flow of the agent is sequentially imaged under a gamma camera. In a normal study, the gallbladder, common bile duct, and small bowel are visualized within 30 to 45 minutes. Nonvisualization of the gallbladder within 90 minutes combined with visualization of the bile ducts and small bowel is highly suggestive of acute cystic duct obstruction (**Fig. 3**).

CT is frequently used in the emergency department for evaluation of patients with abdominal pain (**Fig. 4**). Sensitivity of CT is poor for detecting cystic duct obstruction, but this technique may offer findings similar to those of an ultrasonography, with thickened gallbladder wall, pericholecystic fluid, and gallstones within the gallbladder. MRI is infrequently used in the diagnosis of acute cholecystitis but may be beneficial in patients whose preliminary ultrasonography or CT is indeterminate. MRI may be more useful in diagnosing complications of acute cholecystitis, such as empyema of the gallbladder, gangrenous cholecystitis, or gallbladder hemorrhage.[43]

Management

Medical management focuses on reduction of inflammation in the gallbladder as well as the prevention and treatment of secondary infection. The first course of action is gallbladder rest, which is achieved by fasting and resuscitation with IV fluids. Rest prevents the gallbladder from an obstructed cystic duct, which presumably worsens pain and inflammation. The role of nonsteroidal antiinflammatory drugs has not been examined in the setting of acute cholecystitis, but these drugs do reduce pain in patients with biliary colic.[44]

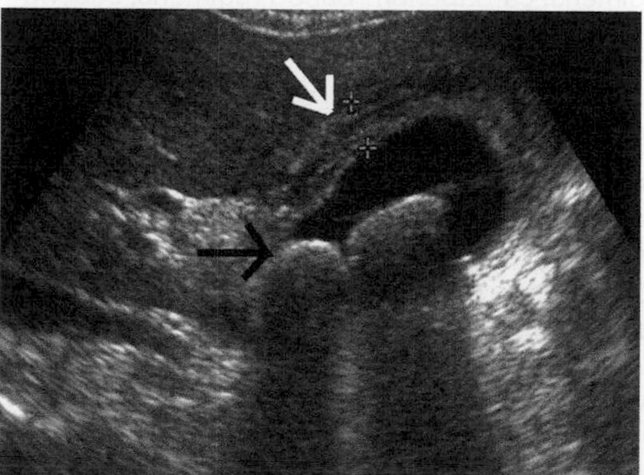

Fig. 2. Ultrasonographic image showing thickened gallbladder wall (*black arrow*) and shadowing gallstones within the gallbladder (*white arrow*) in a patient with acute cholecystitis. (*Courtesy of* Dr Charles Rohrmann Seattle, University of Washington, WA, USA.)

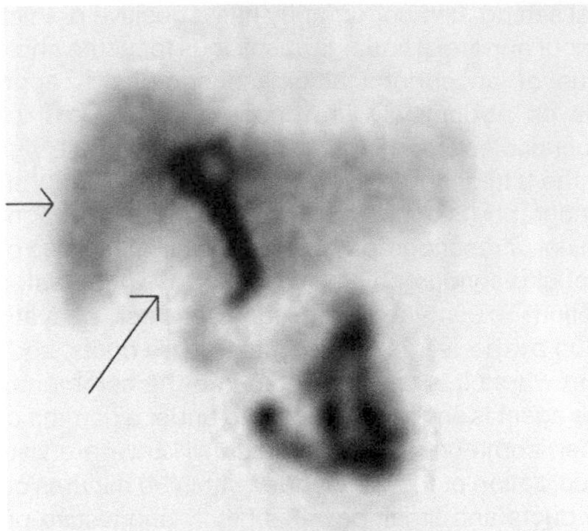

Fig. 3. Hepatobiliary scan, abnormal study. Radiotracer is taken up by the liver (*small arrow*) and excreted into the biliary tract. Absence of gallbladder filling (*large arrow*) with adequate images of the liver, common bile duct, and small bowel is consistent with the diagnosis of acute cholecystitis. (*Courtesy of* Dr David Mankoff, Seattle, University of Washington, WA, USA.)

Antibiotics are often used in the medical management of cholecystitis. As mentioned previously, secondary infection of the gallbladder can occur in acute calculous cholecystitis and may cause increased morbidity and mortality. Choice of antibiotic is dictated by studies that show frequently isolated organisms from bile in patients with acute cholecystitis.[37,38] The Infectious Diseases Society of America recommends that empirical antibiotics should only be given in case of acute cholecystitis and if clinical suspicion is high for an infection.[45] Clinical suspicion is based on clinical and radiological findings. The panel recommended to cover species of the family Enterobacteriaceae but not to routinely cover *Enterococcus* spp, because the latter are not commonly found in biliary flora (grade B level of evidence). Several options exist for empirical treatment of infection, ranging from single-agent regimens (β-lactam/β-lactamase inhibitor regimens, carbapenem-based regimens, second- or third-generation cephalosporins) to combination regimens (quinolone-based regimens plus metronidazole) (grade A level of evidence).

Cholecystectomy and Cholecystostomy

Cholecystectomy is the treatment of choice for acute cholecystitis. For many years there was controversy over the timing of cholecystectomy. In the patient population that is able to tolerate surgery, it seems that early laparoscopic cholecystectomy, within 72 hours of symptom onset, is preferred to delayed cholecystectomy (grade A level of evidence). Delayed cholecystectomy is generally performed weeks later, after a course of antibiotics and a "cooldown" period for the gallbladder. Most evidence suggests that when compared with delayed cholecystectomy, early cholecystectomy is safe and associated with significantly reduced hospital stays, few major complications, and a low rate of conversion to open cholecystectomy.[46–53] Antibiotics may be used before delayed surgery as a bridge to cholecystectomy but not as a curative measure.

Percutaneous cholecystostomy for gallbladder decompression is a treatment typically reserved for patients who are poor operative candidates, such as the elderly or

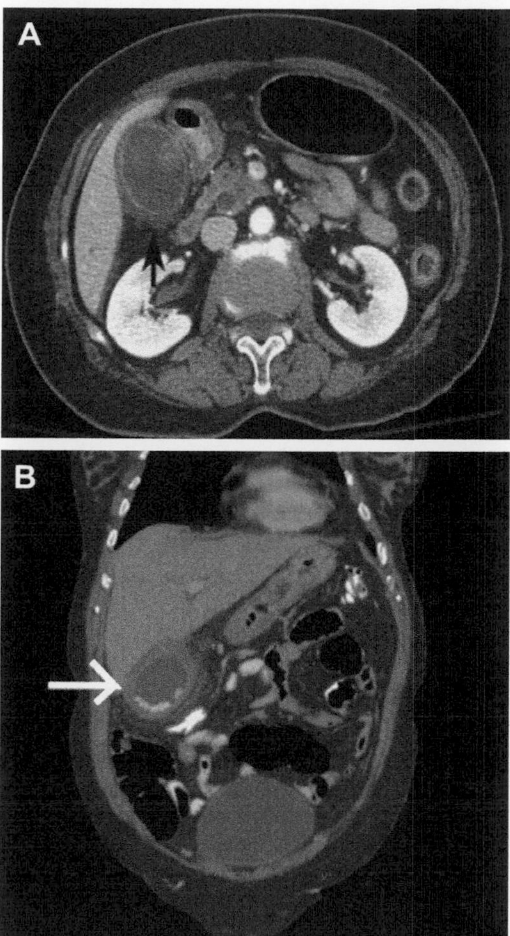

Fig. 4. Abdominal CT scan showing acute cholecystitis. (*A*) Pericholecystic fluid (*black arrow*) around a distended gallbladder with a gallstone. (*B*) Numerous gallstones within the gallbladder (*white arrow*) with a thickened wall. (*Courtesy of* Drs Carlos Cuevas, Seattle, WA, USA and Charles Rohrmann, Seattle, University of Washington, WA, USA.)

critically ill patients. Percutaneous (typically, interventional radiology–guided) cholecystostomy may reduce morbidity when compared with surgery and is an effective technique with few complications. In a randomized trial, placement of a cholecystostomy drain has been proved to be more effective than simple gallbladder aspiration.[54]

Most patients managed with a cholecystostomy drain improve quickly, although long-term prognosis in many of these patients is poor. Cholecystostomy is considered a temporizing measure, and cholecystectomy should be considered if the patient's clinical status improves (grade B level of evidence).[55,56]

ACUTE ACALCULOUS CHOLECYSTITIS

Overview and Pathogenesis

Acute acalculous cholecystitis generally refers to acute cholecystitis that is not caused by gallstone impaction in the cystic duct. This condition represents around 5% to 10%

of all cases of acute cholecystitis.[57,58] Acute acalculous cholecystitis was thought to occur in patients who are hospitalized with critical illness. Predisposing conditions include severe trauma or burns, recent major surgery, or multiorgan failure. Other risk factors include prolonged total parenteral nutrition, prolonged fasting, and sepsis. In addition, acute acalculous cholecystitis has been found to have increased morbidity and mortality when compared with acute calculous cholecystitis. This finding is thought to be secondary to an increased risk of complications, particularly, gangrenous cholecystitis.

A retrospective case series from a tertiary care hospital demonstrated severe outcomes for many of the patients with acalculous cholecystitis, which represented 14% of all cases of acute cholecystitis. Within this group, complicated cholecystitis occurred at high rates, with gangrenous cholecystitis occurring in 63% of patients. Gallbladder perforation occurred in 15%, and 41% of the patients died.[59] Data from a group of patients in a trauma intensive care unit (ICU) demonstrated a 2.6% incidence of acute acalculous cholecystitis within this patient population. Acalculous cholecystitis was more common in patients with more severe trauma injuries, and the investigators concluded that among patients in a trauma ICU, a high index of suspicion was needed to diagnose and manage this condition.[60]

The pathophysiology of acalculous cholecystitis is multifactorial. Biliary stasis along with localized ischemia to the gallbladder mucosa causes chemical inflammation. Biliary stasis is thought to alter the composition of bile, which makes the gallbladder mucosa more susceptible to injury. Systemic hypotension may also contribute and lead to gallbladder ischemia. Cholecystectomy specimens have demonstrated extensive small vessel occlusion, implicating ischemia in the disease process.[61] This finding may explain the increased association of acalculous cholecystitis in older men with atherosclerosis. Case series and studies have shown that patients with acalculous cholecystitis have tended to be men older than 50 years.

Despite the classical teaching that acute acalculous cholecystitis tends to occur in systemically ill patients with severe disease and trauma, it seems that the epidemiology of the disease is changing, which may be because of increased recognition of the disease in other patient populations as opposed to a true evolution in disease epidemiology. A recent retrospective analysis of a database of patients with cholecystitis showed that the prevalence of acute acalculous cholecystitis was similar to that in previously described reports, approximately 8.3%. In this study, all the patients presented as outpatients and none developed cholecystitis as an inpatient. Most patients had no comorbid conditions or critical illness to place them at risk for this condition. This study confirmed a male predominance as previously seen in other studies.[62]

Although the patient population with this disease continues to evolve and include relatively healthy people, patients with acalculous cholecystitis still seem to have a more fulminant outcome than those with calculous cholecystitis. As noted earlier, there seems to be an increased incidence of gallbladder gangrene as well as perforation, empyema, and morbidity and mortality.[63] More recent data demonstrate that although the risk of gangrene remains high, as the disease evolves toward an outpatient population, outcomes and prognosis are starting to improve as well.[64]

Diagnosis

Diagnosis of acute acalculous cholecystitis may prove difficult. One must maintain a high index of suspicion for this diagnosis in critically ill patients with fevers of unclear cause and no other findings. Once again, the noninvasive diagnostic modalities include abdominal ultrasonography, CT, and hepatobiliary scintigraphy. Abdominal ultrasonography tends to be the preferred initial imaging modality, given the lack of

IV contrast and radiation. Findings in acalculous cholecystitis include thickened gallbladder wall, pericholecystic fluid, intramural air, and sonographic Murphy sign. Sensitivity varies from 67% to 92%, and specificity is more than 90% (**Fig. 5**).[65]

CT findings are similar to those of ultrasonography. Sensitivity and specificity of CT are similar to or better than those of ultrasonography, although CT may have an additional risk of IV contrast in a systemically ill patient. The benefit of CT is that it permits evaluation of the entire abdomen rather than just the hepatobiliary system.[65]

Medical Treatment: a Range of Organisms

As seen with acute calculous cholecystitis, acute acalculous cholecystitis can be complicated by secondary bacterial infections. Therefore, early antibiotic therapy should be initiated if there is any evidence of systemic infection. Choice of antibiotic should focus on species of the family Enterobacteriaceae and other anaerobes. Although these are the most common organisms isolated in patients with acute acalculous cholecystitis, many different organisms have been reported in the literature. The type of organism that is identified may vary based on the patient population. For example, an immunocompromised patient may be more susceptible to infection with an opportunistic organism causing primary infection of the gallbladder rather than causing secondary infection related to bile stasis. Immunocompromised patients may be at risk for acute cytomegalovirus (CMV) cholecystitis. This possibility has been reported in the renal transplant population and should be considered as a possibility in posttransplant patients with upper abdominal pain. Acute CMV cholecystitis may be associated with severe outcomes, such as typical acalculous cholecystitis.[66] The individual patient's symptoms, history, and ethnic background must be taken into account when considering antibiotic therapy for acalculous cholecystitis.

Other less common causes of acute acalculous cholecystitis to be considered in the appropriate patients include helminthic infection with *A lumbricoides*. This infection tends to occur in patients from endemic tropical areas and typically affects the intestines and bile ducts. Rarely, the worm can infect the gallbladder and be refractory to standard therapy, leading to cholecystectomy.[67,68] Similar to the liver fluke *C sinensis*, *A lumbricoides* may cause eosinophilic cholecystitis.[69]

Other reported infections causing acute acalculous cholecystitis include leptospirosis,[70] actinomycosis[74,75] as well as the infections caused by dengue virus,[71] *Salmonella enteritidis*,[72] *Staphylococcus aureus*,[73] Epstein-Barr virus,[76] *Candida* sp,[77]

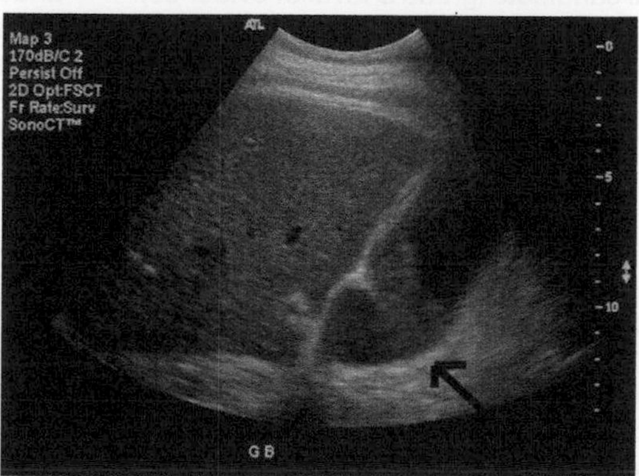

Fig. 5. Acalculous cholecystitis. Ultrasonography shows thickening of gallbladder wall (*arrow*) without stones in the gallbladder. (*Courtesy of* Dr Carlos Cuevas, University of Washington, USA.)

Dolosigranulum pigrum,[78] and *Micrococcus* sp.[79] Noninfectious causes of acute cholecystitis have also been reported. Such causes include infiltration of the gallbladder with malignant leukemia[80] and vasculitis involving the gallbladder.[81,82]

Within the Asian population, chronic biliary parasites must be considered as a cause of the disease. Liver flukes such as *C sinensis* and *O viverrini* have been reported to cause chronic infection of the bile ducts and subsequently lead to chronic acalculous cholecystitis. The flukes may actually be visualized on imaging of the gallbladder with ultrasonography, CT, or MRI. Patients who are chronically infected with these organisms may be at increased risk for cholangiocarcinoma but not carcinoma of the gallbladder. These patients typically have involvement of the bile ducts and may have cholangitis as a presenting symptom rather than acute cholecystitis.[83] Clonorchis infection has been reported to cause eosinophilic cholecystitis.[84]

Although liver flukes may not be associated with increased incidence of gallbladder cancer, other infections of the gallbladder can cause chronic inflammation and predispose to gallbladder cancer. A chronic infection, that is, chronic acalculous cholecystitis, is thought to play a role in transforming a normal gallbladder into one with carcinoma. One of the organisms most strongly linked to the increased risk for gallbladder carcinoma is *Salmonella typhi*. Data from parts of the world where *S typhi* infections are endemic (such as India and Chile) have demonstrated an increased incidence of gallbladder cancer. Direct evidence of salmonella infection of the gallbladder in patients with cancer is lacking, but indirect evidence from polymerase chain reaction assays shows increased rates of salmonella infection in patients with gallbladder cancer when compared with patients with simple gallstones or a normal gallbladder.[85]

Surgical Management

Similar to acute calculous cholecystitis, once acute acalculous cholecystitis is diagnosed prompt treatment is necessary. Treatment consists of either removing or draining the gallbladder. In the inpatient setting, these patients tend to be quite ill, as noted earlier. In this setting, percutaneous cholecystostomy may be the treatment of choice if a patient is not deemed to be a good surgical candidate, secondary to overall acute illness and comorbid conditions. Because there is no obstructive gallstone, percutaneous cholecystostomy has the potential to be the definitive treatment of acalculous cholecystitis and subsequent cholecystectomy may not be necessary. Ultimately, cholecystostomy would be used as a bridge to definitive surgical removal if the patient becomes a surgical candidate (grade B level of evidence).[54–56] Endoscopic retrograde cholangiopancreatography–guided endoscopic drainage of the gallbladder is a potential alternative to percutaneous cholecystostomy, although it is considered technically more difficult with a relapse rate of more than 20% on follow-up.[86] Similar to acute calculous cholecystitis, surgery is generally considered the optimal treatment in appropriately selected patients.

SUMMARY

Infections of the gallbladder can take many different forms. Infection of bile may play a role in the pathogenesis of pigment and cholesterol gallstones, although evidence is still accumulating especially in favor of the latter. A secondary infection may complicate acute calculous cholecystitis, and aggressive antibiotic coverage is indicated. Atypical infections may complicate acalculous cholecystitis, and clinicians need to be aware of these possibilities when treating particular groups of patients. Treatment options can range from surgical cholecystectomy to percutaneous cholecystostomy, but treatment decisions need to be individualized to the particular patient.

REFERENCES

1. Suchy FJ. Anatomy, histology, embryology, developmental anomalies, and pediatric disorders of the biliary tract. In: Feldman M, editor. Sleisenger and Fordtran's gastrointestinal and liver disease. 8th edition. Philadelphia: Saunders Elsevier; 2006. p. 1333–58.
2. Everhart JE, Khare M, Hill M, et al. Prevalence and ethnic differences in gallbladder disease in the United States. Gastroenterology 1999;117:632–9.
3. Shaffer EA. Gallstone disease: epidemiology of gallbladder stone disease. Best Pract Res Clin Gastroenterol 2006;20:981–96.
4. Sampliner RE, Bennett PH, Comers LJ, et al. Gallbladder disease in Pima Indians. Demonstration of high prevalence and early onset by cholecystography. N Engl J Med 1970;283:1358–64.
5. Goodhard GL, Levison ME, Trotman BW, et al. Pigment vs. cholesterol cholelithiasis. Bacteriology of gallbladder stone, bile, and tissue correlated with biliary lipid analysis. Am J Dig Dis 1978;20:735.
6. Schull SD, Wagner CI, Trotman BW, et al. Factors affecting bilirubin excretion in patients with cholesterol or pigment gallstones. Gastroenterology 1977;72: 625–9.
7. Soloway RD, Trotman BW, Maddrey WC, et al. Pigment gallstone composition in patients with hemolysis or infection/stasis. Dig Dis Sci 1986;31:454–60.
8. Trotman BW, Soloway RD. Pigment vs cholesterol cholelithiasis: clinical and epidemiological aspects. Am J Dig Dis 1975;20:735.
9. Nagase M, Tanimura H, Setoyama M, et al. Present features of gallstones in Japan. A collective review of 2144 cases. Am J Surg 1987;135:788.
10. Cetta F. The role of bacteria in pigment gallstones disease. Ann Surg 1991;213: 315–26.
11. Stewart L, Smith AL, Pelligrini CA, et al. Pigment gallstones form as a composite of bacterial microcolonies and pigment solids. Ann Surg 1987;206:242–50.
12. Tabata M, Nakayama F. Bacteria and gallstones. Etiological significance. Dig Dis Sci 1981;26:218.
13. Browning JD. Gallstone disease. In: Feldman LFM, editor. Sleisenger and Fordtran's gastrointestinal and liver disease. Philadelphia: Saunders Elsevier; 2006. p. 1387–418.
14. Skar V, Skar G, Bratlie J, et al. Beta-glucuronidase activity in bile of gallstones patients both with and without duodenal diverticula. Scand J Gastroenterol 1989;24:205.
15. Lee DK, Tarr PI, Haigh WG, et al. Bacterial DNA in mixed cholesterol gallstones. Am J Gastroenterol 1999;94:3502–6.
16. Swidsinski A, Lee SP. The role of bacteria in gallstone pathogenesis. Front Biosci 2001;6:E93–103.
17. Swidsinski A, Ludwig W, Pahlig H, et al. Molecular genetic evidence of bacterial colonization of cholesterol gallstones. Gastroenterology 1995;108:860–4.
18. Ostrow JD. Unconjugated bilirubin and cholesterol gallstone formation. Hepatology 1990;12:219S–26S.
19. Spivak W, DiVenuto D, Yuey W. Non-enzymatic hydrolysis of bilirubin mono- and diglucuronide to unconjugated bilirubin in model and native bile systems. Biochem J 1987;242:323–9.
20. Everson GT, McKinley C, Kern F. Mechanisms of gallstone formation in women. Effects of exogenous estrogen (Premarin) and dietary cholesterol on hepatic lipid metabolism. J Clin Invest 1991;87:237–46.

21. Ito T, Kawata S, Imai Y, et al. Hepatic cholesterol metabolism in patients with cholesterol gallstones: enhanced intracellular transport of cholesterol. Gastroenterology 1996;110:1619–27.
22. Maurer KJ, Carey MC, Fox JG. Roles of infection, inflammation, and the immune system in cholesterol gallstone formation. Gastroenterology 2009;136:425–40.
23. Lee SP, Maher K, Nicholls JF. Origin and fate of biliary sludge. Gastroenterology 1988;94:170–6.
24. Maurer KJ, Ihrig MM, Rogers AB, et al. Identification of cholelithogenic enterohepatic *Helicobacter* species and their role in murine cholesterol gallstone formation. Gastroenterology 2005;128:1023–33.
25. Abeysuriya V, Deen KI, Wijesuriya T, et al. Microbiology of gallbladder bile in uncomplicated symptomatic cholelithiasis. Hepatobiliary Pancreat Dis Int 2008;7:633–7.
26. Hazrah P, Oahn K, Tewari M, et al. The frequency of live bacteria in gallstones. HPB (Oxford) 2004;6:28–32.
27. Bulajic M, Maisonneuve P, Schneider-Brachert W, et al. *Helicobacter pylori* and the risk of benign and malignant biliary tract disease. Cancer 2002;95:1946–53.
28. Chen DF, Hu L, Yi P, et al. *H pylori* are associated with chronic cholecystitis. World J Gastroenterol 2007;13:1119–22.
29. Leong RW, Sung JJ. Review article: *Helicobacter* species and hepatobiliary diseases. Aliment Pharmacol Ther 2002;16:1037–45.
30. Silva CP, Pereira-Lima JC, Oliveira AG, et al. Association of the presence of *Helicobacter* in gallbladder tissue with cholelithiasis and cholecystitis. J Clin Microbiol 2003;41:5615–8.
31. Maurer KJ, Rao VP, Ge Z, et al. T-cell function is critical for murine cholesterol gallstone formation. Gastroenterology 2007;133:1304–15.
32. Indar AA, Beckingham IJ. Acute cholecystitis. BMJ 2002;325:639–43.
33. Roslyn JJ, DenBesten L, Thompson JE Jr, et al. Roles of lithogenic bile and cystic duct occlusion in the pathogenesis of acute cholecystitis. Am J Surg 1980;140:126–30.
34. Strasberg SM. Clinical practice. Acute calculous cholecystitis. N Engl J Med 2008;358:2804–11.
35. Jivegard L, Thornell E, Svanvik J. Pathophysiology of acute obstructive cholecystitis: implications for non-operative management. Br J Surg 1987;74:1084.
36. Thornell E. Mechanisms in the development of acute cholecystitis and biliary pain. A study on the role of prostaglandins and the effects of indomethacin. Scand J Gastroenterol 1982;17:76.
37. Claesson BE, Holmlund DE, Matzsch TW. Biliary microflora in acute cholecystitis and the clinical implications. Acta Chir Scand 1984;150:229.
38. Claesson BE, Holmlund DE, Matzsch TW. Microflora of the gallbladder related to duration of acute cholecystitis. Surg Gynecol Obstet 1986;62:531.
39. Turner MA, Fulcher AS. The cystic duct: normal anatomy and disease processes. Radiographics 2001;21:3–22 questionnaire 288–94.
40. Ralls PW, Colletti PM, Lapin SA, et al. Real-time sonography in suspected acute cholecystitis. Prospective evaluation of primary and secondary signs. Radiology 1985;155:767–71.
41. Carroll BA. Preferred imaging techniques for the diagnosis of cholecystitis and cholelithiasis. Ann Surg 1989;210:1–12.
42. Chatziioannou SN, Moore WH, Ford PV, et al. Hepatobiliary scintigraphy is superior to abdominal ultrasonography in suspected acute cholecystitis. Surgery 2000;127:609–13.
43. Watanabe Y, Nagayama M, Okumura A, et al. MR imaging of acute biliary disorders. Radiographics 2007;27:477–95.

44. Akriviadis EA, Hatzigavriel M, Kapnias D, et al. Treatment of biliary colic with diclofenac: a randomized, double-blind, placebo-controlled study. Gastroenterology 1997;113:225–31.
45. Solomkin JS, Mazuski JE, Baron EJ, et al. Guidelines for the selection of anti-infective agents for complicated intra-abdominal infections. Clin Infect Dis 2003;37:997–1005.
46. Avrutis O, Friedman SJ, Meshoulm J, et al. Safety and success of early laparoscopic cholecystectomy for acute cholecystitis. Surg Laparosc Endosc Percutan Tech 2000;10:200–7.
47. Casillas RA, Yegiyants S, Collins JC. Early laparoscopic cholecystectomy is the preferred management of acute cholecystitis. Arch Surg 2008;143:533–7.
48. Chandler CF, Lane JS, Ferguson P, et al. Prospective evaluation of early versus delayed laparoscopic cholecystectomy for treatment of acute cholecystitis. Am Surg 2000;66:896–900.
49. Deziel DJ, Millikan KW, Economou SG, et al. Complications of laparoscopic cholecystectomy: a national survey of 4,292 hospitals and an analysis of 77,604 cases. Am J Surg 1993;165:9–14.
50. Eldar S, Sabo E, Nash E, et al. Laparoscopic cholecystectomy for acute cholecystitis: prospective trial. World J Surg 1997;21:540–5.
51. Kane RL, Lurie N, Borbas C, et al. The outcomes of elective laparoscopic and open cholecystectomies. J Am Coll Surg 1995;180:136–45.
52. Pessaux P, Tuech JJ, Rouge C, et al. Laparoscopic cholecystectomy in acute cholecystitis. A prospective comparative study in patients with acute vs. chronic cholecystitis. Surg Endosc 2000;14:358–61.
53. Tzovaras G, Zacharoulis D, Liakou P, et al. Timing of laparoscopic cholecystectomy for acute cholecystitis: a prospective non randomized study. World J Gastroenterol 2006;12:5528–31.
54. Ito K, Fujita N, Noda Y, et al. Percutaneous cholecystostomy versus gallbladder aspiration for acute cholecystitis: a prospective randomized controlled trial. AJR Am J Roentgenol 2004;183:193–6.
55. Chang L, Moonka R, Stelzner M. Percutaneous cholecystostomy for acute cholecystitis in veteran patients. Am J Surg 2000;180:198–202.
56. Li JC, Lee DW, Lai CW, et al. Percutaneous cholecystostomy for the treatment of acute cholecystitis in the critically ill and elderly. Hong Kong Med J 2004;10:389–93.
57. Barie PS, Fischer E. Acute acalculous cholecystitis. J Am Coll Surg 1995;180:232–44.
58. Howard R. Acute acalculous cholecystitis. Am J Surg 1981;141:194.
59. Kalliafas S, Ziegler DW, Flancbaum L, et al. Acute acalculous cholecystitis: incidence, risk factors, diagnosis, and outcome. Am Surg 1998;64:471–5.
60. Hamp T, Fridrich P, Mauritz W, et al. Cholecystitis after trauma. J Trauma 2009;66:400–6.
61. Warren BL. Small vessel occlusion in acute acalculous cholecystitis. Surgery 1992;111:163–8.
62. Shridhar Ganpathi I, Diddapur RK, Eugene H, et al. Acute acalculous cholecystitis: challenging the myths. HPB (Oxford) 2007;9:131–4.
63. Johndon L. The importance of early diagnosis of acute acalculous cholecystitis. Surg Gynecol Obstet 1987;164:197.
64. Ryu JK, Ryu KH, Kim KH. Clinical features of acute acalculous cholecystitis. J Clin Gastroenterol 2003;36:166–9.
65. Mirvis SE, Vainright JR, Nelson AW, et al. The diagnosis of acute acalculous cholecystitis: a comparison of sonography, scintigraphy, and CT. AJR Am J Roentgenol 1986;147:1171–775.

66. Drage M, Reid A, Callaghan CJ, et al. Acute cytomegalovirus cholecystitis following renal transplantation. Am J Transplant 2009;9:1249–52.
67. Elaldi N, Turan M, Arslan M, et al. An unusual cause of cholecystitis: a worm in the bag. Emerg Med J 2003;20:489–90.
68. Shetty B, Shetty PK, Sharma P. Ascariasis cholecystitis: an unusual cause. J Minim Access Surg 2008;4:108–10.
69. Kaji K, Yoshiji H, Yoshikawa M, et al. Eosinophilic cholecystitis along with pericarditis caused by *Ascaris lumbricoides*: a case report. World J Gastroenterol 2007; 13:3760–2.
70. Chong VH, Goh SK. Leptospirosis presenting as acute acalculous cholecystitis and pancreatitis. Ann Acad Med Singapore 2007;36:215–6.
71. Berrington WR, Hitti J, Casper C. A case report of dengue virus infection and acalculous cholecystitis in a pregnant returning traveler. Travel Med Infect Dis 2007;5:251–3.
72. Ruiz-Rebollo ML, Sanchez-Antolin G, Garcia-Pajares F, et al. Acalculous cholecystitis due to *Salmonella enteritidis*. World J Gastroenterol 2008;14:6408–9.
73. Merchant SS, Falsey AR. *Staphylococcus aureus* cholecystitis: a report of three cases with review of the literature. Yale J Biol Med 2002;75:285–91.
74. Acevedo F, Baudrand R, Letelier LM, et al. Actinomycosis: a great pretender. Case reports of unusual presentations and a review of the literature. Int J Infect Dis 2008;12:358–62.
75. Hefny AF, Torab FC, Joshi S, et al. Actinomycosis of the gallbladder: case report and review of the literature. Asian J Surg 2005;28:230–2.
76. Chalupa P, Kaspar M, Holub M. Acute acalculous cholecystitis with pericholecystitis in a patient with Epstein-Barr virus infectious mononucleosis. Med Sci Monit 2009;15:CS30–3.
77. Yildirim M, Ozaydin I, Sahin I, et al. Acute calculous cholecystitis caused by *Candida lusitaniae*: an unusual causative organism in a patient without underlying malignancy. Jpn J Infect Dis 2008;61:138–9.
78. Lin JC, Hou SJ, Huang LU, et al. Acute cholecystitis accompanied by acute pancreatitis potentially caused by *Dolosigranulum pigrum*. J Clin Microbiol 2006;44:2298–9.
79. Ma ES, Wong CL, Lai KT, et al. *Kocuria kristinae* infection associated with acute cholecystitis. BMC Infect Dis 2005;5:60.
80. Shimizu T, Tajiri T, Akimaru K, et al. Cholecystitis caused by infiltration of immature myeloid cells: a case report. J Nippon Med Sch 2006;73:97–100.
81. Francescutti V, Ellis AK, Bourgeois JM, et al. Acute acalculous cholecystitis: an unusual presenting feature of Churg-Strauss vasculitis. Can J Surg 2008;51: E129–30.
82. Shin SJ, Na KS, Jung SS, et al. Acute acalculous cholecystitis associated with systemic lupus erythematosus with Sjogren's syndrome. Korean J Intern Med 2002;17:61–4.
83. Lim JH, Mairiang E, Ahn GH. Biliary parasitic diseases including clonorchiasis, opisthorchiasis and fascioliasis. Abdom Imaging 2008;33(2):157–65.
84. Lai CH, Chin C, Chung HC, et al. Clonorchiasis-associated perforated eosinophilic cholecystitis. Am J Trop Med Hyg 2007;76:396–8.
85. Kumar S, Kumar S, Kumar S. Infection as a risk factor for gallbladder cancer. J Surg Oncol 2006;93:633–9.
86. Mutignani M, Iacopini F, Perri V, et al. Endoscopic gallbladder drainage for acute cholecystitis: technical and clinical results. Endoscopy 2009;41:539–46.

Epidemiology and Management of Hepatocellular Carcinoma

Ju Dong Yang, MD, Lewis R. Roberts, MBChB, PhD*

KEYWORDS

• Hepatitis B • Hepatitis C • Pathogenesis • Liver transplantation
• Transarterial chemoembolization • Radiofrequency ablation

EPIDEMIOLOGY

Hepatocellular carcinoma (HCC) is the seventh most common cancer and the third leading cause of cancer-related death worldwide, with an estimated 748,000 new liver cancer cases and 696,000 liver cancer deaths caused in 2008, which increased from 626,000 incident liver cancers and 598,000 deaths in 2002.[1] The incidence of HCC varies across the world. More than 80% of HCCs develop in Asian and African countries, where between 40% and 90% of HCCs are attributable to chronic hepatitis B (**Fig. 1**).[2,3] The incidence of HCC in the United States and Europe is relatively low and up to two-thirds of HCCs in these regions are attributable to chronic hepatitis C virus (HCV) infection (see **Fig. 1**).[3] The incidence of HCC has been rapidly increasing in Western countries because of the increased prevalence of HCV infection contracted within the 20 to 40 years before testing for HCV was available. In the United States, the incidence of HCC has tripled, from 1.6 per 100,000 in 1975 to 4.9 per 100,000 in 2005.[4] It is expected that the incidence of HCC will continue to increase in the next decade because of the 20 to 40 year lag time between virus acquisition and the development of HCC and the peak incidence of HCV infection in the 1980s.[5] HCC is 2 to 4 times more frequent in men than in women. Exposure to hepatocarcinogens and a higher prevalence of hepatitis infection partially explain this gender difference; however, intrinsic protection of women, which has been partially attributed to suppression of interleukin (IL)-6 signaling by estrogens and increased androgen receptor signaling in men, seems to contribute to the gender difference in the risk of HCC.[6–8] In Western

Financial disclosure: This work was supported by grant no. CA100882 from the National Institutes of Health.

Miles and Shirley Fiterman Center for Digestive Diseases, Division of Gastroenterology and Hepatology, College of Medicine, Mayo Clinic, 200 First Street South West, Rochester, MN 55905, USA
* Corresponding author.
E-mail address: Roberts.lewis@mayo.edu

Infect Dis Clin N Am 24 (2010) 899–919
doi:10.1016/j.idc.2010.07.004 id.theclinics.com

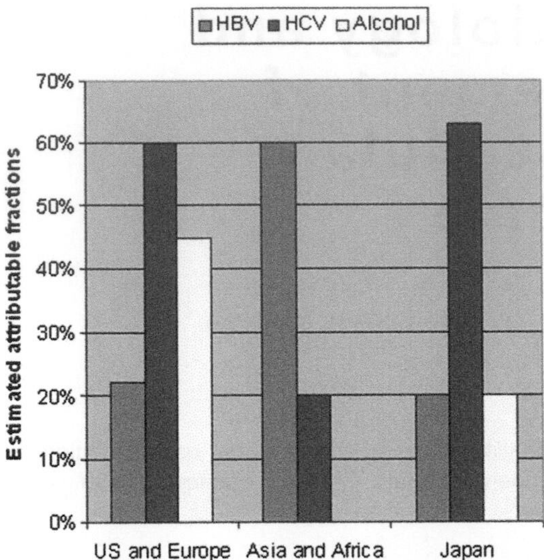

Fig. 1. Risk factors of primary liver cancer and estimated attributable fractions in different parts of the world. (*From* Bosch FX, Ribes J, Diaz M, et al. Primary liver cancer: worldwide incidence and trends. Gastroenterology 2004;127:S5; with permission.)

countries where HCV and hepatitis B virus (HBV) infection are typically acquired in adolescence, early adulthood, or later, HCC rarely develops before the age of 45 years, but incidence rates continue to increase with age.[9] However, in Africa and Asia, because of the early exposure to hepatitis viruses and hepatocarcinogens such as dietary aflatoxins, HCC tends to develop at an earlier age.

CAUSES OF HCC

Chronic Hepatitis B

Chronic HBV infection is the most common cause of HCC. Mother-to-infant vertical transmission is the usual route of HBV acquisition in HBV hyperendemic regions in Asia, whereas horizontal transmission in early life is most frequent in Africa. In the United States and other Western countries, where the prevalence of HBV infection is low, it is usually acquired through high-risk behaviors such as intravenous drug use, sexual exposure, or iatrogenically through blood transfusion, hemodialysis, or organ transplantation.

Causal associations between HBV and HCC have been shown in several studies. In a population-based, large, prospective study of 22,708 Taiwanese men with 8.9 years of follow-up, the incidence of HCC was 98.4 times higher in HBV carriers than in noncarriers.[10] The overall incidence of HCC in hepatitis B carriers seems to depend on race/ethnicity. In one prospective study from Canada of 1069 hepatitis B carriers (71% Asian) with 26 months of follow-up, the incidence of HCC was 0.47% per year.[11] However, in another study of 371 asymptomatic hepatitis B carriers, most of whom were French Canadian, no HCCs developed in 16 years of follow-up.[12] White hepatitis B carriers tend to develop HCC at an older age in a background of underlying liver cirrhosis, whereas Asians and Africans tend to develop HCC at a relatively early age with less cirrhotic change of the liver. This difference seems to be caused by the difference in age at which HBV infection is acquired in the different populations. The risk of HCC is much higher in patients who are hepatitis B e antigen (HBeAg) positive than in those who are hepatitis B surface antigen (HBsAg) positive but HBeAg negative.[13–15] In a large, prospective study of 11,893 Taiwanese men with a mean follow-up of 10 years, compared with those who were both HBeAg and HBsAg negative, the relative risk for HCC was 9.6 for individuals who were positive for HBsAg alone and 60.2 for individuals who were positive for both HBsAg and HBeAg.[15] The HBV DNA level also influences the risk of HCC. In a large, prospective study of 3653 patients with a mean of 11.4 years follow-up, the HBV DNA level was significantly correlated with the incidence of HCC.[16] A previous history of HBV infection (HBsAg−, HBcAb+) also increases the risk of HCC. In patients with HCC who were HBsAg negative, 29% had detectable HBV DNA in either serum or liver tissue. Previous HBV infection was the only risk factor for HCC in 12% of the patients.[17]

HBV has a circular DNA genome that encodes structural and replicative proteins, and contains DNA regulatory elements. After entry into the hepatocyte, viral messenger RNAs are transcribed and translated into viral proteins. New viral genomic DNA is also synthesized by reverse transcription from viral messenger RNA. These new viral genomes, core protein, and polymerase assemble into the complete structures called Dane particles, which are released from the hepatocyte. Viral DNA is able to integrate into host genomic DNA in infected hepatocytes during this process. HBV infection results in chronic inflammation of the liver with the release of inflammatory cytokines that induce liver fibrosis and enhance cell proliferation and the generation of genotoxic reactive oxygen species. Rapid cell cycling of hepatocytes within this oncogenic microenvironment facilitates carcinogenesis.[18] Integration of viral DNA into the host genome may itself generate genomic instability.[19] HBV DNA may insert into or adjacent to cellular genes that encode proteins important in carcinogenesis.[20–23] The hepatitis B X gene encodes an important oncogenic viral protein. HBx protein transactivates cellular promoters through protein-protein interactions,[24] leading to activation of oncogenic signaling pathways. HBx can also modulate proteasome and mitochondrial function and calcium homeostasis, resulting in effects on cell proliferation and viability (**Fig. 2**).[25–28] The HBV preS2 and S proteins may also enhance cell proliferation.[29]

Chronic Hepatitis C

HCV is the most common blood-borne infection and the leading cause of chronic liver disease and HCC in the United States.[30] The incidence of HCV-related HCC has tripled in the past 40 years.[31] HCV is commonly acquired through direct exposure to blood. Needle sharing during injection drug use and intranasal cocaine use seem to be the most common routes of HCV infection.[30] Individuals with multiple sexual contacts are at increased risk of HCV infection, but transmission rates between individuals in monogamous sexual relationships are low.[30] Blood transfusion used to account for 15% to 20% of HCV infection, but is now less than 0.03% per unit transfused since the implementation of donor blood screening for HCV in 1994.[32,33] Vertical transmission from mother to infant occurs in less than 10% of cases; a high HCV titer in the mother increases the frequency of HCV transmission.[34,35]

In a large population-based study of 12,008 Taiwanese men with a mean follow-up of 9.2 years, a 20-fold increased risk of HCC was found in anti-HCV–positive compared with anti-HCV–negative individuals.[36] Concomitant heavy alcohol use, diabetes mellitus, latent HBV infection, older age, black race, lower platelet count, high alkaline phosphatase, presence of varices, and smoking seem to increase the risk of HCV-induced HCC.[37–41]

HCV is a positive-sense RNA virus with a 9400-nucleotide RNA. It has structural and nonstructural genes that encode at least 10 different proteins. There are at least 6 major HCV genotypes. Frequent mutation of HCV genomic RNA because of an error-prone

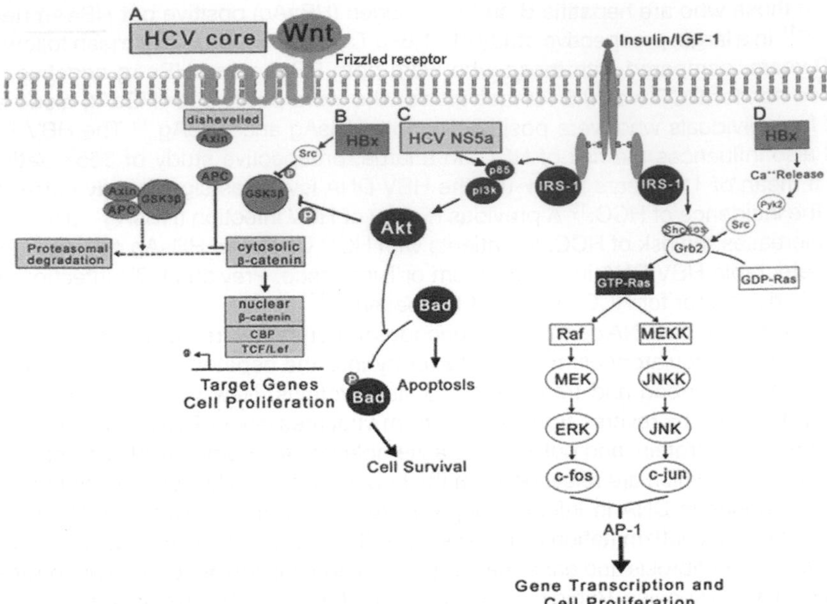

Fig. 2. Two major signaling pathways activated by HBV and HCV in hepatocarcinogenesis. Cytosolic β-catenin is normally phosphorylated by a complex of adenomatous polyposis coli (APC), Axin, and glycogen synthase kinase 3β(GSK3β) and then degraded by the proteasome (*dotted lines*). Increased Wnt expression by HCV core protein activates Wnt/β-catenin pathway. GSK3β, APC, Axin complex is dissociated by Dishevelled and this results in the accumulation of cytosolic and nuclear β-catenin, which interacts with T-cell factor (TCF) and lymphoid enhancer binding protein (Lef), leading to the expression of target genes that stimulate liver cell proliferation. (*A*) HBx protein inactivates GSK3β via Src. This inactivation eventually results in the accumulation of nuclear β-catenin and increases the expression of genes involved in liver cell proliferation. (*B*) HCV NS5a protein interacts with p85. This interaction leads to the activation of Akt. Activated Akt phosphorylates Bad and decreases apoptosis of liver cells. At the same time, Akt phosphorylates GSK3β, thereby preventing proteasomal degradation of β-catenin. (*C*) HBx protein increases the cytosolic calcium level, leading to activation of the Ras-Raf-ERK and Ras-MEKK-JNK cascades. AP-1, activator protein-1; ERK, extracellular signal-regulated kinase; IRS-1, insulin receptor substrate-1; JNK, jun, N-terminal kinase; PI3K, phosphatidylinositol-3 kinase. (*Modified from* Branda M, Wands JR. Signal transduction cascades and Hepatitis B and C related hepatocellular carcinoma. Hepatology 2006;43(5):891; with permission.)

RNA polymerase enables HCV to escape host immune responses, resulting in persistent viral infection.[42] HCV causes chronic liver inflammation with increased oxidative stress, leading to cycles of death and regeneration of hepatocytes. In this context of increased cell turnover and reactive oxygen species, hepatocytes are susceptible to genetic mutations. The accumulation of these genetic changes eventually results in malignant transformation of hepatocytes. In addition to this indirect role of HCV in carcinogenesis, viral proteins seem to play direct roles in promoting tumorigenesis. The core, NS3, NS4B, and NS5A proteins have been implicated in apoptosis, signal transduction, transcriptional activation, and cellular transformation (see **Fig. 2**).[28,43–45]

Chronic Hepatitis and Cirrhosis

The incidence of HCC among cirrhotic patients is 2% to 4% per year.[46,47] Alcoholic liver disease is the most common cause of liver cirrhosis other than viral hepatitis.

In a large case control study, alcohol intake increased the risk of HCC in a linear manner and this risk was greater in patients with viral hepatitis.[48] Cirrhosis from nonalcoholic steatohepatitis is emerging as a major risk factor for HCC. Primary biliary cirrhosis, genetic hemochromatosis, autoimmune hepatitis, and α1-antitrypsin deficiency are less common, but important, risk factors for liver cirrhosis and HCC.[49,50]

Other Risk and Protective Factors

A case control study suggested that hypothyroidism is more frequent in patients with HCC with an unknown cause than in patients with HCC with a known cause.[51] Recently, a larger study confirmed a significant association between hypothyroidism and HCC in women, with an adjusted odds ratio (OR) of 2.9.[52]

Coffee consumption has a protective effect from HCC. A meta-analysis estimated that 2 or more cups of coffee per day results in a 43% risk reduction for HCC.[53] In a recent large case control study, statin use also showed a protective effect against HCC in a diabetic population with an adjusted OR of 0.74.[54]

Preventive Measures

Prevention of HBV infection is the most effective measure to prevent HBV-induced HCC. Universal vaccination was implemented in 164 out of 190 World Health Organization member states as of 2006, and has resulted in dramatic decreases in the incidence of HBV infection. After the introduction of HBV vaccination in 1984, the prevalence of HBsAg+ carrier status in Taiwanese children younger than 15 years old decreased from 9.8% in 1984 to 0.7% in 1999.[55] At the same time, the incidence of HCC in Taiwanese children decreased by 50% from 0.7 per 100,000 between 1981 and 1986 to 0.36 per 100,000 between 1990 and 1994.[56] Recently, a large population-based study in Taiwan has shown that the age- and sex-adjusted relative risk for HCC was 0.31 among children aged 6 to 19 years in vaccinated, compared with unvaccinated, birth cohorts.[57] Global vaccination of newborns, especially in HBV-hyperendemic populations, should lead to a substantial reduction in the incidence of HBV-related HCC within the next few decades.

For patients who have already contracted chronic HBV infection, it is important to avoid modifiable risk factors.[37,41] It seems that the risk of HCC is decreased in patients responding to treatment with interferon (INF).[58–60] In a large, prospective, randomized, controlled trial of 651 patients with a median follow-up of 32 months, lamivudine decreased progression from cirrhosis to HCC with a hazard ratio of 0.49 (P = .047).[61] Risk reductions for HCC have been also observed in patients with HBV without cirrhosis in several case control studies.[62,63]

There is no vaccination available for HCV, partly because of its high propensity for genomic mutation during viral replication. Therefore, it is important to avoid modifiable risk factors for HCC. Studies investigating the role of antiviral treatment of HCV in the prevention of HCC in cirrhotic patients have been inconclusive. In a prospective, randomized, controlled trial of 90 patients with HCV-related cirrhosis with an average of 8.2 years of follow-up, HCC developed in 73% of untreated, but in only 27% of INF-treated, patients.[64] Multiple other retrospective studies and several meta-analyses have reached similar conclusions. The magnitude of the effect seems to be largest in sustained responders.[65,66] In contrast, prospective controlled trials from France and Italy showed no evidence that INF monotherapy decreases the risk of HCC among patients with HCV-related cirrhosis.[67,68] INF treatment in patients with HCV who are noncirrhotic seems to decrease the risk for HCC. In a large, retrospective Japanese study of 2890 patients with chronic HCV with 4.3 years of follow-up, the incidence of HCC in patients treated with INF was 1.1% per year, compared with 3.1% per year in the untreated group. This effect was most significant among patients responding to INF and those with stage 2 and 3 fibrosis.[69] There has been a question whether INF treatment may reduce the risk for HCC because of its antiproliferative action, even in patients who do not achieve sustained virologic responses; however, the Hepatitis C Antiviral Long-term Treatment Against Cirrhosis (HALT-C) Trial has recently shown that long-term maintenance therapy with pegylated INF does not decrease the risk for HCC in patients with advanced liver fibrosis.[40,70]

CLINICAL FEATURES OF HCC

Aside from symptoms related to chronic liver disease, patients are usually asymptomatic at HCC diagnosis. Active surveillance for HCC in high-risk populations has increased the frequency of diagnosis of HCC in asymptomatic patients. Symptoms occurring in patients with advanced disease include abdominal pain, weight loss, pleuritic chest pain from subcapsular masses, or bone pain from distant metastases. HCC development may result in rapid worsening of liver function because of replacement of functioning liver tissue or invasion of the portal vein. Increased ascites, spontaneous bacterial peritonitis, variceal bleeding, jaundice, and hepatic encephalopathy should therefore raise the suspicion for HCC. Intra-abdominal hemorrhage from ruptured HCC or paraneoplastic syndromes manifesting as hypoglycemia, erythrocytosis, or hypercalcemia are uncommon. Physical examination usually shows signs of cirrhosis with portal hypertension, including spider angiomas, jaundice, gynecomastia, palmar erythema, ascites, and caput medusae. A bruit is occasionally present over the liver because of the highly vascular nature of HCCs. Laboratory findings are usually nonspecific. Anemia, thrombocytopenia, and abnormal liver tests are commonly found.

DIAGNOSIS OF HCC

Surveillance

Regular surveillance is recommended for individuals at high risk for HCC development (**Table 1**). In a randomized controlled trial of 18,816 Chinese patients with chronic hepatitis, surveillance for HCC with ultrasound (US) and serum α-fetoprotein (AFP) level every 6 months increased the detection of small HCCs, the frequency of surgical resection, and improved overall survival with a mortality reduction of 37%.[71] US examination is the most important screening tool for HCC. Despite several limitations of US, such as operator-dependent interpretation, poor diagnostic performance in obese patients, and impaired detection of nodules in the cirrhotic liver, its sensitivity and specificity are 65% to 80% and 90% respectively.[72] One retrospective study has reported no difference in HCC stage at detection and 5-year survival between groups

Table 1
Group of patients for whom surveillance is recommended

Hepatitis B Carrier	Cirrhosis from Other Causes
Cirrhotic HBV carriers	Hepatitis C
Family history of HCC	Alcoholic liver disease
Africans >20 years old	Genetic hemochromatosis
Asian men >40 years old	Primary biliary cirrhosis
Asian women >50 years old High viral load (HBV DNA >2000 IU/mL) High transaminases	Potentially cirrhosis from any cause including nonalcoholic steatohepatitis, α1-antitrypsin deficiency, autoimmune hepatitis

undergoing US surveillance at intervals of 6 versus 12 months; however, most hepatologists use a 6-month interval.[73] The routine use of computed tomography (CT) in place of US for surveillance is not recommended because of the high cost and repeated radiation and contrast exposure. However, screening by CT was associated with the greatest gain in life expectancy in patients on a waiting list for liver transplantation.[74] The serum AFP level is used for surveillance in combination with US in most high-incidence countries. In one study, at a cutoff value of 20 ng/mL, the sensitivity of AFP was 60%, with a specificity of 90.6%. With a cutoff value of 200 ng/mL, the specificity of AFP increased to 99.4%, but sensitivity dropped to 22.4%.[75] Therefore, the use of AFP alone for HCC surveillance is discouraged. Other tumor markers such as des-γ-carboxyprothrombin (DCP) and lectin-bound AFP (AFP-L3) are used in Asia as adjunctive diagnostic and prognostic markers to AFP because of their correlation with tumor size and high specificity respectively. However, their routine use for surveillance is not yet formally recommended in Europe and North America. A recent multicenter study in the United States has shown that AFP had the best area under the receiver operating characteristic curve for early-stage HCC, followed by DCP and AFP-L3% and suggested an optimal cutoff value of 10.9 ng/mL (sensitivity of 66% and specificity of 82%) for surveillance.[76]

DIAGNOSTIC APPROACH TO HCC

Triple phase contrast-enhanced helical CT or dynamic magnetic resonance imaging (MRI) are the diagnostic modalities of choice once suspicious lesions are found by surveillance US. The presence of arterial enhancement followed by portal venous washout has an overall sensitivity and specificity of 90% and 95% respectively, with a specificity of 98% for lesions greater than 2 cm in size. The overall performance of MRI is slightly better than CT.[77]

The American Association for the Study of Liver Diseases has recommended a diagnostic approach for HCC that depends on lesion size (**Fig. 3**).[78] If a new lesion in a cirrhotic liver is larger than 2 cm, the presence of arterial enhancement followed by portal venous washout on 1 dynamic imaging modality is diagnostic for HCC. An AFP more than 200 ng/mL may substitute for dynamic imaging criteria. For lesions between 1 and 2 cm in a cirrhotic liver, characteristic imaging findings are less reliable and should be present on both CT and MRI scans to diagnose HCC. If the lesion is smaller than 1 cm, it should be followed with US at intervals of 3 to 6 months. If there is no change in the lesion during a close follow-up period of 2 years, patients can return to routine surveillance.

Percutaneous liver biopsy is indicated when dynamic imaging modalities show inconclusive results. Specifically, biopsy is usually required when lesions (>1 cm) develop without background liver cirrhosis, lesions are larger than 2 cm without a characteristic vascular profile on either of the dynamic imaging studies with AFP less than 200 ng/mL, or the lesions are between 1 and 2 cm and show an inconsistent vascular profile on 2 dynamic imaging studies. The sensitivity of US-guided percutaneous needle biopsy has been reported to be 90%.[79] Therefore, a negative result from percutaneous liver biopsy does not rule out HCC. Close follow-up of such lesions at 3- to 6-month intervals is required until the nodules disappear or acquire the typical radiologic features of HCC. There is a risk of biopsy complications such as bleeding or seeding of tumor along the needle track.[80] A recent meta-analysis has reported that the incidence of needle track tumor seeding is 2.7% overall, or 0.9% per year after biopsy.[81] Therefore, percutaneous biopsy should be used with caution and due consideration, particularly in patients who are eligible for curative therapies.

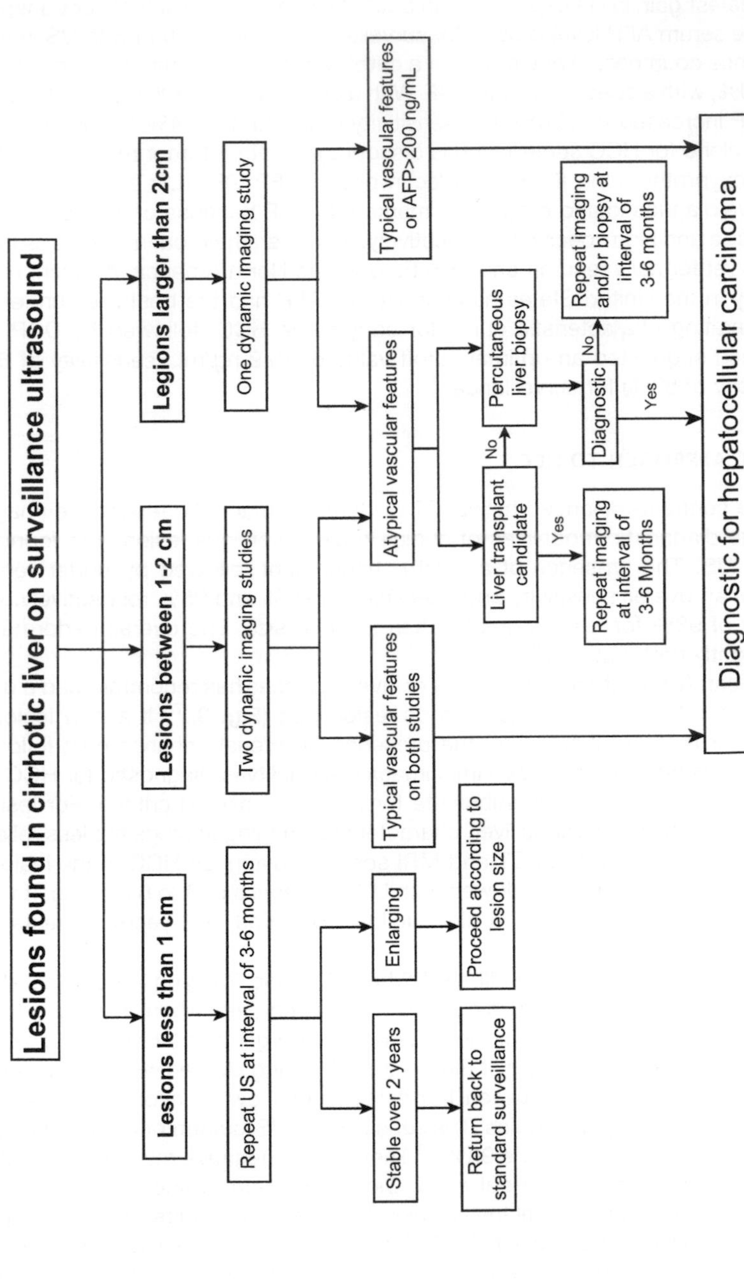

Fig. 3. Algorithm for HCC diagnosis suggested by the American Association for the Study of Liver Disease. (*Modified from* Bruix J, Sherman M. Management of hepatocellular carcinoma. Hepatology 2005;42:1208; with permission.)

TREATMENT APPROACH FOR HCC

Stage of HCC

HCC staging systems usually include tumor characteristics such as tumor size, number, vascular invasion and metastasis. The severity of underlying liver disease is also incorporated in some models because of the effect of cirrhosis with portal hypertension on survival of patients with HCC. The tumor, node, metastasis (TNM); Barcelona Clinic Liver Cancer (BCLC), Cancer of the Liver Italian Program (CLIP), and Japan Integrated Scoring System (JIS) are the most widely used staging systems for HCC (**Table 2**). TNM staging classifies patients into 4 groups based on tumor size, number, lymph node, vascular invasion, and distant metastasis. Its role in the prediction of

Table 2
Commonly used HCC staging systems

TNM Staging

Stage I	Stage II	Stage IIIA	Stage IIIB	Stage IIIC	Stage IV
T1, N0, M0	T2, N0, M0	T3, N0, M0	T4, N0, M0	Any T, N1, M0	Any T, N, M1
T1	Solitary tumor without vascular invasion				
T2	Solitary tumor with vascular invasion, or multiple tumors none more than 5 cm				
T3	Multiple tumors more than 5 cm or tumor involving a major branch of the portal or hepatic vein(s)				
T4	Tumors with direct invasion of adjacent organs other than the gallbladder or with perforation of the visceral peritoneum				
N0	No regional lymph node metastasis; N1, regional lymph node metastasis				
M0	No distant metastasis; M1, distant metastasis				

CLIP Staging

Score	0	1	2
Child-Pugh stage	A	B	C
Tumor morphology	Uninodular and extension ≤50%	Multinodular and extension ≤50%	Massive or extension >50%
AFP	<400 ng/dL	≤400 ng/dL	
Portal vein thrombosis	No	Yes	
The total score is derived by adding each of the subscores			
Early stage (0 point); intermediate stage (1–3 points); advanced stage (4–6 points)			

The BCLC Staging Classification

BCLC stage	Performance status	Tumor stage	Liver function
A0	0	Single, <2 cm	Child-Pugh A
A	0	Single tumor or no more than 3 tumors, each <3 cm	Child-Pugh A-B
B	0	Multinodular (≥4 lesions or largest lesion ≥3 cm)	Child-Pugh A-B
C	1–2	Vascular invasion or extrahepatic spread	Child-Pugh A-B
D	3–4	Any stage	Child-Pugh C

Stage 0, very early stage; stage A, early stage; stage B, intermediate stage; stage C, advanced stage; stage D, terminal stage survival has been validated in a large cohort of patients undergoing liver transplantation.[82] TNM staging does not account for the severity of underlying chronic liver disease, which is a major prognostic factor in patients who are not eligible for curative treatment. The CLIP score incorporates severity of liver disease (Child-Turcotte-Pugh score) and tumor characteristics (tumor morphology, AFP, portal vein thrombosis) and classifies patients with HCC into 6 groups. This system is useful for patients undergoing nonsurgical treatment, but provides limited stratification of patients with early-stage HCC.[83,84]

The BCLC staging system classifies patients into 5 groups based on tumor characteristics, severity of liver disease and performance status, and cancer-related symptoms to predict prognosis and guide the treatment approach (**Fig. 4**). The performance of the BCLC system has been validated in several independent studies.[85,86] The biggest advantage of this system is its ability to link stage of HCC to a recommended treatment modality. Very early HCC can be treated with resection or radiofrequency ablation (RFA) depending on tumor location and medical comorbidities. Patients with early-stage HCC are eligible for resection, ablation, or liver transplantation. Intermediate-stage HCCs are managed by palliative transarterial chemoembolization (TACE) or radioembolization. Sorafenib is the only available FDA-approved treatment for patients with advanced-stage HCC and symptomatic management is most appropriate in patients with terminal-stage HCC.

Surgical Resection

Surgical resection is a potentially curative treatment for HCC. Resection is restricted to patients without cirrhosis or those with cirrhosis and well-preserved liver function because of the risk of liver decompensation after resection. In Asian countries, the indocyanin green retention test is performed to assure the safety of surgical resection. In Western countries, clinical assessment of portal hypertension and bilirubin are used to confirm candidacy for surgical resection. A hepatic vein pressure gradient less than 10 mm Hg and normal serum bilirubin level were the best predictors of a good outcome after surgery. No decompensation was found in this group and the 5-year

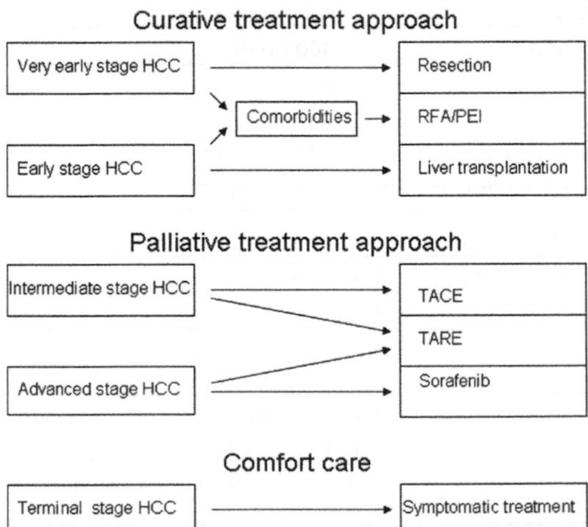

Fig. 4. Treatment recommendation according to the modified BCLC staging classification. PEI, percutaneous ethanol injection; RFA, radiofrequency ablation; TACE, transarterial chemoembolization; TARE, transarterial radioembolization.

survival was greater than 70%.[87,88] In contrast, most patients with significant portal hypertension and normal bilirubin developed postoperative decompensation with a 5-year survival of less than 50%. Patients with portal hypertension and an increased serum bilirubin level had a 5-year survival of less than 30%. Clinically significant portal hypertension can also be presumed from the presence of thrombocytopenia (platelet count <100,000) and splenomegaly. Therefore, resection is considered in patients with a normal bilirubin and a platelet count higher than 100,000 without varices or other signs of clinically significant portal hypertension. A Model for End-Stage Liver Disease (MELD) score of 8 or less is functionally equivalent to these criteria.[89]

Resection is recommended for single tumors or multiple tumors confined to 1 lobe of the liver. In a study of 12,118 Japanese patients with HCC, the 5-year survival was 57% after resection of a single lesion, 45% for patients with 2 lesions, and 26% in patients with 3 or more lesions.[90] Five-year survival after resection decreased as tumor size increased, with a range of 53% to 66% for tumors less than 5 cm, and 32% to 38% for tumors larger than 5 cm.[90] Because some tumors with less aggressive biology present as a single large lesion without microvascular invasion, the size of the tumor alone should not preclude surgical resection. In patients with cirrhosis, the remaining liver continues to be at risk of development of cancer after surgical resection, and the risk of recurrence at 5 years exceeds 70%.[91] Microvascular invasion is a strong predictor of recurrence.[92] A narrow resection margin also increases the risk of recurrent HCC.[93] There is no known adjuvant treatment that decreases the risk of tumor recurrence after resection.

Liver Transplantation

Liver transplantation is the most definitive treatment of HCC because it removes not only the malignancy but also the underlying diseased liver with its high risk of recurrence. The selection criteria for liver transplantation were initially broad and patient outcomes were poor, with 5-year survival of less than 20%.[94,95] This rate changed after adoption of the Milan criteria for selection of candidates with HCC for liver transplantation, which restrict transplantation to patients with 1 tumor 5 cm or less in diameter or up to 3 lesions with the largest no more than 3 cm in diameter. These criteria resulted in 4-year overall survival and recurrence-free survival rates of 75% and 83% respectively after liver transplantation, making long-term survival of patients transplanted for HCC similar to that of patients receiving liver transplants for non-HCC indications.[96] Among patients who met the Milan criteria on pathologic examination of the explanted liver, the 4-year overall survival and recurrence-free survival rates increased to 85% and 92%.[96] The University of California in San Francisco (UCSF) has proposed expanded selection criteria for liver transplantation.[97] The UCSF criteria (1 tumor no more than 6.5 cm or up to 3 lesions with each lesion no more than 4 cm with a total tumor diameter 8 cm or less) are more inclusive but maintain a 75% 5-year survival comparable with the overall survival with Milan criteria. The UCSF criteria are yet to be implemented by the United Network for Organ Sharing (UNOS), except on appeal as an exception to standard criteria. For patients with HCC meeting UNOS criteria for liver transplantation, a MELD exception score, which is based on the probability of death within 3 months, is awarded so that transplantation can be accomplished in a reasonable timeframe. Patients receive a MELD score of 22 unless their calculated MELD is greater. Patients with HCC receive additional MELD points every 3 months while on the waiting list because of the increased risk of pretransplantation mortality.

For HCCs initially beyond UNOS criteria, downstaging using local or locoregional therapy has been used to decrease the size or number of tumors into the range of the UNOS criteria to allow listing for liver transplantation.[98–100] This approach has achieved some success with reduction of the tumor size and number in 70% of patients, eventually resulting in successful liver transplantation in 53% of patients with an intention-to-treat survival of 81.8% at 2 years among 30 patients.[99] A validation study with a larger sample size and longer follow-up has shown similar rates of success in downstaging tumors (70%) and in achieving liver transplantation (57.4%), with an intention-to-treat survival of 69.3% at 4 years.[100]

Living donor liver transplantation (LDLT) entails a significant morbidity and mortality to donors.[101] In spite of the known donor risk, given the shortage of deceased donors, LDLT has been used to shorten the waiting time or broaden the selection criteria for liver transplantation. This treatment modality may be effective for selected patients given that tumor progression beyond UNOS criteria or death while on a waiting list results in a cumulative dropout rate of 15% to 25% at 12 months.[102]

Percutaneous Ablation

Percutaneous ablation is effective for treatment of small tumors in patients who are not eligible for liver transplantation or resection. In percutaneous ethanol injection (PEI), ethanol is injected directly into the tumor under US guidance. PEI has an excellent treatment effect, resulting in complete necrosis of small tumors; however, as the tumor nodule gets larger, the treatment effect is impaired because the injected ethanol cannot access the entire volume of tumor. As a result, the necrosis rate decreases from 90% to 100% for HCCs smaller than 2 cm to 70% for tumors between 2 and 3 cm, and 50% for tumors between 3 and 5 cm.[103–105]

For RFA, an electrode is inserted into the tumor and excited by a radiofrequency generator, thus delivering heat into the tumor and leading to tumor necrosis. RFA is now more frequently used than PEI because of the ability to completely ablate larger tumors in fewer treatment sessions. Several randomized controlled trials have reported that RFA has better efficacy than PEI.[106,107] In a randomized controlled trial of treatment of HCCs less than 4 cm in size, RFA was superior to PEI in rate of complete tumor necrosis (96% in RFA vs 88% in PEI), 3 year overall survival (62%–78% in RFA vs 36%–72% in PEI), and recurrence-free survival (34%–49% in RFA vs 12%–43% in PEI).[107] RFA seems to have similar efficacy to surgical resection in the treatment of very early-stage HCCs, with a lower complication rate and cost.[108–110]

TACE

TACE is a dual treatment process that includes (1) intraarterial delivery of chemotherapeutic agent(s) directly into the tumor, and (2) embolization of the hepatic artery that feeds the tumor. TACE is currently recommended in patients with large multifocal HCCs and preserved liver function without cancer-related symptoms, vascular invasion, or metastasis. Patients with poor liver function or portal vein thrombosis are not candidates because of the high risk of acute liver decompensation, which occurs after 20% of sessions and is irreversible in 3% of cases.[111] Randomized controlled trials have shown the benefit of TACE in selected patients with unresectable HCC.[112,113] The TACE groups had better overall survival than the conservative management groups (2-year survival of 31%–64% and 11%–27% in the TACE and control groups respectively). In a prospective cohort study of 8510 patients who underwent TACE for unresectable HCC, median survival was 34 months with a 5-year overall survival of 26%.[114] TACE is also used in patients with early-stage HCC when ablative treatment cannot be safely performed because of the tumor location. TACE is frequently used for downsizing the tumor or as a bridging treatment before liver transplantation.[99,115] An additive effect of TACE to RFA has been reported, but a recent randomized controlled trial with 89 patients with a single HCC nodule less than 3 cm showed no additive effect of TACE compared with RFA alone.[116–118] Postembolization syndrome is the most common complication of TACE and results in abdominal pain, nausea, vomiting, and fever caused by hepatic arterial occlusion and tumor ischemia. Postembolization syndrome usually resolves within a week with conservative management. The treatment effect of TACE is evaluated by comparison of vascular enhancement of the tumor in dynamic imaging studies rather than tumor size because most tumor nodules do not decrease in size even after successful treatment.[119,120] TACE may be repeated at 2- to 6-month intervals if there is tumor progression.[121]

Radionuclide Yttrium 90 Radioembolization

Delivery of yttrium 90–impregnated glass microspheres (TheraSphere) or resin beads (SirSphere) by transarterial radioembolization (TARE) has been shown to be effective in patients with intermediate- to advanced-stage HCC (**Fig. 5**).[122–124] Potential radiation exposure to the gastrointestinal tract is managed by embolization of hepatic artery branches to the stomach or small intestine. Lung exposure is assessed by infusion of technetium 99 macroaggregated albumin into the hepatic artery followed by a radionuclide scan before treatment to identify candidates with significant intratumoral vascular shunting that precludes radioembolization. Additional randomized studies are required to evaluate the long-term efficacy and side effect profile of TARE.

Systemic Chemotherapy and Targeted Treatments

Most HCCs are resistant to chemotherapeutics and patients usually have poor tolerance of systemic chemotherapy because of the underlying portal hypertension with resultant pancytopenia. Hence, there have been sustained efforts to understand the basic molecular pathogenesis of HCC to develop targeted therapies. Molecular pathways implicated in liver carcinogenesis include receptor tyrosine kinases, Wnt/β-catenin, ubiquitin-proteasome, epigenetic promoter methylation and histone acetylation, PI3 kinase/AKT/MTOR, proangiogenic molecules, and telomerase.[125] Sorafenib, an oral multikinase inhibitor that targets the Raf kinase, vascular endothelial growth factor receptor, and platelet-derived growth factor receptor signaling pathways involved in

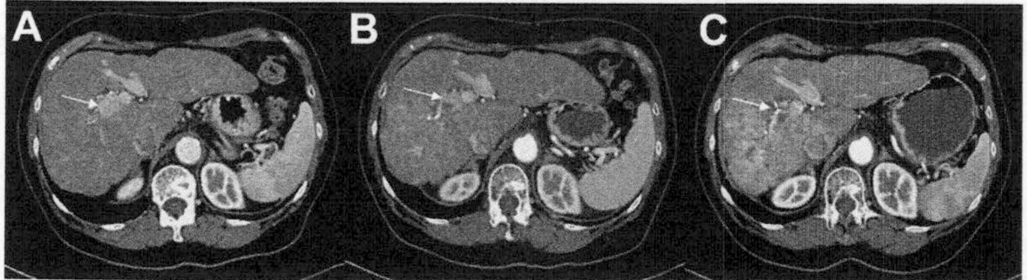

Fig. 5. Treatment effect of radioembolization (TheraSphere treatment). (*A*) Contrast-enhanced CT of the abdomen with biphasic imaging of the liver found a 2.6×1.9-cm mass (*white arrow*) located near the portal vein bifurcation. This mass was treated with radioembolization because of the patient's older age, tumor location, and increased bilirubin. (*B*) One month after the treatment, the mass immediately adjacent to the right portal vein has decreased to 1.4 cm (*white arrow*). (*C*) Three months after the treatment, the previously noted hepatic mass adjacent to the right portal vein has decreased further in size (*white arrow*) and is difficult to differentiate from the background heterogeneous enhancement. Patient has survived for more than 3 years since the treatment without any evidence of recurrence.

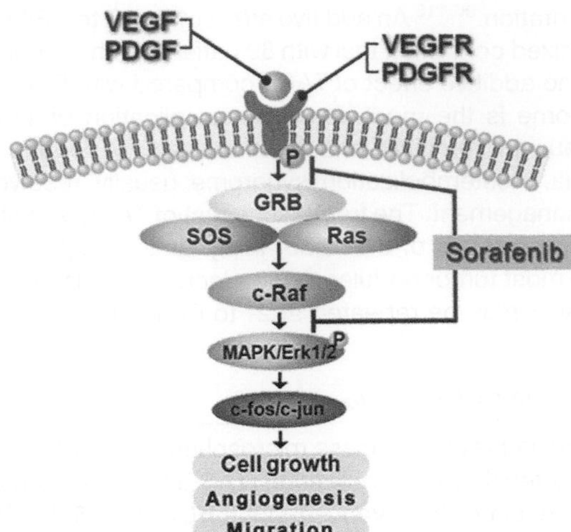

Fig. 6. Mechanism of the antitumor effect of sorafenib. Sorafenib has dual antitumor effects. (1) Inhibition of vascular endothelial growth factor/platelet-derived growth factor signaling; (2) inhibition of Raf kinase-1 activities.

tumor cell proliferation and angiogenesis (**Fig. 6**), is the only agent currently approved for treatment of advanced HCC. In a multicenter, randomized, placebo-controlled trial of 602 patients with advanced HCC, overall survival was 10.7 months in the sorafenib group compared with 7.9 months in the placebo group: a highly significant difference.[126] Median time to progression was 5.5 months in the sorafenib group and 2.8 months in the placebo group. Diarrhea, hypertension, and hand-foot skin reaction are the most significant side effects.

SUMMARY

Chronic hepatitis B and C remain the most important risk factors for HCC. Primary prevention of HBV and HCV infection is the most effective way to decrease the worldwide disease burden of HCC. Global vaccination of infants against HBV will eventually decrease the incidence of HBV-related HCCs. A decreased incidence of transfusion-related HCV infection and increased awareness of the risks of behaviors such as needle sharing, intranasal cocaine use, and nonsanitary injection practices will contribute to the decreased incidence of HBV- and HCV-related HCC.

The incidence of HCC is expected to continue to increase for the next several years. New antivirals that can effectively treat chronic viral hepatitis will be important for the prevention of HCC in patients with chronic HBV or HCV infections. In spite of much effort directed toward the early detection of HCC, it is still diagnosed at an advanced stage in most cases. Continued efforts are needed to improve the early detection of HCC through development of new tumor markers or imaging tools and by encouraging more widespread implementation of existing surveillance modalities, particularly ultrasonography. Liver transplantation, surgical resection, and RFA are effective therapies for early-stage HCC. Recent advances in understanding molecular and signaling pathways in hepatocarcinogenesis have ushered in a new era of targeted therapies for treatment of HCC. The hope is that the convergence of advances in cancer biology and therapeutic technologies will eventually result in the development of highly effective therapies against intermediate- to advanced-stage HCC.

ACKNOWLEDGMENTS

Secretarial support from Victoria Campion is gratefully acknowledged.

REFERENCES

1. Yang JD, Roberts LR. Hepatocellular carcinoma: a global view. Nat Rev Gastroenterol Hepatol 2010;7(8):448–58.
2. Parkin DM, Bray F, Ferlay J, et al. Global cancer statistics, 2002. CA Cancer J Clin 2005;55(2):74–108.
3. Bosch FX, Ribes J, Diaz M, et al. Primary liver cancer: worldwide incidence and trends. Gastroenterology 2004;127(5 Suppl 1):S5–16.
4. Altekruse SF, McGlynn KA, Reichman ME. Hepatocellular carcinoma incidence, mortality, and survival trends in the United States from 1975 to 2005. J Clin Oncol 2009;27(9):1485–91.
5. Armstrong GL, Alter MJ, McQuillan GM, et al. The past incidence of hepatitis C virus infection: implications for the future burden of chronic liver disease in the United States. Hepatology 2000;31(3):777–82.
6. Ma WL, Hsu CL, Wu MH, et al. Androgen receptor is a new potential therapeutic target for the treatment of hepatocellular carcinoma. Gastroenterology 2008; 135(3):947–55, 955, e941–5.
7. Naugler WE, Sakurai T, Kim S, et al. Gender disparity in liver cancer due to sex differences in MyD88-dependent IL-6 production. Science 2007;317(5834): 121–4.
8. Yu MW, Chen CJ. Elevated serum testosterone levels and risk of hepatocellular carcinoma. Cancer Res 1993;53(4):790–4.
9. El-Serag HB, Rudolph KL. Hepatocellular carcinoma: epidemiology and molecular carcinogenesis. Gastroenterology 2007;132(7):2557–76.
10. Beasley RP. Hepatitis B virus. The major etiology of hepatocellular carcinoma. Cancer 1988;61(10):1942–56.
11. Sherman M, Peltekian KM, Lee C. Screening for hepatocellular carcinoma in chronic carriers of hepatitis B virus: incidence and prevalence of hepatocellular carcinoma in a North American urban population. Hepatology 1995;22(2):432–8.
12. Villeneuve JP, Desrochers M, Infante-Rivard C, et al. A long-term follow-up study of asymptomatic hepatitis B surface antigen-positive carriers in Montreal. Gastroenterology 1994;106(4):1000–5.
13. Chen CJ, Liang KY, Chang AS, et al. Effects of hepatitis B virus, alcohol drinking, cigarette smoking and familial tendency on hepatocellular carcinoma. Hepatology 1991;13(3):398–406.
14. Lu SN, Lin TM, Chen CJ, et al. A case-control study of primary hepatocellular carcinoma in Taiwan. Cancer 1988;62(9):2051–5.
15. Yang HI, Lu SN, Liaw YF, et al. Hepatitis B e antigen and the risk of hepatocellular carcinoma. N Engl J Med 2002;347(3):168–74.
16. Chen CJ, Yang HI, Su J, et al. Risk of hepatocellular carcinoma across a biological gradient of serum hepatitis B virus DNA level. JAMA 2006;295(1):65–73.
17. Liang TJ, Jeffers LJ, Reddy KR, et al. Viral pathogenesis of hepatocellular carcinoma in the United States. Hepatology 1993;18(6):1326–33.
18. Chisari FV. Rous-Whipple Award Lecture. Viruses, immunity, and cancer: lessons from hepatitis B. Am J Pathol 2000;156(4):1117–32.
19. Dandri M, Burda MR, Burkle A, et al. Increase in de novo HBV DNA integrations in response to oxidative DNA damage or inhibition of poly(ADP-ribosyl)ation. Hepatology 2002;35(1):217–23.

20. Bonilla Guerrero R, Roberts LR. The role of hepatitis B virus integrations in the pathogenesis of human hepatocellular carcinoma. J Hepatol 2005;42(5):760–77.
21. Ferber MJ, Montoya DP, Yu C, et al. Integrations of the hepatitis B virus (HBV) and human papillomavirus (HPV) into the human telomerase reverse transcriptase (hTERT) gene in liver and cervical cancers. Oncogene 2003;22(24):3813–20.
22. Horikawa I, Barrett JC. *cis*-Activation of the human telomerase gene (hTERT) by the hepatitis B virus genome. J Natl Cancer Inst 2001;93(15):1171–3.
23. Paterlini-Brechot P, Saigo K, Murakami Y, et al. Hepatitis B virus-related insertional mutagenesis occurs frequently in human liver cancers and recurrently targets human telomerase gene. Oncogene 2003;22(25):3911–6.
24. Yen TS. Hepadnaviral X protein: review of recent progress. J Biomed Sci 1996; 3(1):20–30.
25. Bouchard MJ, Wang LH, Schneider RJ. Calcium signaling by HBx protein in hepatitis B virus DNA replication. Science 2001;294(5550):2376–8.
26. Chami M, Ferrari D, Nicotera P, et al. Caspase-dependent alterations of Ca2+ signaling in the induction of apoptosis by hepatitis B virus X protein. J Biol Chem 2003;278(34):31745–55.
27. Rahmani Z, Huh KW, Lasher R, et al. Hepatitis B virus X protein colocalizes to mitochondria with a human voltage-dependent anion channel, HVDAC3, and alters its transmembrane potential. J Virol 2000;74(6):2840–6.
28. Branda M, Wands JR. Signal transduction cascades and hepatitis B and C related hepatocellular carcinoma. Hepatology 2006;43(5):891–902.
29. Brechot C. Pathogenesis of hepatitis B virus-related hepatocellular carcinoma: old and new paradigms. Gastroenterology 2004;127(5 Suppl 1):S56–61.
30. Alter MJ, Kruszon-Moran D, Nainan OV, et al. The prevalence of hepatitis C virus infection in the United States, 1988 through 1994. N Engl J Med 1999;341(8): 556–62.
31. Kiyosawa K, Tanaka E. Characteristics of hepatocellular carcinoma in Japan. Oncology 2002;62(Suppl 1):5–7.
32. Donahue JG, Munoz A, Ness PM, et al. The declining risk of post-transfusion hepatitis C virus infection. N Engl J Med 1992;327(6):369–73.
33. Schreiber GB, Busch MP, Kleinman SH, et al. The risk of transfusion-transmitted viral infections. The Retrovirus Epidemiology Donor Study. N Engl J Med 1996; 334(26):1685–90.
34. Lam JP, McOmish F, Burns SM, et al. Infrequent vertical transmission of hepatitis C virus. J Infect Dis 1993;167(3):572–6.
35. Ohto H, Terazawa S, Sasaki N, et al. Transmission of hepatitis C virus from mothers to infants. The Vertical Transmission of Hepatitis C Virus Collaborative Study Group. N Engl J Med 1994;330(11):744–50.
36. Sun CA, Wu DM, Lin CC, et al. Incidence and cofactors of hepatitis C virus-related hepatocellular carcinoma: a prospective study of 12,008 men in Taiwan. Am J Epidemiol 2003;157(8):674–82.
37. Hassan MM, Hwang LY, Hatten CJ, et al. Risk factors for hepatocellular carcinoma: synergism of alcohol with viral hepatitis and diabetes mellitus. Hepatology 2002;36(5):1206–13.
38. Ikeda K, Marusawa H, Osaki Y, et al. Antibody to hepatitis B core antigen and risk for hepatitis C-related hepatocellular carcinoma: a prospective study. Ann Intern Med 2007;146(9):649–56.
39. Ohki T, Tateishi R, Sato T, et al. Obesity is an independent risk factor for hepatocellular carcinoma development in chronic hepatitis C patients. Clin Gastroenterol Hepatol 2008;6(4):459–64.

40. Lok AS, Seeff LB, Morgan TR, et al. Incidence of hepatocellular carcinoma and associated risk factors in hepatitis C-related advanced liver disease. Gastroenterology 2009;136(1):138–48.
41. Chen CL, Yang HI, Yang WS, et al. Metabolic factors and risk of hepatocellular carcinoma by chronic hepatitis B/C infection: a follow-up study in Taiwan. Gastroenterology 2008;135(1):111–21.
42. Pawlotsky JM. Genetic heterogeneity and properties of hepatitis C virus. Acta Gastroenterol Belg 1998;61(2):189–91.
43. Lai MM, Ware CF. Hepatitis C virus core protein: possible roles in viral pathogenesis. Curr Top Microbiol Immunol 2000;242:117–34.
44. Park JS, Yang JM, Min MK. Hepatitis C virus nonstructural protein NS4B transforms NIH3T3 cells in cooperation with the Ha-ras oncogene. Biochem Biophys Res Commun 2000;267(2):581–7.
45. Sakamuro D, Furukawa T, Takegami T. Hepatitis C virus nonstructural protein NS3 transforms NIH 3T3 cells. J Virol 1995;69(6):3893–6.
46. Colombo M, de Franchis R, Del Ninno E, et al. Hepatocellular carcinoma in Italian patients with cirrhosis. N Engl J Med 1991;325(10):675–80.
47. Tsukuma H, Hiyama T, Tanaka S, et al. Risk factors for hepatocellular carcinoma among patients with chronic liver disease. N Engl J Med 1993;328(25):1797–801.
48. Donato F, Tagger A, Gelatti U, et al. Alcohol and hepatocellular carcinoma: the effect of lifetime intake and hepatitis virus infections in men and women. Am J Epidemiol 2002;155(4):323–31.
49. Caballeria L, Pares A, Castells A, et al. Hepatocellular carcinoma in primary biliary cirrhosis: similar incidence to that in hepatitis C virus-related cirrhosis. Am J Gastroenterol 2001;96(4):1160–3.
50. Elmberg M, Hultcrantz R, Ekbom A, et al. Cancer risk in patients with hereditary hemochromatosis and in their first-degree relatives. Gastroenterology 2003; 125(6):1733–41.
51. Reddy A, Dash C, Leerapun A, et al. Hypothyroidism: a possible risk factor for liver cancer in patients with no known underlying cause of liver disease. Clin Gastroenterol Hepatol 2007;5(1):118–23.
52. Hassan MM, Kaseb A, Li D, et al. Association between hypothyroidism and hepatocellular carcinoma: a case-control study in the United States. Hepatology 2009;49(5):1563–70.
53. Larsson SC, Wolk A. Coffee consumption and risk of liver cancer: a meta-analysis. Gastroenterology 2007;132(5):1740–5.
54. El-Serag HB, Johnson ML, Hachem C, et al. Statins are associated with a reduced risk of hepatocellular carcinoma in a large cohort of patients with diabetes. Gastroenterology 2009;136(5):1601–8.
55. Ni YH, Chang MH, Huang LM, et al. Hepatitis B virus infection in children and adolescents in a hyperendemic area: 15 years after mass hepatitis B vaccination. Ann Intern Med 2001;135(9):796–800.
56. Chang MH, Chen CJ, Lai MS, et al. Universal hepatitis B vaccination in Taiwan and the incidence of hepatocellular carcinoma in children. N Engl J Med 1997; 336(26):1855–9.
57. Chang MH, You SL, Chen CJ, et al. Decreased incidence of hepatocellular carcinoma in hepatitis B vaccinees: a 20-year follow-up study. J Natl Cancer Inst 2009;101(19):1348–55.
58. Lin SM, Sheen IS, Chien RN, et al. Long-term beneficial effect of interferon therapy in patients with chronic hepatitis B virus infection. Hepatology 1999; 29(3):971–5.

59. Papatheodoridis GV, Manesis E, Hadziyannis SJ. The long-term outcome of interferon-alpha treated and untreated patients with HBeAg-negative chronic hepatitis B. J Hepatol 2001;34(2):306–13.
60. van Zonneveld M, Honkoop P, Hansen BE, et al. Long-term follow-up of alpha-interferon treatment of patients with chronic hepatitis B. Hepatology 2004;39(3): 804–10.
61. Liaw YF, Sung JJ, Chow WC, et al. Lamivudine for patients with chronic hepatitis B and advanced liver disease. N Engl J Med 2004;351(15):1521–31.
62. Matsumoto A, Tanaka E, Rokuhara A, et al. Efficacy of lamivudine for preventing hepatocellular carcinoma in chronic hepatitis B: a multicenter retrospective study of 2795 patients. Hepatol Res 2005;32(3):173–84.
63. Yuen MF, Seto WK, Chow DH, et al. Long-term lamivudine therapy reduces the risk of long-term complications of chronic hepatitis B infection even in patients without advanced disease. Antivir Ther 2007;12(8):1295–303.
64. Nishiguchi S, Shiomi S, Nakatani S, et al. Prevention of hepatocellular carcinoma in patients with chronic active hepatitis C and cirrhosis. Lancet 2001;357(9251):196–7.
65. Camma C, Giunta M, Andreone P, et al. Interferon and prevention of hepatocellular carcinoma in viral cirrhosis: an evidence-based approach. J Hepatol 2001; 34(4):593–602.
66. Papatheodoridis GV, Papadimitropoulos VC, Hadziyannis SJ. Effect of interferon therapy on the development of hepatocellular carcinoma in patients with hepatitis C virus-related cirrhosis: a meta-analysis. Aliment Pharmacol Ther 2001; 15(5):689–98.
67. Bernardinello E, Cavalletto L, Chemello L, et al. Long-term clinical outcome after beta-interferon therapy in cirrhotic patients with chronic hepatitis C. TVVH Study Group. Hepatogastroenterology 1999;46(30):3216–22.
68. Valla DC, Chevallier M, Marcellin P, et al. Treatment of hepatitis C virus-related cirrhosis: a randomized, controlled trial of interferon alfa-2b versus no treatment. Hepatology 1999;29(6):1870–5.
69. Yoshida H, Shiratori Y, Moriyama M, et al. Interferon therapy reduces the risk for hepatocellular carcinoma: national surveillance program of cirrhotic and noncirrhotic patients with chronic hepatitis C in Japan. IHIT Study Group. Inhibition of Hepatocarcinogenesis by Interferon Therapy. Ann Intern Med 1999;131(3): 174–81.
70. Di Bisceglie AM, Shiffman ML, Everson GT, et al. Prolonged therapy of advanced chronic hepatitis C with low-dose peginterferon. N Engl J Med 2008;359(23):2429–41.
71. Zhang BH, Yang BH, Tang ZY. Randomized controlled trial of screening for hepatocellular carcinoma. J Cancer Res Clin Oncol 2004;130(7):417–22.
72. Bolondi L, Sofia S, Siringo S, et al. Surveillance programme of cirrhotic patients for early diagnosis and treatment of hepatocellular carcinoma: a cost effectiveness analysis. Gut 2001;48(2):251–9.
73. Trevisani F, De NS, Rapaccini G, et al. Semiannual and annual surveillance of cirrhotic patients for hepatocellular carcinoma: effects on cancer stage and patient survival (Italian experience). Am J Gastroenterol 2002;97(3):734–44.
74. Saab S, Ly D, Nieto J, et al. Hepatocellular carcinoma screening in patients waiting for liver transplantation: a decision analytic model. Liver Transpl 2003;9(7): 672–81.
75. Trevisani F, D'Intino PE, Morselli-Labate AM, et al. Serum alpha-fetoprotein for diagnosis of hepatocellular carcinoma in patients with chronic liver disease: influence of HBsAg and anti-HCV status. J Hepatol 2001;34(4):570–5.

76. Marrero JA, Feng Z, Wang Y, et al. Alpha-fetoprotein, des-gamma carboxyprothrombin, and lectin-bound alpha-fetoprotein in early hepatocellular carcinoma. Gastroenterology 2009;137(1):110–8.
77. Burrel M, Llovet JM, Ayuso C, et al. MRI angiography is superior to helical CT for detection of HCC prior to liver transplantation: an explant correlation. Hepatology 2003;38(4):1034–42.
78. Bruix J, Sherman M. Management of hepatocellular carcinoma. Hepatology 2005;42(5):1208–36.
79. Durand F, Regimbeau JM, Belghiti J, et al. Assessment of the benefits and risks of percutaneous biopsy before surgical resection of hepatocellular carcinoma. J Hepatol 2001;35(2):254–8.
80. Huang GT, Sheu JC, Yang PM, et al. Ultrasound-guided cutting biopsy for the diagnosis of hepatocellular carcinoma–a study based on 420 patients. J Hepatol 1996;25(3):334–8.
81. Silva MA, Hegab B, Hyde C, et al. Needle track seeding following biopsy of liver lesions in the diagnosis of hepatocellular cancer: a systematic review and meta-analysis. Gut 2008;57(11):1592–6.
82. Vauthey JN, Ribero D, Abdalla EK, et al. Outcomes of liver transplantation in 490 patients with hepatocellular carcinoma: validation of a uniform staging after surgical treatment. J Am Coll Surg 2007;204(5):1016–27 [discussion: 1027–8].
83. Prospective validation of the CLIP score: a new prognostic system for patients with cirrhosis and hepatocellular carcinoma. The Cancer of the Liver Italian Program (CLIP) Investigators. Hepatology 2000;31(4):840–5.
84. Ueno S, Tanabe G, Sako K, et al. Discrimination value of the new western prognostic system (CLIP score) for hepatocellular carcinoma in 662 Japanese patients. Cancer of the Liver Italian Program. Hepatology 2001;34(3):529–34.
85. Marrero JA, Fontana RJ, Barrat A, et al. Prognosis of hepatocellular carcinoma: comparison of 7 staging systems in an American cohort. Hepatology 2005;41(4):707–16.
86. Llovet JM, Bru C, Bruix J. Prognosis of hepatocellular carcinoma: the BCLC staging classification. Semin Liver Dis 1999;19(3):329–38.
87. Bruix J, Castells A, Bosch J, et al. Surgical resection of hepatocellular carcinoma in cirrhotic patients: prognostic value of preoperative portal pressure. Gastroenterology 1996;111(4):1018–22.
88. Llovet JM, Fuster J, Bruix J. Intention-to-treat analysis of surgical treatment for early hepatocellular carcinoma: resection versus transplantation. Hepatology 1999;30(6):1434–40.
89. Teh SH, Christein J, Donohue J, et al. Hepatic resection of hepatocellular carcinoma in patients with cirrhosis: Model of End-Stage Liver Disease (MELD) score predicts perioperative mortality. J Gastrointest Surg 2005;9(9):1207–15 [discussion: 1215].
90. Ikai I, Arii S, Kojiro M, et al. Reevaluation of prognostic factors for survival after liver resection in patients with hepatocellular carcinoma in a Japanese nationwide survey. Cancer 2004;101(4):796–802.
91. Imamura H, Matsuyama Y, Tanaka E, et al. Risk factors contributing to early and late phase intrahepatic recurrence of hepatocellular carcinoma after hepatectomy. J Hepatol 2003;38(2):200–7.
92. Okada S, Shimada K, Yamamoto J, et al. Predictive factors for postoperative recurrence of hepatocellular carcinoma. Gastroenterology 1994;106(6):1618–24.

93. Shi M, Guo RP, Lin XJ, et al. Partial hepatectomy with wide versus narrow resection margin for solitary hepatocellular carcinoma: a prospective randomized trial. Ann Surg 2007;245(1):36–43.
94. Penn I. Hepatic transplantation for primary and metastatic cancers of the liver. Surgery 1991;110(4):726–34 [discussion: 734–5].
95. Ringe B, Pichlmayr R, Wittekind C, et al. Surgical treatment of hepatocellular carcinoma: experience with liver resection and transplantation in 198 patients. World J Surg 1991;15(2):270–85.
96. Mazzaferro V, Regalia E, Doci R, et al. Liver transplantation for the treatment of small hepatocellular carcinomas in patients with cirrhosis. N Engl J Med 1996; 334(11):693–9.
97. Yao FY, Ferrell L, Bass NM, et al. Liver transplantation for hepatocellular carcinoma: expansion of the tumor size limits does not adversely impact survival. Hepatology 2001;33(6):1394–403.
98. Chapman WC, Majella Doyle MB, Stuart JE, et al. Outcomes of neoadjuvant transarterial chemoembolization to downstage hepatocellular carcinoma before liver transplantation. Ann Surg 2008;248(4):617–25.
99. Yao FY, Hirose R, LaBerge JM, et al. A prospective study on downstaging of hepatocellular carcinoma prior to liver transplantation. Liver Transpl 2005; 11(12):1505–14.
100. Yao FY, Kerlan RK Jr, Hirose R, et al. Excellent outcome following down-staging of hepatocellular carcinoma prior to liver transplantation: an intention-to-treat analysis. Hepatology 2008;48(3):819–27.
101. Trotter JF, Wachs M, Everson GT, et al. Adult-to-adult transplantation of the right hepatic lobe from a living donor. N Engl J Med 2002;346(14):1074–82.
102. Yao FY, Bass NM, Nikolai B, et al. Liver transplantation for hepatocellular carcinoma: analysis of survival according to the intention-to-treat principle and dropout from the waiting list. Liver Transpl 2002;8(10):873–83.
103. Ishii H, Okada S, Nose H, et al. Local recurrence of hepatocellular carcinoma after percutaneous ethanol injection. Cancer 1996;77(9):1792–6.
104. Livraghi T, Bolondi L, Lazzaroni S, et al. Percutaneous ethanol injection in the treatment of hepatocellular carcinoma in cirrhosis. A study on 207 patients. Cancer 1992;69(4):925–9.
105. Vilana R, Bruix J, Bru C, et al. Tumor size determines the efficacy of percutaneous ethanol injection for the treatment of small hepatocellular carcinoma. Hepatology 1992;16(2):353–7.
106. Lencioni RA, Allgaier HP, Cioni D, et al. Small hepatocellular carcinoma in cirrhosis: randomized comparison of radio-frequency thermal ablation versus percutaneous ethanol injection. Radiology 2003;228(1):235–40.
107. Lin SM, Lin CJ, Lin CC, et al. Radiofrequency ablation improves prognosis compared with ethanol injection for hepatocellular carcinoma < or =4 cm. Gastroenterology 2004;127(6):1714–23.
108. Chen MS, Li JQ, Zheng Y, et al. A prospective randomized trial comparing percutaneous local ablative therapy and partial hepatectomy for small hepatocellular carcinoma. Ann Surg 2006;243(3):321–8.
109. Livraghi T, Meloni F, Di Stasi M, et al. Sustained complete response and complications rates after radiofrequency ablation of very early hepatocellular carcinoma in cirrhosis: Is resection still the treatment of choice? Hepatology 2008; 47(1):82–9.
110. Lau WY, Lai EC. The current role of radiofrequency ablation in the management of hepatocellular carcinoma: a systematic review. Ann Surg 2009;249(1):20–5.

111. Chan AO, Yuen MF, Hui CK, et al. A prospective study regarding the complications of transcatheter intraarterial lipiodol chemoembolization in patients with hepatocellular carcinoma. Cancer 2002;94(6):1747–52.
112. Llovet JM, Real MI, Montana X, et al. Arterial embolisation or chemoembolisation versus symptomatic treatment in patients with unresectable hepatocellular carcinoma: a randomised controlled trial. Lancet 2002;359(9319):1734–9.
113. Lo CM, Ngan H, Tso WK, et al. Randomized controlled trial of transarterial lipiodol chemoembolization for unresectable hepatocellular carcinoma. Hepatology 2002;35(5):1164–71.
114. Takayasu K, Arii S, Ikai I, et al. Prospective cohort study of transarterial chemoembolization for unresectable hepatocellular carcinoma in 8510 patients. Gastroenterology 2006;131(2):461–9.
115. Alba E, Valls C, Dominguez J, et al. Transcatheter arterial chemoembolization in patients with hepatocellular carcinoma on the waiting list for orthotopic liver transplantation. AJR Am J Roentgenol 2008;190(5):1341–8.
116. Takaki H, Yamakado K, Nakatsuka A, et al. Radiofrequency ablation combined with chemoembolization for the treatment of hepatocellular carcinomas 5 cm or smaller: risk factors for local tumor progression. J Vasc Interv Radiol 2007;18(7): 856–61.
117. Yamakado K, Nakatsuka A, Ohmori S, et al. Radiofrequency ablation combined with chemoembolization in hepatocellular carcinoma: treatment response based on tumor size and morphology. J Vasc Interv Radiol 2002;13(12):1225–32.
118. Shibata T, Isoda H, Hirokawa Y, et al. Small hepatocellular carcinoma: is radiofrequency ablation combined with transcatheter arterial chemoembolization more effective than radiofrequency ablation alone for treatment? Radiology 2009;252(3):905–13.
119. Castrucci M, Sironi S, De Cobelli F, et al. Plain and gadolinium-DTPA-enhanced MR imaging of hepatocellular carcinoma treated with transarterial chemoembolization. Abdom Imaging 1996;21(6):488–94.
120. Forner A, Ayuso C, Varela M, et al. Evaluation of tumor response after locoregional therapies in hepatocellular carcinoma: are response evaluation criteria in solid tumors reliable? Cancer 2009;115(3):616–23.
121. Tezuka M, Hayashi K, Okada Y, et al. Therapeutic results of computed-tomography-guided transcatheter arterial chemoembolization for local recurrence of hepatocellular carcinoma after initial transcatheter arterial chemoembolization: the results of 85 recurrent tumors in 35 patients. Dig Dis Sci 2009;54(3):661–9.
122. Geschwind JF, Salem R, Carr BI, et al. Yttrium-90 microspheres for the treatment of hepatocellular carcinoma. Gastroenterology 2004;127(5 Suppl 1):S194–205.
123. Sangro B, Bilbao JI, Boan J, et al. Radioembolization using 90Y-resin microspheres for patients with advanced hepatocellular carcinoma. Int J Radiat Oncol Biol Phys 2006;66(3):792–800.
124. Vente MA, Wondergem M, van der Tweel I, et al. Yttrium-90 microsphere radioembolization for the treatment of liver malignancies: a structured meta-analysis. Eur Radiol 2009;19(4):951–9.
125. Roberts LR, Gores GJ. Hepatocellular carcinoma: molecular pathways and new therapeutic targets. Semin Liver Dis 2005;25(2):212–25.
126. Llovet JM, Ricci S, Mazzaferro V, et al. Sorafenib in advanced hepatocellular carcinoma. N Engl J Med 2008;359(4):378–90.

Acute Pancreatitis with an Emphasis on Infection

Lutz Schneider, MD[a], Markus W. Büchler, MD[a], Jens Werner, MD[b,*]

KEYWORDS

- Acute pancreatitis • Guidelines • Review • Pathophysiology
- Diagnostics • Treatment • Surgery • Interventions

Acute pancreatitis (AP) is an inflammatory disease of the pancreas. Severe cases can cause systemic inflammatory response, distant organ injury, and death.[1] The earliest pathophysiologic theory was stated by Bernard[2] in 1856. He assumed that biliary reflux into the common pancreatic duct as the main cause of AP. In 1901 Opie[3] described a common channel theory, and hypothesized that gallstone migration with occlusion of the biliopancreatic and subsequent biliary reflux into the pancreas causes AP. Until today, multiple pathophysiologic and etiologic theories have been developed and are discussed in the literature.

The differentiation of a mild and severe form of AP was described by Woosley[4] in 1903. A mild edematous pancreatitis is self-limiting without any mortality. The patients only need supportive therapy and recover without persisting complications. However, in 20% of cases, severe necrotizing pancreatitis occurs. Irrespective of a differentiated multimodal therapy, the mortality is up to 30% even today.[5] For these patients, intensive research has been performed in the past century to optimize diagnostics and management. This article reviews pathophysiologic theories as well as the diagnostics and management of severe necrotizing pancreatitis. This review emphasizes the effect of infectious agents initiating AP and the concepts for treatment of infected pancreatic necrosis.

EPIDEMIOLOGY

The incidence of AP has increased in the past decades and varies in different countries.[6–11] In the United States there are more than 200,000 hospital admissions because of AP every year.[10] Thus the disease is an important medical, surgical, and

[a] Department of General Surgery, University of Heidelberg, Im Neuenheimer Feld 110, 69120 Heidelberg, Germany
[b] Division of Pancreatic Surgery, Department of General Surgery, University of Heidelberg, Im Neuenheimer Feld 110, 69120 Heidelberg, Germany
* Corresponding author.
E-mail address: Jens.Werner@med.uni-heidelberg.de

Infect Dis Clin N Am 24 (2010) 921–941
doi:10.1016/j.idc.2010.07.011
id.theclinics.com
0891-5520/10/$ – see front matter

financial problem.[12] Potential causes are the increase of alcohol consumption, obesity, and gallstones.[13,14]

The cause can be identified in 75% to 85% of cases of AP in Western countries.[7] The mean age of the first attack is the sixth decade.[14] This may be caused by the high incidence of gallstones in women more than 60 years of age.[15,16] Worldwide, infectious agents are responsible for AP in less than 1% of cases. Nevertheless, in India, AP induced by *Ascaris lumbricoides* is the second most frequent cause (23%) after gallstones.[17] This shows the regional relevance of infectious causes of AP. Only 20% of patients develop a severe necrotizing disease. In these cases, the mortality (up to 30%) is still high, despite improved intensive care treatment.[5]

PATHOPHYSIOLOGY

Regardless of the cause of AP, the pathophysiologic pathways are identical. AP is triggered by intrapancreatic trypsinogen activation to trypsin as well as other enzymes. Intrapancreatic trypsin leads to autodigestion and inflammation of the pancreas. AP occurs when uncontrolled regulatory mechanisms lead to overwhelming trypsinogen production or inactivating mechanisms are defective. These inactivating mechanisms include autolysis of activated trypsin, enzyme compartmentation, synthesis of specific trypsin inhibitors such as serine protease inhibitor Kazal type 1 (SPINK1), low intracellular ionized calcium concentration, or reduced pancreatic fluid secretion with subsequent increased intrapancreatic trypsin as observed in patients with cystic fibrosis.[7,10,14]

Intracellular trypsin activates several pancreatic proenzymes including phospholipase A2, elastase, and the kinin and complement pathways.[18] Moreover, neutrophiles, lymphocytes, and macrophages release inflammatory mediators such as interleukin (IL)-1, IL-6, IL-8, and tumor necrosis factor (TNF) α, which increase local inflammation, and might conduct systemic inflammation including the systemic inflammatory response syndrome (SIRS).[7,19]

In addition, the released inflammatory mediators activate the vascular endothelium and induce pancreatic microcirculatory disturbances. These disturbances are characterized by reduced pancreatic blood flow, with subsequent reduced oxygen saturation and increased transmigration of activated leukocytes into the pancreatic tissue.[20–22] Transmigrated neutrophiles release inflammatory mediators, supporting the ongoing inflammatory process irrespective of the initial trigger. The inflammatory mediator release may lead to SIRS[19] and might result in an acute respiratory distress syndrome (ARDS) or multiorgan dysfunction syndrome (MODS). This inflammatory cascade is not only induced by local pancreatic inflammatory mediator release but also indirectly by mediators released from the liver. Increased inflammatory cytokines released from the pancreas induce a hepatic inflammatory mediator release and seem to be partly responsible for the development of ARDS and MODS.[23] Tonsi and colleagues[14] classify this as the first or early phase of AP caused by the inflammatory mediator release and characterizes day 1 to 14 after onset of symptoms where SIRS, ARDS and MODS are the main clinical problems.[24] In this early phase, usually no infectious problems occur. Local complications such as infected necrosis, abscess, or cyst formation appear in the late phase of AP, which starts 14 days after onset of disease. In this late phase, infected pancreatic necrosis and septic complications are the main clinical problems leading to the high mortality.[25]

CAUSES

The United Kingdom guidelines[26] for management of AP arrogate to find the causation for AP in at least 80% of the cases. Not more than 20% should be defined as idiopathic. In developed countries the most common causes for AP are gallstones (38%) and alcohol abuse (36%).[26]

Biliary Pancreatitis

Gallstone migration leads to obstruction of the common biliary and pancreatic duct, with subsequent increased pressure in the pancreatic duct leading to unregulated activation of pancreatic enzymes. The highest risk of migration is associated with gallstones of less than 5 mm in size. Gallstones with a diameter of 8 mm or more usually remain in the gallbladder.[27,28] If there is a previous history of biliary colic and an increase of hepatic enzymes 3 times higher than normal serum concentrations, a biliary pancreatitis is likely.[29] However, 1 out of 4 patients with biliary pancreatitis has normal serum concentrations of hepatic enzymes.[30] Transabdominal ultrasound is the gold standard for detection of gallstones. With this technique, dilatation of the common bile duct may be visible as well as any remaining gallstones in the gallbladder. If there is no gallstone visible, it may still be a biliary pancreatitis without any stone remaining in the bladder. Magnetic resonance cholagiopancreatography or endoscopic ultrasound should be performed to visualize the presence of microlithiasis or other causes of duct obstruction in the absence of stones.[7] If there is any doubt for the diagnosis of abdominal pain, further diagnostic imaging studies, such as computed tomography (CT) or magnetic resonance imaging (MRI) should be performed.

Alcoholic Pancreatitis

The second most frequent cause of AP is chronic alcohol abuse.[7] The pathogenesis of alcoholic pancreatitis remains unclear. AP develops in less than 10% of heavy drinkers (>80 g daily intake).[31] Alcohol itself could not induce AP in experimental settings.[23] Development of alcoholic pancreatitis seems to be triggered by both genetic and environmental factors.[31] Thus, failure to inhibit trypsin activity (gene mutation and absence of SPINK1), or failure to wash active trypsin into pancreatic ducts (gene mutation with dysfunction of the cystic fibrosis transmembrane conductance regulator gene, CFRT) might promote alcoholic pancreatits.[7] There are different theories for how alcohol may lead to AP. Toxic metabolites of alcohol, such as fatty ethyl esters (nonoxidative pathway) and acetaldehyde (oxidative pathway), may directly induce pancreatic damage.[32–34] Another explanation is based on reflux of biliary or duodenal juice into the pancreas induced by alcohol-related dysmotility of the sphincter oddi.[35] Guy and colleagues[36] hypothesized that precipitated proteins lead to pancreatic duct obstruction and alcoholic pancreatitis. Alcoholic pancreatitis may also develop as a consequence of pancreatic ischemia induced by alcohol itself.[37–39]

Pancreatitis After Endoscopic Retrograde Cholangiopancreaticography

In a cohort of 2347 patients undergoing endoscopic retrograde cholangiopancreaticography (ERCP) Freeman and colleagues[40] showed a postinterventional AP in 5.4% of patients and an asymptomatic hyperamylasemia in 35% to 70%. The risk of this postinterventional pancreatitis is higher when it is performed for dysfunction of the sphincter rather than removal of gallstones.[41] Further risk factors for postinterventional pancreatitis are young age, female sex, number of cannulation attempts of the papilla, and poor emptying of the pancreatic duct after opacification.[7] Prevention in high-risk patients may be achieved with a temporary pancreatic stent.[42,43]

Infectious Pancreatitis

Less than 1% of APs are induced by infectious agents.[44] However, in most of these cases, other potential causes (eg, gallstones) have not been excluded in a standardized fashion. Several infectious causes have been described to initiate AP.

Viral infections including measles,[45,46] Coxsackie B virus,[47–49] Hepatitis B virus,[50,51] cytomegalovirus,[52–55] Herpes simplex virus,[56] varicella-zoster,[57,58] and human immunodeficiency virus[59–61] might induce AP. Other viruses, such as Epstein-Barr, vaccinia, rubella, adenovirus, and rubeola have been believed to be associated with AP in several reports, but the evidence for causality is weak and questionable.[44]

Bacteria may cause AP by ascending from the small bowel, descending from the biliary tree, or via hematogenous or lymphatic spread. Identified bacteria include *Mycoplasma pneumoniae*,[62,63] *Salmonella thyphi*,[64] *Leptospira*,[65] *Yersinia enterocolica*, *Yersinia pseudotuberculosis*,[66,67] *Campylobacter jejuni*, *Mycobacterium tuberculosis*,[68] and *Mycobacterium avium*.[69] There are also reports about AP being caused by legionellosis, brucellosis, *Actinomyces*, and *Nocardia*.[70–73]

Fungal infections rarely affect the pancreas and are classified as molds or yeasts. Among the molds, *Aspergillus* has been detected in a patient with lymphoma, causing thrombotic infarction, necrosis, and inflammation of the pancreas.[74] The yeasts *Cryptococcus neoformans*, *Coccidioiodes immitis*, *Paracoccidioides brasiliensis*, *Histoplasma capsulatum*, and *Pneumocytis carinii* have been detected in patients with AP, but a causal association with AP has not been proved.[44,59,75,76]

Parasites might cause AP. Among those parasites, *A lumbricoides* and *Echinococcus granulosus* cause AP by pancreatic duct obstruction. *A lumbricoides* can cause AP by migration of worms into the duodenal papilla,[14] and this is the second most common cause of AP in India.[17] The worms cause AP by migrating into, and obstructing, the pancreatic duct. In cases of migration into the distal parts of the pancreatic duct, abscess formation is frequently observed. However, *E granulosus* may appear as a space-occupying pancreatic lesion leading to AP by indirect pancreatic duct obstruction.[77]

Anatomic Abnormalities

A pancreas divisum is observed in about 7% of autopsies. This embryologic abnormality is the consequence of a missing fusion of the dorsal and ventral pancreatic duct systems.[78] The lack of the ductal fusion can lead to insufficient drainage of the pancreatic duct in some cases, with a subsequent increase of pancreatic pressure and attacks of AP. Whether anatomic abnormalities or sphincter dysfunctions may cause pancreatitis is a matter of controversy in the literature.[7]

Miscellaneous other causes of AP are metabolic disorders such as hypertriglyceridemia and hypercalcemia, pancreatic tumors with duct obstruction, several drugs (eg, azathioprine, thiazides, and estrogens), and trauma.[10] Major surgery, especially cardiac surgery, with subsequent pancreatic hypoperfusion and ischemia, might also induce AP.[79]

There are several hereditary forms of AP. The inability to inhibit active intrapancreatic trypsin, as observed in patients with SPINK1 mutations, as well as premature trypsinogen activation into trypsin by mutations of the cationic trypsinogen gene (*PRSS1*), and CFTR gene mutations, can lead to acute and chronic pancreatitis in children and adults.[14,80,81]

Another rare form of AP is autoimmune pancreatitis. Patients with this condition frequently present with an inflammatory mass in the pancreas that is often difficult to differentiate from a pancreatic malignancy. The diagnosis of autoimmune pancreatitis can be suspected by MRI, histology, and serum analyses. Patients may present with increased serum immunoglobulin (Ig) G4 levels. The therapy is the application of steroids, which may also be used as a diagnostic short-term treatment of 2 weeks.[14,82]

DIAGNOSIS

Typical clinical presentation of AP is a sudden upper abdominal pain that often radiates to the back. Patients often suffer severe nausea and vomiting. In some patients, clinical examination shows ecchymoses in the flanks (Gray-Turner sign) or in the periumbilical region (Cullen sign). These patients usually have severe AP and a high mortality.[83] Serum analysis shows an early increase of pancreatic amylase and lipase.[84] Amylase or lipase levels more than 3 times higher than normal hint at the diagnosis of AP. However, a lack of increased amylase or lipase levels does not exclude a diagnosis of AP. Amylase levels may reduce to normal 4 days after onset of clinical symptoms. Nineteen percent of patients with AP show normal amylase levels at hospital admission, and there are various other diseases leading to hyperamylasemia.[7,85,86] Lipase, which has a longer half-life than amylase in serum, has a higher sensitivity, specificity, and overall accuracy for the diagnosis of AP.[26,84,87] Other diagnostic markers are not routinely available and include trypsinogen activation peptide (TAP) and trypsinogen-2.[81,88]

Imaging procedures can be used to diagnose AP if other abdominal disease is certain or biliary pancreatitis is suspected. Transabdominal ultrasound may detect gallstones, sludge, or dilatation of the cystic duct. Contrast medium–enhanced computed tomography (CM-CT) can be used to confirm the diagnosis of AP (sensitivity 87%–90%, specificity 90%–92%) in the early phase or may detect local complications after more than 4 days.[89] CM-CT is useful to rule out other diseases causing severe abdominal pain.

PREDICTION OF SEVERITY

Eighty percent of patients with AP show mild self-limiting courses of the disease with no need for special intensive therapy. Supportive therapy, including analgesia, fluid supplementation, and temporary cessation of enteral nutrition, leads to a restitutio ad integrum. Nevertheless, 20% of patients develop a severe AP with a mortality of up to 30%.[5] The need for early aggressive treatment in these patients in intensive care units (ICUs) by a team of specialized physicians shows the importance of early separation between patients with mild disease and those with severe disease.[88] Several scores have been developed to predict the course of AP. The Ranson score, including 11 items, and the Glasgow severity scoring system, including 9 items, can be completed 48 hours after hospital admission (**Table 1**; **Box 1**).[90,91] The Acute Physiology and Chronic Health Evaluation II (APACHEII) score includes 12 items, and a daily measurement allows an assessment of disease progression.[92,93] Because obesity has been demonstrated to be an additional factor predicting severe disease, the APACHEII score has been modified to the APACHE-O score, including 2 items of obesity.[94] Brown and colleagues[95] published a Panc 3 score predicting the clinical course of severe AP by hematocrit greater than 44 mg/dL, body mass index more than 30, and pleural effusion on chest radiograph. Future studies will establish the clinical effectiveness of these scoring systems.

An important predictive factor for the outcome of severe pancreatitis is the assessment of organ failure. Johnson and Abu-Hilal[96] showed that organ failure for more than 48 hours is associated with a mortality of up to 50%, whereas mortality was 0% when

Table 1
Ranson criteria for prediction of severity of AP

On Admission	During Initial 48 h
Age>55 years	Hemoglobin falls to less than 10 mg/dL
White cell count <16,000/L	Blood urea nitrogen increases by >5 mg/dL
Lactate dehydrogenase >350 units/L	Calcium <8 mg/dL
Aspartate aminotransferase >250 units/L	Pao_2 <60 mm Hg (8 kPa)
Glucose >200 mg/dL, base deficit >4 mEq/L	Base deficit >4 mEq/L
	Fluid sequestration >6 L

organ failure was present for less than 48 hours after admission. This finding shows the importance of clinical evaluation including organ failure. The sequential organ failure assessment (SOFA) score helps clinicians to assess organ injury and SIRS. It should be performed daily for assessment of disease progression (**Table 2**).

If pancreatic necrosis is present in AP, the mortality increases from 1% to between 10% and 23%, showing the importance of early detection of pancreatic necrosis.[89] CM-CT is the gold standard for detecting pancreatic necrosis and should be performed if necrosis is suspected on day 5 after onset of clinical symptoms, because CM-CT might underestimate the complete extend of necrosis and the final severity of the disease if performed earlier (**Fig. 1**A). The radiological findings can be categorized by a CT severity index (CTSI) as proposed by Balthazar[89] (**Table 3**). If the CTSI is 5 or higher, patients have a higher mortality, longer hospital stay, and a higher risk for undergoing surgical necrosectomy.[24] Usually no follow-up CT is required because the local situation in severe AP remains stable in most cases. Nevertheless, follow-up CT may be useful for detection of local complications, including cysts, abscess, or gas bubbles, indicating infected necrosis.

Serum parameters may also be used for predicting severity of the disease. C-reactive protein (cutoff 150 mg/L) predicts pancreatic necrosis at 48 to 72 hours after onset of symptoms with a sensitivity and specificity of 80%.[97–99] Other special markers can predict severe disease earlier but are not commonly available. Serum procalcitonin, urinary TAP, and trypsinogen-2 may be useful to discriminate between mild and severe disease directly at hospital admission.[88,100]

Box 1
Glasgow (Imrie) severity scoring system for AP

Age more than 55 years

White cell count more than 15×10^9/L

Arterial partial pressure of oxygen (Pao_2) less than 60 mm Hg (8 kPa)

Serum lactate dehydrogenase more than 600 units/L

Serum aspartate aminotransferase more than 200 units/L

Serum albumin less than 32 g/L

Serum calcium less than 2 mmol/L

Serum glucose more than 10 mmol/L

Serum urea more than 16 mmol/L

Table 2
SOFA score

Organ System Involved	Score				
	1	2	3	4	5
Cardiovascular	No hypotension	MAP <70 mm Hg	Dopamine or dobutamine (any dose)	Dopamine >5 μg per kg per min or adrenaline (epinephrine) <0.1 μg per kg per min or noradrenaline (norepinephrine) <0.1 μg per kg per min	<0.1 μg per kg per min dopamine >15 μg per kg per min or adrenaline >0.1 μg per kg per min or noradrenaline >0.1 μg per kg per min
Respiratory Pao_2/Fio_2 (mm Hg)	>400	400–300	300–200	200–100[a]	≤100[a]
Renal creatinine (μmol/L)	<100	100–200	200–350	350–500	>500
Neurologic Glasgow Coma Score	15	14–13	12–10	9–7	≤6
Hematological platelet count (×109/L)	>150	150–100	100–50	20–50	≤20
Hepatic bilirubin (μmol/L)	<20	20–60	60–120	120–240	>240

The SOFA score is calculated as the sum of the scores for the individual organs.[14]
Abbreviations: Fio_2, fraction of inspired oxygen; MAP, mean arterial pressure.
[a] These values are calculated with ventilatory support.

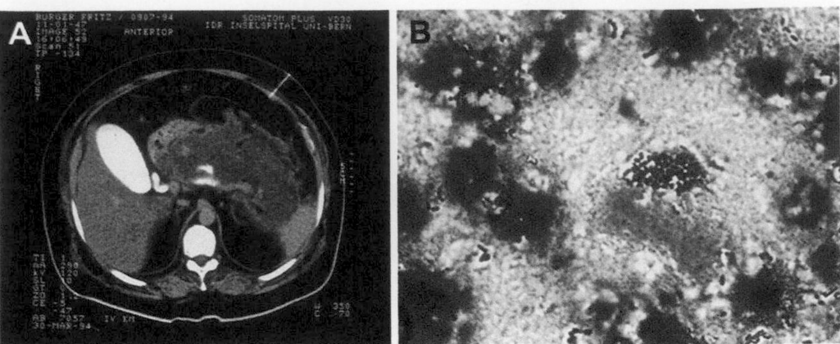

Fig. 1. (*A*) Contrast medium–enhanced CT of necrotizing pancreatitis. Gas bubbles indicate infected necrosis. (*B*) Gram staining of aspirates after fine needle aspiration biopsy showing gram-negative bacteria in infected necrosis.

CLINICAL MANAGEMENT OF AP

Mild forms of AP are usually treated with analgesia, fluid resuscitation, antiemetics, and oxygen administration. Enteral nutrition should be continued if tolerated. Causative therapy may be cholecystectomy for biliary pancreatitis, and is recommended to be performed during the same hospital stay before hospital discharge.[101] Prophylaxis of recurrent pancreatitis include restriction of alcohol in alcoholic pancreatitis or change of medications when medication-induced AP is suspected.

Severe AP still has a high mortality and requires a specialized multidisciplinary team including intensivists, gastroenterologists, interventional radiologists, and surgeons. For these patients, rigorous fluid resuscitation, close monitoring, nutritional support, and management of pancreatic necrosis are essential.

During fluid application, fluid loss into the third space makes it important to keep an adequate intravascular fluid volume. Cardiovascular, respiratory, and renal monitoring is mandatory to manage organ dysfunctions adequately. For suppression of exocrine pancreatic function, parenteral nutrition has been advocated in the early phase of severe AP.[102] However, intestinal mucosal atrophy is a complication of parenteral nutrition and promotes bacterial translocation from the gut as well as enhanced

Table 3
CTSI (score greater than 5 is associated with higher mortality)

			Necrosis		
Grade	**CT Finding**	**Points**	**Percentage**	**Additional Points**	**Severity Index**
A	Normal pancreas	0	0	0	0
B	Pancreatic enlargement	1	0	0	1
C	Pancreatic inflammation and/or peripancreatic fat	2	<30	2	4
D	Single peripancreatic fluid collection	3	30–50	4	7
E	Two or more fluid collections and/or retroperitoneal air	4	>50	6	10

proinflammatory response.[103,104] Moreover, surgical interventions, infections, and noninfectious complications are reduced when early enteral nutrition is applied. However, there is no proven reduction of mortality compared with parenteral nutrition.[104] Thus, early enteral nutrition is recommended in the treatment of AP. In addition, some studies suggest that enteral feeding can be applied by nasogastric or nasojejunal tube.[105]

The prophylactic use of probiotics has been advocated. However, a recent multicenter randomized controlled trial showed not only no improvement of the disease by the application of probiotics, but an increased mortality.[106] Therefore, probiotics should not be used in patients with severe AP, although the reason for the increased mortality remains unclear.

The use of prophylactic antibiotics to prevent infection of pancreatic necrosis is highly controversial. Bacteria infecting pancreatic necrosis are usually gut derived.[107] They translocate via the impaired gut mucosal barrier and reach the pancreatic necrosis by lymphatic vessels. Before prophylactic antibiotics were used routinely, gut-derived infectious agents usually included *Escherichia coli* and *Bacteroides*. *Candida* species were found in 2.6%.[25] Nevertheless, the clinical role of fungal contamination is controversial because it may be only a colocalization phenomenon without clinical evidence.[108] Because prophylactic antibiotics are widely used, a shift from gram-negative to gram-positive bacteria is observed. However, no increased resistance to antibiotics or increasing fungal contamination was reported.[109] Despite the low accumulation of antibiotics in pancreatic necrotic tissue, a potential advantage is the avoidance of systemic septic complications.[110] This is supported by recent randomized controlled trials.[111] Various studies and meta-analyses recommend the use of prophylactic antibiotics, whereas others do not.[103,111–116] There is no clear evidence for the benefit of prophylactic antibiotics in severe AP. Most of the studies are underpowered. The authors do not expect a new, adequately powered, randomized controlled trial to definitively answer the question of whether prophylactic antibiotics should be applied to patients. It will be an individual decision of the treating centers, the local guidelines, and economic possibilities.[117] The International Association of Pancreatology (IAP) guideline from 2002 recommends prophylactic broad-spectrum antibiotics for prevention of infected necrosis. Patients with pancreatic necrosis of more than 50% may profit from this approach. However, there seems to be no benefit regarding patients' survival.[101] The available evidence supports the use of prophylactic imipenem, with or without clistatin, to address infected pancreatic necrosis.[114,118]

The first 14 days after onset of symptoms are mainly dominated by conservative ICU management. Only for biliary AP the United Kingdom guidelines recommend an early intervention by ERCP, including endoscopic sphincterotomy (ES), within the first 72 hours after onset of symptoms.[26] In contrast, the 2007 guidelines of the American Gastroenterology Association advocate no early ERCP for patients with biliary AP when cholangitis signs are absent.[119] For these patients with severe biliary AP, a delayed cholecystectomy is recommended after full recovery of acute inflammation and AP.[101]

There is increasing incidence of infected pancreatic necrosis with potential need of interventions after day 14 of the disease. In cases of infected pancreatic necrosis, there is a significant increase in morbidity and mortality.[7] Infected necrosis may be suspected when gas bubbles appear in CM-CT. The IAP guidelines advocate a fine needle aspiration biopsy of pancreatic necrosis to verify infection for patients with clinical signs or symptoms of sepsis.[101] If infection is proved, interventional drainage or surgical therapy is needed (see **Fig. 1**).

INTERVENTIONAL/SURGICAL THERAPY FOR INFECTED PANCREATIC NECROSIS

The time point for surgical or interventional procedures has changed in the last decades. There was a mortality of up to 65% for patients undergoing early surgical necrosectomy.[120,121] Today, delayed surgical interventions are advocated and interventions and surgery should be postponed for as long as possible. Ideally, necrosectomy should be performed on day 30 after onset of symptoms.[122] Delayed necrosectomy allows demarcation of the necrotic tissue from surrounding vital tissue and offers an organ-saving surgical approach. This concept has reduced the mortality significantly.[123,124]

There are multiple possible ways to perform a necrosectomy, including interventional drainage, endoscopic necrosectomy, minimally invasive surgery, and open surgery.[125]

Percutaneous, CT-guided, interventional drainage of infected pancreatic necrosis seems to be a bridging procedure in instable patients before surgical necrosectomy is performed in a second procedure. The drainages are suitable for draining abscesses, but an extended necrosectomy is rarely possible or only performed in multiple sessions.[126–128]

Endoscopic necrosectomy is usually performed with the assistance of endoscopic ultrasound. The most common approach is through the dorsal side of the stomach into the necrotic cavity. It is performed as an interventional endoscopic procedure, but may be called natural orifice transluminal endoscopic surgery. A nasocystic catheter is left after necrosectomy for continuous lavage until the necrotic tissue is removed.[129,130] The procedure usually needs repetitive sessions until the necrosectomy is completed. The largest study available today has recently been published by Seifert and colleagues[131] and includes 93 patients undergoing endoscopic necrosectomy for pancreatic necrosis. There was an average of 6 sessions per patient to achieve complete necrosectomy. There was proven infected necrosis only in 54% of the patients, which makes the need for intervention in this cohort of patients doubtful. The mortality of 7.5% in this context is significant. Endoscopic necrosectomy requires an excellent endoscopic technique. Whether morbidity and mortality is comparable with conventional surgical approaches needs to be evaluated in prospective randomized studies. One problem of the transgastric or transduodenal approach is that necrotic areas on the left side might not be reached safely. Thus, a combined approach together with the percutaneous intervention (as described later) may be a solution in these cases.

Surgical procedures for necrosectomy focus on elimination of necrotic tissue and removal of postoperative debris and exudates. The aim of organ-saving necrosectomy is to preserve the exocrine and endocrine function of the pancreas. There are 4 conventional surgical procedures described in the literature: (1) open necrosectomy with open packing and planed relaparotomy, (2) open necrosectomy with planned relaparotomies, (3) open necrosectomy with continuous postoperative lavage of the lesser sac and retroperitoneum, and (4) open necrosectomy with closed packing.

The open necrosectomy with open packing and planed relaparotomies includes repetitive laparotomies every 48 hours after primary necrosectomy until necrotic tissue has been completely removed and infection is controlled. The abdominal cavity is not closed between the laparotomies and the repetitive lavage procedures.[132–138]

When open necrosectomy with staged and repeated lavages is performed, planned relaparotomies are performed on alternate days in the operating theater until all infected necrosis has been eliminated. Some surgeons use abdominal wall zips for easier access to the abdominal cavity in some cases.[139–142]

The following 2 surgical procedures (open necrosectomy combined with continuous postoperative lavage of the lesser sac and retroperitoneum, and open necrosectomy with closed packing) differ from the techniques mentioned earlier because of the aim to explore the abdominal cavity only once without repeated laparotomies. A continuous drainage of debris via the placed drains is essential. The advantage of a single exploration of the abdominal cavity is the avoidance of further contamination and the reduction of operative trauma. Thus, fistula and bleeding complications are reduced by these techniques compared with the open packing and staged relaparotomies.[125]

Open necrosectomy with continuous lavage of the lesser sac and retroperitoneum is performed over 2 to 4 flushing drains. A lavage with 10 to 15 l/24 hours is performed in the first days for sufficient drainage of debris and exudates. This procedure seems to have the lowest mortality and is advocated by the authors.[143–150]

Open necrosectomy with closed packing includes placing of gauze-filled Penrose drains and suction drains after primary necrosectomy. These drains can usually be removed after 7 days.[125,151] The currently available data concerning the 4 techniques of open necrosectomy are listed in **Table 4**.

Apart from the classic open necrosectomy, minimally invasive procedures for necrosectomy have been developed in the last decades. The rationale was to minimize operative trauma and to avoid bacterial contamination and translocation by

Table 4
Mortality of open necrosectomy procedures

Technique	Patients (n)	Infected Necrosis, n (%)	Mortality, n (%)	Relaparotomy (n)
Open Packing				
Bradley 1993[133]	71	71 (100)	15	1–5/patient
Branum et al 1998[134]	50	42 (84)	6 (12)	2–13/patient
Bosscha et al 1998[132]	28	28 (100)	11 (39)	17 (mean)/ patient
Nieuwenhuijs et al 2003[135]	38	–	18 (47)	
Planned Relaparotomies				
Sarr et al 1991[141]	23	18 (75)	4 (17)	2–>5/patient
Tsiotos et al 1998[142]	72	57 (79)	18 (25)	1–7/patient
Closed Packing				
Fernandez-del Castillo et al 1998[151]	64	36 (56)	4 (6)	11 (17)
Rodriguez et al[169]	167	120 (72)	19 (11.4)	21 (12.6)
Closed Continuous Lavage				
Beger et al 1988[143]	95	37 (39)	8 (8)	26 (27)
Farkas 1996[170]	123	123 (100)	9 (7)	
Büchler et al 2000[145]	29	27 (93)	7 (24)	6 (22)
Nieuwenhuijs 2003[135]	21	–	7 (33)	

the surgical procedure. Today, several minimally invasive techniques are known.[125] The most common gateways to the necrotic area are either transperitoneal laparoscopic or the retroperitoneal approach. The advantage of the retroperitoneal approach is the avoidance of peritoneal contamination during necrosectomy. The access to the necrotic tissue usually follows preoperative CT-guided placement of interventional drains. After debridement, drains are placed in the cavity for postinterventional lavage.[152–158] The potential disadvantage is that any complications, including colonic ischemia, cannot be seen. There is also no opportunity to perform a simultaneous cholecystectomy or placement of a jejunal feeding catheter.[159] The transperitoneal laparoscopic approach usually explores the lesser sac via a transmesocolic route.[160–164] This procedure is also performed by a hand-assisted laparoscopic approach, to allow manual preparation.[163] However, the retroperitoneal approach seems to be the most widely accepted today. It seems to be a safer procedure; it was advocated first by Carter and colleagues,[165] and since then has been applied by many centers.[125,165] The potential disadvantage of the minimally invasive procedures is an incomplete necrosectomy and potentially an increased local complication rate. The current data on success and complication rates of minimally invasive approaches are outlined in **Table 5**. A theoretic advantage of a reduced systemic injury is being evaluated in a randomized multicenter trial (the PANTER trial). The results of the PANTER trial are anticipated soon (open necrosectomy vs minimally invasive necrosectomy).[166]

Irrespective of the procedure performed, complications such as pancreatic or enterocutaneous fistula remain common and seem to be associated with extended necrotic areas.[167] These fistulas are recommended to be treated conservatively until pancreatitis is resolved. A further severe complication may be postoperative bleeding. If bleeding occurs, the primary treatment approach should include embolization by an interventional radiologist rather than a surgical approach. Late complications may be organized sterile necrosis, or cysts, as well as pancreatic insufficiency.[168] Today, no advantage of minimally invasive surgery compared with open surgery has been shown in a randomized controlled trial.

Table 5
Current knowledge of success and complication rates of minimally invasive necrosectomy in AP

Series	n	Infection (%)	Mortality (%)	Success (%)	Complications (%)
Laparoscopy					
Zhu 2001[172]	10	0	10	90	0
Parekh 2006[163]	19	64	13	84	79
Bücher et al 2008[153]	8	100	0	100	0
Retroperitoneoscopy					
Gambiez 1998[173]	20	65	10	75	60
Carter et al 2000[165]	10	100	20	80	28
Horvath et al 2001[157]	6	100	0	66	33
Castellanos 2002[174]	15	100	27	N/A	40
Connor et al 2003[155]	24	58	25	67	20
Risse et al 2004[158]	6	100	0	100	17
Castellanos 2005[175]	11	100	0	100	0
Chang 2006[171]	19	80	16	N/A	11

Abbreviation: N/A, not available.

In summary, severe necrotizing pancreatitis is a disease with high mortality, even today. It should be managed by an interdisciplinary specialized team. Diagnostic CM-CT is still the gold standard for staging the local situation and should be performed at 5 days after onset of the disease. The SOFA score offers a good evaluation of organ dysfunction in severe disease, which is associated with increased mortality. In severe biliary AP, an early ERCP with ES within 72 hours is advocated when cholangitis signs are present. The primary treatment of AP is conservative. If surgery is needed for infected necrosis, the ideal time point is 3 to 4 weeks after onset of the disease. Today, minimally invasive or open surgical approaches, as well as endoscopic or radiological interventions, might be used, depending on the expertise in the center.

REFERENCES

1. Bradley EL 3rd. A clinically based classification system for acute pancreatitis. Summary of the International Symposium on Acute Pancreatitis, Atlanta, GA, September 11 through 13, 1992. Arch Surg 1993;128:586.
2. Bernard Cln: Lecons de physiologie experimentale, 2. Paris: Bailliere; 1856. 278.
3. Opie E. The etiology of acute hemorrhagic pancreatitis. Johns Hopks Hosp Bull 1901;12:182.
4. Woolsey G. Viii. The diagnosis and treatment of acute pancreatitis. Ann Surg 1903;38:726.
5. McKay CJ, Imrie CW. The continuing challenge of early mortality in acute pancreatitis. Br J Surg 2004;91:1243.
6. Frey CF, Zhou H, Harvey DJ, et al. The incidence and case-fatality rates of acute biliary, alcoholic, and idiopathic pancreatitis in California, 1994–2001. Pancreas 2006;33:336.
7. Frossard JL, Steer ML, Pastor CM. Acute pancreatitis. Lancet 2008;371:143.
8. Jaakkola M, Nordback I. Pancreatitis in Finland between 1970 and 1989. Gut 1993;34:1255.
9. Lindkvist B, Appelros S, Manjer J, et al. Trends in incidence of acute pancreatitis in a Swedish population: is there really an increase? Clin Gastroenterol Hepatol 2004;2:831.
10. Whitcomb DC. Clinical practice. Acute pancreatitis. N Engl J Med 2006;354: 2142.
11. Yadav D, Lowenfels AB. Trends in the epidemiology of the first attack of acute pancreatitis: a systematic review. Pancreas 2006;33:323.
12. Neoptolemos JP, Raraty M, Finch M, et al. Acute pancreatitis: the substantial human and financial costs. Gut 1998;42:886.
13. Skipworth JR, Pereira SP. Acute pancreatitis. Curr Opin Crit Care 2008;14:172.
14. Tonsi AF, Bacchion M, Crippa S, et al. Acute pancreatitis at the beginning of the 21st century: the state of the art. World J Gastroenterol 2009;15:2945.
15. Chwistek M, Roberts I, Amoateng-Adjepong Y. Gallstone pancreatitis: a community teaching hospital experience. J Clin Gastroenterol 2001;33:41.
16. Levy P, Boruchowicz A, Hastier P, et al. Diagnostic criteria in predicting a biliary origin of acute pancreatitis in the era of endoscopic ultrasound: multicentre prospective evaluation of 213 patients. Pancreatology 2005;5:450.
17. Khuroo MS, Zargar SA, Yattoo GN, et al. Ascaris-induced acute pancreatitis. Br J Surg 1992;79:1335.
18. Frossard JL, Hadengue A. [Acute pancreatitis: new physiopathological concepts]. Gastroenterol Clin Biol 2001;25:164 [in French].

19. Norman J. The role of cytokines in the pathogenesis of acute pancreatitis. Am J Surg 1998;175:76.
20. Klar E, Werner J. [New pathophysiologic knowledge about acute pancreatitis]. Chirurg 2000;71:253 [in German].
21. Schneider L, Pietschmann M, Hartwig W, et al. Inosine reduces microcirculatory disturbance and inflammatory organ damage in experimental acute pancreatitis in rats. Am J Surg 2006;191:510.
22. Werner J, Z'Graggen K, Fernandez-del Castillo C, et al. Specific therapy for local and systemic complications of acute pancreatitis with monoclonal antibodies against ICAM-1. Ann Surg 1999;229:834.
23. Schneider L, Pietschmann M, Hartwig W, et al. Alcohol pretreatment increases hepatic and pulmonary injury in experimental pancreatitis. Pancreatology 2009;9:258.
24. Werner J, Uhl W, Hartwig W, et al. Modern phase-specific management of acute pancreatitis. Dig Dis 2003;21:38.
25. Beger HG, Bittner R, Block S, et al. Bacterial contamination of pancreatic necrosis. A prospective clinical study. Gastroenterology 1986;91:433.
26. UK Working Party on Acute Pancreatitis. UK guidelines for the management of acute pancreatitis. Gut 2005;54(Suppl 3):iii1.
27. Diehl AK, Holleman DR Jr, Chapman JB, et al. Gallstone size and risk of pancreatitis. Arch Intern Med 1997;157:1674.
28. Frossard JL, Hadengue A, Amouyal G, et al. Choledocholithiasis: a prospective study of spontaneous common bile duct stone migration. Gastrointest Endosc 2000;51:175.
29. Tenner S, Dubner H, Steinberg W. Predicting gallstone pancreatitis with laboratory parameters: a meta-analysis. Am J Gastroenterol 1994;89:1863.
30. Dholakia K, Pitchumoni CS, Agarwal N. How often are liver function tests normal in acute biliary pancreatitis? J Clin Gastroenterol 2004;38:81.
31. Whitcomb DC. Genetic polymorphisms in alcoholic pancreatitis. Dig Dis 2005; 23:247.
32. Werner J, Laposata M, Fernandez-del Castillo C, et al. Pancreatic injury in rats induced by fatty acid ethyl ester, a nonoxidative metabolite of alcohol. Gastroenterology 1997;113:286.
33. Werner J, Saghir M, Fernandez-del Castillo C, et al. Linkage of oxidative and nonoxidative ethanol metabolism in the pancreas and toxicity of nonoxidative ethanol metabolites for pancreatic acinar cells. Surgery 2001;129:736.
34. Werner J, Saghir M, Warshaw AL, et al. Alcoholic pancreatitis in rats: injury from nonoxidative metabolites of ethanol. Am J Physiol Gastrointest Liver Physiol 2002;283:G65.
35. Pirola RC, Davis AE. Effects of ethyl alcohol on sphincteric resistance at the choledocho-duodenal junction in man. Gut 1968;9:557.
36. Guy O, Robles-Diaz G, Adrich Z, et al. Protein content of precipitates present in pancreatic juice of alcoholic subjects and patients with chronic calcifying pancreatitis. Gastroenterology 1983;84:102.
37. Foitzik T, Fernandez-del Castillo C, Rattner DW, et al. Alcohol selectively impairs oxygenation of the pancreas. Arch Surg 1995;130:357.
38. Hartwig W, Werner J, Ryschich E, et al. Cigarette smoke enhances ethanol-induced pancreatic injury. Pancreas 2000;21:272.
39. Horwitz LD, Myers JH. Ethanol-induced alterations in pancreatic blood flow in conscious dogs. Circ Res 1982;50:250.
40. Freeman ML, Nelson DB, Sherman S, et al. Complications of endoscopic biliary sphincterotomy. N Engl J Med 1996;335:909.

41. Cheng CL, Sherman S, Watkins JL, et al. Risk factors for post-ERCP pancreatitis: a prospective multicenter study. Am J Gastroenterol 2006;101:139.
42. Harewood GC, Pochron NL, Gostout CJ. Prospective, randomized, controlled trial of prophylactic pancreatic stent placement for endoscopic snare excision of the duodenal ampulla. Gastrointest Endosc 2005;62:367.
43. Nelson DB, Jarvis WR, Rutala WA, et al. Multi-society guideline for reprocessing flexible gastrointestinal endoscopes. Dis Colon Rectum 2004;47:413.
44. Parenti DM, Steinberg W, Kang P. Infectious causes of acute pancreatitis. Pancreas 1996;13:356.
45. Feldstein JD, Johnson FR, Kallick CA, et al. Acute hemorrhagic pancreatitis and pseudocyst due to mumps. Ann Surg 1974;180:85.
46. Witte CL, Schanzer B. Pancreatitis due to mumps. JAMA 1968;203:1068.
47. Fechner RE, Smith MG, Middlekamp JN. Coxsackie B virus infection of the newborn. Am J Pathol 1963;42:493.
48. Iwasaki T, Monma N, Satodate R, et al. An immunofluorescent study of generalized Coxsackie virus B3 infection in a newborn infant. Acta Pathol Jpn 1985;35:741.
49. Lal SM, Fowler D, Losasso CJ, et al. Coxsackie virus-induced acute pancreatitis in a long-term dialysis patient. Am J Kidney Dis 1988;11:434.
50. Alexander JA, Demetrius AJ, Gavaler JS, et al. Pancreatitis following liver transplantation. Transplantation 1988;45:1062.
51. Joshi RA, Probstein JG, Blumenthal HT. A survey of experiences with three hundred clinical and one hundred and eight autopsy cases of acute pancreatitis. Am Surg 1957;23:34.
52. Iwasaki T, Tashiro A, Satodate R, et al. Acute pancreatitis with cytomegalovirus infection. Acta Pathol Jpn 1987;37:1661.
53. Parham DM. Post-transplantation pancreatitis associated with cytomegalovirus (report of a case). Hum Pathol 1981;12:663.
54. Peterson PK, Balfour HH Jr, Marker SC, et al. Cytomegalovirus disease in renal allograft recipients: a prospective study of the clinical features, risk factors and impact on renal transplantation. Medicine (Baltimore) 1980;59:283.
55. Teixidor HS, Honig CL, Norsoph E, et al. Cytomegalovirus infection of the alimentary canal: radiologic findings with pathologic correlation. Radiology 1987;163:317.
56. Zimmerli W, Bianchi L, Gudat F, et al. Disseminated herpes simplex type 2 and systemic Candida infection in a patient with previous asymptomatic human immunodeficiency virus infection. J Infect Dis 1988;157:597.
57. Cheatham WJ, Dolan TF Jr, Dower JC, et al. Varicella: report of two fatal cases with necropsy, virus isolation, and serologic studies. Am J Pathol 1956;32:1015.
58. Miliauskas JR, Webber BL. Disseminated varicella at autopsy in children with cancer. Cancer 1984;53:1518.
59. Bonacini M. Pancreatic involvement in human immunodeficiency virus infection. J Clin Gastroenterol 1991;13:58.
60. Bricaire F, Marche C, Zoubi D, et al. HIV and the pancreas. Lancet 1988;1:65.
61. Brivet F, Coffin B, Bedossa P, et al. Pancreatic lesions in AIDS. Lancet 1987;2:570.
62. Herbaut C, Tielemans C, Burette A, et al. *Mycoplasma pneumoniae* infection and acute pancreatitis. Acta Clin Belg 1983;38:186.
63. Mardh PA, Ursing B. The occurrence of acute pancreatitis in *Mycoplasma pneumoniae* infection. Scand J Infect Dis 1974;6:167.
64. Kune GA, Coster D. Typhoid pancreatic abscess. Med J Aust 1972;1:417.

65. Edwards CN, Evarard CO. Hyperamylasemia and pancreatitis in leptospirosis. Am J Gastroenterol 1991;86:1665.
66. Lindholt J, Teglgaard Hansen P. Yersiniosis as a possible cause of acute pancreatitis. Acta Chir Scand 1985;151:703.
67. Pettersson T, Gordin R. *Yersinia enterocolitica* infection as a possible cause of gallbladder and pancreatic disease. Ann Clin Res 1970;2:157.
68. Stambler JB, Klibaner MI, Bliss CM, et al. Tuberculous abscess of the pancreas. Gastroenterology 1982;83:922.
69. Uchiyama N, Greene GR, Warren BJ, et al. Possible monocyte killing defect in familial atypical mycobacteriosis. J Pediatr 1981;98:785.
70. al-Awadhi NZ, Ashkenani F, Khalaf ES. Acute pancreatitis associated with brucellosis. Am J Gastroenterol 1989;84:1570.
71. Halevy A, Blenkharn JI, Christodoloupolous J, et al. Actinomycosis of the pancreas. Br J Surg 1987;74:150.
72. Larsen MC, Diamond HD, Collins HS. *Nocardia asteroides* infection; a report of seven cases. AMA Arch Intern Med 1959;103:712.
73. Michel O, Naeije N, Csoma M, et al. Acute pancreatitis in Legionnaires' disease. Eur J Respir Dis 1985;66:62.
74. Guice KS, Lynch M, Weatherbee L. Invasive aspergillosis: an unusual cause of hemorrhagic pancreatitis. Am J Gastroenterol 1987;82:563.
75. Awen CF, Baltzan MA. Systemic dissemination of *Pneumocystis carinii* pneumonia. Can Med Assoc J 1971;104:809.
76. Goodwin RA Jr, Shapiro JL, Thurman GH, et al. Disseminated histoplasmosis: clinical and pathologic correlations. Medicine (Baltimore) 1980;59:1.
77. Morton PC, Terblanche JT, Bornman PC, et al. Obstructive jaundice caused by an intrapancreatic hydatid cyst. Br J Surg 1981;68:474.
78. Stern CD. A historical perspective on the discovery of the accessory duct of the pancreas, the ampulla 'of Vater' and pancreas divisum. Gut 1986;27:203.
79. Hackert T, Hartwig W, Fritz S, et al. Ischemic acute pancreatitis: clinical features of 11 patients and review of the literature. Am J Surg 2009;197:450.
80. Schneider A, Barmada MM, Slivka A, et al. Clinical characterization of patients with idiopathic chronic pancreatitis and SPINK1 mutations. Scand J Gastroenterol 2004;39:903.
81. Teich N, Mossner J. Hereditary chronic pancreatitis. Best Pract Res Clin Gastroenterol 2008;22:115.
82. Moon SH, Kim MH, Park DH, et al. Is a 2-week steroid trial after initial negative investigation for malignancy useful in differentiating autoimmune pancreatitis from pancreatic cancer? A prospective outcome study. Gut 2008;57:1704.
83. Meyers MA, Feldberg MA, Oliphant M. Grey Turner's sign and Cullen's sign in acute pancreatitis. Gastrointest Radiol 1989;14:31.
84. Matull WR, Pereira SP, O'Donohue JW. Biochemical markers of acute pancreatitis. J Clin Pathol 2006;59:340.
85. Clavien PA, Robert J, Meyer P, et al. Acute pancreatitis and normoamylasemia. Not an uncommon combination. Ann Surg 1989;210:614.
86. Winslet M, Hall C, London NJ, et al. Relation of diagnostic serum amylase levels to aetiology and severity of acute pancreatitis. Gut 1992;33:982.
87. Malka D, Rosa-Hezode I. [Positive and etiological diagnosis of acute pancreatitis]. Gastroenterol Clin Biol 2001;25:1S153 [in French].
88. Werner J, Hartwig W, Uhl W, et al. Useful markers for predicting severity and monitoring progression of acute pancreatitis. Pancreatology 2003;3:115.

89. Balthazar EJ. Acute pancreatitis: assessment of severity with clinical and CT evaluation. Radiology 2002;223:603.
90. Blamey SL, Imrie CW, O'Neill J, et al. Prognostic factors in acute pancreatitis. Gut 1984;25:1340.
91. Ranson JH, Rifkind KM, Roses DF, et al. Prognostic signs and the role of operative management in acute pancreatitis. Surg Gynecol Obstet 1974;139:69.
92. Knaus WA, Draper EA, Wagner DP, et al. APACHE II: a severity of disease classification system. Crit Care Med 1985;13:818.
93. Wilson C, Heath DI, Imrie CW. Prediction of outcome in acute pancreatitis: a comparative study of APACHE II, clinical assessment and multiple factor scoring systems. Br J Surg 1990;77:1260.
94. Johnson CD, Toh SK, Campbell MJ. Combination of APACHE-II score and an obesity score (APACHE-O) for the prediction of severe acute pancreatitis. Pancreatology 2004;4:1.
95. Brown A, James-Stevenson T, Dyson T, et al. The Panc 3 score: a rapid and accurate test for predicting severity on presentation in acute pancreatitis. J Clin Gastroenterol 2007;41:855.
96. Johnson CD, Abu-Hilal M. Persistent organ failure during the first week as a marker of fatal outcome in acute pancreatitis. Gut 2004;53:1340.
97. Al-Bahrani AZ, Ammori BJ. Clinical laboratory assessment of acute pancreatitis. Clin Chim Acta 2005;362:26.
98. Dervenis C, Johnson CD, Bassi C, et al. Diagnosis, objective assessment of severity, and management of acute pancreatitis. Santorini consensus conference. Int J Pancreatol 1999;25:195.
99. Uhl W, Büchler M, Malfertheiner P, et al. PMN-elastase in comparison with CRP, antiproteases, and LDH as indicators of necrosis in human acute pancreatitis. Pancreas 1991;6:253.
100. Rau BM, Kemppainen EA, Gumbs AA, et al. Early assessment of pancreatic infections and overall prognosis in severe acute pancreatitis by procalcitonin (PCT): a prospective international multicenter study. Ann Surg 2007;245:745.
101. Uhl W, Warshaw A, Imrie C, et al. IAP guidelines for the surgical management of acute pancreatitis. Pancreatology 2002;2:565.
102. Nathens AB, Curtis JR, Beale RJ, et al. Management of the critically ill patient with severe acute pancreatitis. Crit Care Med 2004;32:2524.
103. Heinrich S, Schafer M, Rousson V, et al. Evidence-based treatment of acute pancreatitis: a look at established paradigms. Ann Surg 2006;243:154.
104. Marik PE, Zaloga GP. Meta-analysis of parenteral nutrition versus enteral nutrition in patients with acute pancreatitis. BMJ 2004;328:1407.
105. Eatock FC, Chong P, Menezes N, et al. A randomized study of early nasogastric versus nasojejunal feeding in severe acute pancreatitis. Am J Gastroenterol 2005;100:432.
106. Besselink MG, van Santvoort HC, Buskens E, et al. Probiotic prophylaxis in predicted severe acute pancreatitis: a randomised, double-blind, placebo-controlled trial. Lancet 2008;371:651.
107. Garg PK, Khanna S, Bohidar NP, et al. Incidence, spectrum and antibiotic sensitivity pattern of bacterial infections among patients with acute pancreatitis. J Gastroenterol Hepatol 2001;16:1055.
108. Gloor B, Muller CA, Worni M, et al. Pancreatic infection in severe pancreatitis: the role of fungus and multiresistant organisms. Arch Surg 2001;136:592.
109. Howard TJ, Temple MB. Prophylactic antibiotics alter the bacteriology of infected necrosis in severe acute pancreatitis. J Am Coll Surg 2002;195:759.

110. Barie PS. A critical review of antibiotic prophylaxis in severe acute pancreatitis. Am J Surg 1996;172:38S.
111. Isenmann R, Runzi M, Kron M, et al. Prophylactic antibiotic treatment in patients with predicted severe acute pancreatitis: a placebo-controlled, double-blind trial. Gastroenterology 2004;126:997.
112. Büchler M, Uhl W, Beger HG. Complications of acute pancreatitis and their management. Curr Opin Gen Surg 1993;282.
113. Delcenserie R, Yzet T, Ducroix JP. Prophylactic antibiotics in treatment of severe acute alcoholic pancreatitis. Pancreas 1996;13:198.
114. Nordback I, Sand J, Saaristo R, et al. Early treatment with antibiotics reduces the need for surgery in acute necrotizing pancreatitis–a single-center randomized study. J Gastrointest Surg 2001;5:113.
115. Pederzoli P, Bassi C, Vesentini S, et al. A randomized multicenter clinical trial of antibiotic prophylaxis of septic complications in acute necrotizing pancreatitis with imipenem. Surg Gynecol Obstet 1993;176:480.
116. Sainio V, Kemppainen E, Puolakkainen P, et al. Early antibiotic treatment in acute necrotising pancreatitis. Lancet 1995;346:663.
117. Werner J, Hartwig W, Büchler MW. Antibiotic prophylaxis: an ongoing controversy in the treatment of severe acute pancreatitis. Scand J Gastroenterol 2007;42:667.
118. Villatoro E, Bassi C, Larvin M. Antibiotic therapy for prophylaxis against infection of pancreatic necrosis in acute pancreatitis. Cochrane Database Syst Rev 2006;4:CD002941.
119. Forsmark CE, Baillie J. AGA Institute technical review on acute pancreatitis. Gastroenterology 2007;132:2022.
120. Fernandez-Cruz L, Navarro S, Valderrama R, et al. Acute necrotizing pancreatitis: a multicenter study. Hepatogastroenterology 1994;41:185.
121. Kivilaakso E, Fraki O, Nikki P, et al. Resection of the pancreas for acute fulminant pancreatitis. Surg Gynecol Obstet 1981;152:493.
122. Besselink MG, Verwer TJ, Schoenmaeckers EJ, et al. Timing of surgical intervention in necrotizing pancreatitis. Arch Surg 2007;142:1194.
123. Hartwig W, Maksan SM, Foitzik T, et al. Reduction in mortality with delayed surgical therapy of severe pancreatitis. J Gastrointest Surg 2002;6:481.
124. Mier J, Leon EL, Castillo A, et al. Early versus late necrosectomy in severe necrotizing pancreatitis. Am J Surg 1997;173:71.
125. Werner J, Feuerbach S, Uhl W, et al. Management of acute pancreatitis: from surgery to interventional intensive care. Gut 2005;54:426.
126. Echenique AM, Sleeman D, Yrizarry J, et al. Percutaneous catheter-directed debridement of infected pancreatic necrosis: results in 20 patients. J Vasc Interv Radiol 1998;9:565.
127. Freeny PC, Hauptmann E, Althaus SJ, et al. Percutaneous CT-guided catheter drainage of infected acute necrotizing pancreatitis: techniques and results. AJR Am J Roentgenol 1998;170:969.
128. Gouzi JL, Bloom E, Julio C, et al. [Percutaneous drainage of infected pancreatic necrosis: an alternative to surgery]. Chirurgie 1999;124:31 [in French].
129. Mathew A, Biswas A, Meitz KP. Endoscopic necrosectomy as primary treatment for infected peripancreatic fluid collections (with video). Gastrointest Endosc 2008;68:776.
130. Schrover IM, Weusten BL, Besselink MG, et al. EUS-guided endoscopic transgastric necrosectomy in patients with infected necrosis in acute pancreatitis. Pancreatology 2008;8:271.

131. Seifert H, Biermer M, Schmitt W, et al. Transluminal endoscopic necrosectomy after acute pancreatitis: a multicentre study with long-term follow-up (the GEPARD Study). Gut 2009;58:1260.
132. Bosscha K, Hulstaert PF, Hennipman A, et al. Fulminant acute pancreatitis and infected necrosis: results of open management of the abdomen and "planned" reoperations. J Am Coll Surg 1998;187:255.
133. Bradley EL 3rd. A fifteen year experience with open drainage for infected pancreatic necrosis. Surg Gynecol Obstet 1993;177:215.
134. Branum G, Galloway J, Hirchowitz W, et al. Pancreatic necrosis: results of necrosectomy, packing, and ultimate closure over drains. Ann Surg 1998;227:870.
135. Nieuwenhuijs VB, Besselink MG, van Minnen LP, et al. Surgical management of acute necrotizing pancreatitis: a 13-year experience and a systematic review. Scand J Gastroenterol Suppl 2003;239:111.
136. Nordback I, Paajanen H, Sand J. Prospective evaluation of a treatment protocol in patients with severe acute necrotising pancreatitis. Eur J Surg 1997;163:357.
137. Orlando R 3rd, Welch JP, Akbari CM, et al. Techniques and complications of open packing of infected pancreatic necrosis. Surg Gynecol Obstet 1993; 177:65.
138. Pemberton JH, Nagorney DM, Becker JM, et al. Controlled open lesser sac drainage for pancreatic abscess. Ann Surg 1986;203:600.
139. Garcia-Sabrido JL, Tallado JM, Christou NV, et al. Treatment of severe intra-abdominal sepsis and/or necrotic foci by an 'open-abdomen' approach. Zipper and zipper-mesh techniques. Arch Surg 1988;123:152.
140. van Goor H, Sluiter WJ, Bleichrodt RP. Early and long term results of necrosectomy and planned re-exploration for infected pancreatic necrosis. Eur J Surg 1997;163:611.
141. Sarr MG, Nagorney DM, Mucha P Jr, et al. Acute necrotizing pancreatitis: management by planned, staged pancreatic necrosectomy/debridement and delayed primary wound closure over drains. Br J Surg 1991;78:576.
142. Tsiotos GG, Luque-de Leon E, Sarr MG. Long-term outcome of necrotizing pancreatitis treated by necrosectomy. Br J Surg 1998;85:1650.
143. Beger HG, Büchler M, Bittner R, et al. Necrosectomy and postoperative local lavage in necrotizing pancreatitis. Br J Surg 1988;75:207.
144. Besselink MG, de Bruijn MT, Rutten JP, et al. Surgical intervention in patients with necrotizing pancreatitis. Br J Surg 2006;93:593.
145. Büchler MW, Gloor B, Muller CA, et al. Acute necrotizing pancreatitis: treatment strategy according to the status of infection. Ann Surg 2000; 232:619.
146. Farkas G, Marton J, Mandi Y, et al. Surgical management and complex treatment of infected pancreatic necrosis: 18-year experience at a single center. J Gastrointest Surg 2006;10:278.
147. Larvin M, Chalmers AG, Robinson PJ, et al. Debridement and closed cavity irrigation for the treatment of pancreatic necrosis. Br J Surg 1989;76:465.
148. Nicholson ML, Mortensen NJ, Espiner HJ. Pancreatic abscess: results of prolonged irrigation of the pancreatic bed after surgery. Br J Surg 1988;75:89.
149. Pederzoli P, Bassi C, Vesentini S, et al. Retroperitoneal and peritoneal drainage and lavage in the treatment of severe necrotizing pancreatitis. Surg Gynecol Obstet 1990;170:197.
150. Rau B, Bothe A, Beger HG. Surgical treatment of necrotizing pancreatitis by necrosectomy and closed lavage: changing patient characteristics and outcome in a 19-year, single-center series. Surgery 2005;138:28.

151. Fernandez-del Castillo C, Rattner DW, Makary MA, et al. Debridement and closed packing for the treatment of necrotizing pancreatitis. Ann Surg 1998;228:676.
152. Alverdy J, Vargish T, Desai T, et al. Laparoscopic intracavitary debridement of peripancreatic necrosis: preliminary report and description of the technique. Surgery 2000;127:112.
153. Bücher P, Pugin F, Morel P. Minimally invasive necrosectomy for infected necrotizing pancreatitis. Pancreas 2008;36:113.
154. Cheung MT, Ho CN, Siu KW, et al. Percutaneous drainage and necrosectomy in the management of pancreatic necrosis. ANZ J Surg 2005;75:204.
155. Connor S, Ghaneh P, Raraty M, et al. Minimally invasive retroperitoneal pancreatic necrosectomy. Dig Surg 2003;20:270.
156. Haan JM, Scalea TM. Laparoscopic debridement of recurrent pancreatic abscesses in the hostile abdomen. Am Surg 2006;72:511.
157. Horvath KD, Kao LS, Ali A, et al. Laparoscopic assisted percutaneous drainage of infected pancreatic necrosis. Surg Endosc 2001;15:677.
158. Risse O, Auguste T, Delannoy P, et al. Percutaneous video-assisted necrosectomy for infected pancreatic necrosis. Gastroenterol Clin Biol 2004;28:868.
159. Bradley EL 3rd, Howard TJ, van Sonnenberg E, et al. Intervention in necrotizing pancreatitis: an evidence-based review of surgical and percutaneous alternatives. J Gastrointest Surg 2008;12:634.
160. Adamson GD, Cuschieri A. Multimedia article. Laparoscopic infracolic necrosectomy for infected pancreatic necrosis. Surg Endosc 2003;17:1675.
161. Ammori BJ. Laparoscopic transgastric pancreatic necrosectomy for infected pancreatic necrosis. Surg Endosc 2002;16:1362.
162. Cuschieri A. Pancreatic necrosis: pathogenesis and endoscopic management. Semin Laparosc Surg 2002;9:54.
163. Parekh D. Laparoscopic-assisted pancreatic necrosectomy: a new surgical option for treatment of severe necrotizing pancreatitis. Arch Surg 2006;141:895.
164. Zhou ZG, Zheng YC, Shu Y, et al. Laparoscopic management of severe acute pancreatitis. Pancreas 2003;27:e46.
165. Carter CR, McKay CJ, Imrie CW. Percutaneous necrosectomy and sinus tract endoscopy in the management of infected pancreatic necrosis: an initial experience. Ann Surg 2000;232:175.
166. Besselink MG, van Santvoort HC, Nieuwenhuijs VB, et al. Minimally invasive 'step-up approach' versus maximal necrosectomy in patients with acute necrotising pancreatitis (PANTER trial): design and rationale of a randomised controlled multicenter trial [ISRCTN13975868]. BMC Surg 2006;6:6.
167. Lau ST, Simchuk EJ, Kozarek RA, et al. A pancreatic ductal leak should be sought to direct treatment in patients with acute pancreatitis. Am J Surg 2001; 181:411.
168. Haney JC, Pappas TN. Necrotizing pancreatitis: diagnosis and management. Surg Clin North Am 2007;87:1431.
169. Rodriguez JR, Razo AO, Targarona J, et al. Debridement and closed packing for sterile or infected necrotizing pancreatitis: insights into indications and outcomes in 167 patients. Ann Surg 2008;247(2):294–9.
170. Farkas G, Marton J, Mandi Y, et al. Surgical strategy and management of infected pancreatic necrosis. The British Journal of Surgery 1996;83(7):930–3.
171. Chang YC, Tsai HM, Lin XZ, et al. No debridement is necessary for symptomatic or infected acute necrotizing pancreatitis: delayed, mini-retroperitoneal drainage for acute necrotizing pancreatitis without debridement and irrigation. Dig Dis Sci 2006;51(8):1388–95.

172. Zhu JF, Fan XH, Zhang XH. Laparoscopic treatment of severe acute pancreatitis. Surgical endoscopy 2001;15(2):146–8.
173. Gambiez LP, Denimal FA, Porte HL, et al. Retroperitoneal approach and endoscopic management of peripancreatic necrosis collections. Arch Surg 1998; 133(1):66–72.
174. Castellanos G, Pinero A, Serrano A, et al. Infected pancreatic necrosis: translumbar approach and management with retroperitoneoscopy. Arch Surg 2002; 137(9):1060–3 [discussion: 1063].
175. Castellanos G, Pinero A, Serrano A, et al. Translumbar retroperitoneal endoscopy: an alternative in the follow-up and management of drained infected pancreatic necrosis. Arch Surg 2005;140(10):952–5.

Small Intestinal Bacterial Overgrowth

Eamonn M.M. Quigley, MD, FRCP, FRCPI*,
Ahmed Abu-Shanab, MB BCh, MSc, MRCP

KEYWORDS

• Bacterial overgrowth • Intestine • Microbiota

THE NORMAL ENTERIC FLORA

In the healthy host, enteric bacteria colonize the alimentary tract soon after birth, and the composition of the intestinal microflora remains relatively constant throughout life. Because of peristalsis and the antimicrobial effects of gastric acidity, the stomach and proximal small intestine contain small numbers of bacteria in healthy individuals. Jejunal cultures may not detect any bacteria in as many as 33% of healthy people. When bacterial species are present, they are usually lactobacilli, enterococci, oral streptococci, and other gram-positive aerobic or facultative anaerobes reflecting the bacterial flora of the oropharynx. The bacterial counts of coliforms rarely exceed 10^3 colony-forming units (CFU)/mL in jejunal juice. The microbiology of the terminal ileum represents a transition zone between the sparse bacterial flora of the jejunum, containing predominantly aerobic species and the dense population of anaerobes found in the colon. Bacterial colony counts may be as high as 10^9 CFU/mL in the terminal ileum immediately proximal to the ileocecal valve, with a predominance of gram-negative organisms and anaerobes. On crossing into the colon, the concentration and variety of enteric flora change dramatically. Concentrations as high as 10^{12} CFU/mL may be found, comprised mainly of anaerobes such as bacteroides, porphyromonas, bifidobacteria, lactobacilli, and clostridia.[1] In contrast, contaminating flora in small intestinal bacterial overgrowth (SIBO) commonly features both oropharyngeal and colonic-type bacteria such as *Streptococcus* (71%), *Escherichia coli* (69%), *Staphylococcus* (25%), *Micrococcus* (22%), and *Klebsiella* (20%).[2]

The normal enteric bacteria influence a variety of intestinal functions. Unabsorbed dietary sugars are salvaged by bacterial dissacaridases, converted into short-chain fatty acids, and used as an energy source by the colonic mucosa. Vitamins and nutrients such as folate and vitamin K are produced by enteric bacteria. The relationship between the host's immune system and nonpathogenic flora is important in protecting

Supported in part, by grants from Science Foundation Ireland.
Alimentary Pharmabiotic Centre, University College Cork, Cork, Ireland
* Corresponding author. Department of Medicine, Clinical Sciences Building, Cork University Hospital, Cork, Ireland.
E-mail address: e.quigley@ucc.ie

Infect Dis Clin N Am 24 (2010) 943–959
doi:10.1016/j.idc.2010.07.007 id.theclinics.com
0891-5520/10/$ – see front matter

the host from colonization by pathogenic species. Bacterial metabolism of some medications (such as sulfasalazine), within the intestinal lumen, is essential for the release of active moieties.

SIBO: DEFINITION

The human gastrointestinal microflora is a complex ecosystem of approximately 400 bacterial species. Because the small intestine is the site of digestion and absorption of food, bacterial flora are largely excluded from the small intestine to prevent unwanted competition with the host and abnormal entry of bacteria across the more permeable epithelium of the small intestine. In addition, gas production from bacterial fermentation of food is minimized.

Although SIBO is usually defined in quantitative terms, as the number of CFU per milliliter, the interpretation of such definitions must be mindful, first, of the location, in the intestine, from where the sample was obtained and, second, that most bacterial species in the gut remain unculturable. Thus molecular techniques such as genomics and metabolomics suggest that as much as 60% of the normal flora is not identified by culture-based methods. Alternatively, the diagnosis may be based on the presence of such consequences of SIBO as malabsorption combined with a positive result from such noninvasive diagnostic methods as breath tests. These reservations notwithstanding, SIBO is usually, and pending the validation of a more accurate methodology based on molecular microbiology, defined as the presence of 10^5 or more CFU/mL of bacteria in the proximal small bowel.[3,4] Other investigators have entertained the diagnosis of SIBO in the presence of lower colony counts ($\geq 10^3$ CFU/mL), provided that the species of bacteria isolated in the jejunal aspirate is one that normally colonizes the large bowel or that the same species is absent from saliva and gastric juice.[4]

PREVALENCE

The true prevalence of SIBO and its relationship to several clinical disorders remains contentious and unclear largely because of continuing uncertainty with respect to its detection and definition.[5] Its contribution to the pathogenesis of purportedly associated disorders is further complicated by overlap in symptoms between SIBO and a variety of gastrointestinal disorders and with other causes of malabsorption, in particular.[6] Although the diagnosis of SIBO has traditionally been entertained in the context of a malabsorption syndrome, and SIBO is recognized as an important cause of chronic diarrhea,[7] interest in this entity has been augmented of late by suggestions of a role for SIBO in the pathogenesis of symptoms in conditions as diverse as celiac disease,[8,9] inflammatory bowel disease (IBD)[10,11] and, most recently, and most controversially, irritable bowel syndrome (IBS).[12–14] In these and other situations in which biochemical and pathologic findings that can be plausibly linked to SIBO are lacking, it is often unclear whether SIBO is a cause, a consequence, or an epiphenomenon in relation to the other supposedly associated disorder. These issues will remain unresolved until progress is made and consensus reached on the diagnosis of SIBO, whether encountered in the context of predisposing conditions or in the absence of any obvious cause or typical symptoms.[15]

The prevalence of SIBO is directly dependent on the characteristics of the study population and the diagnostic method used to detect or define bacterial overgrowth. If a breath test is used as the diagnostic method, prevalence varies further depending on the nature and dose of substrate used. In healthy people, SIBO has been described in 0% to 12.5% by the glucose breath test, 20% to 22% by the lactulose breath test, and 0% to 35% by the ^{14}C D-xylose breath test. Elderly patients may be especially susceptible to SIBO because of both a lack of gastric acid and the consumption of a disproportionately large number of drugs that can cause hypomotility. Although SIBO has been diagnosed in up to 35% of apparently healthy elderly patients with hypochlorhydria by the ^{14}C D-xylose breath test, others have described SIBO as an important cause of occult malabsorption in elderly patients.[16]

PATHOGENESIS

The most important defensive factors are gastric acid and small intestinal motility. In the stomach, acid kills and suppresses the growth of most organisms that enter from the oropharynx. In the small bowel, the cleansing action of aborad propulsive forces and, especially, phase III of the interdigestive migrating motor complex (MMC), limits the ability of bacteria to colonize the small intestine.[17] Other protective factors include the integrity of the intestinal mucosa and its protective mucus layer, the enzymatic activities of intestinal, pancreatic, and biliary secretions, the protective effects of some of the commensal flora, such as lactobacilli, and the mechanical and physiologic properties of the ileocecal valve.[18] Small intestinal dysmotility, rather than fasting hypochlorhydria or immunodeficiency, is probably the major contributor to SIBO in elderly patients.

Disorders leading to alterations in one of more of these defensive systems may be associated with SIBO (**Box 1**). The most common disorders associated with SIBO are intestinal dysmotility syndromes and chronic pancreatitis. Because dysmotility predisposes to an increase in colonic bacteria in the small intestine, diseases resulting in impaired intestinal motility are likely to have SIBO as a complication. The cause of SIBO in chronic pancreatitis is multifactorial and includes a decrease in intestinal motility consequent on the inflammatory process, the effects of narcotics on gut motility, and intestinal obstruction. Stagnation and/or recirculation of intestinal contents resulting from fistulas, enterostomies, and anastomoses also predispose to SIBO, thus explaining the frequent association of SIBO with Crohn disease, radiation enteropathy, and reconstructive surgery.

SIBO is common in scleroderma and was documented in 43% to 56% of patients in 2 recent studies.[19,20] The prevalence of SIBO was higher among those with a higher global symptom score and, especially, among those with a high score for digestive symptoms. Other risk factors for SIBO included the presence of diarrhea and constipation. Eradication of SIBO, successful in 52% to 73%, resulted in symptom improvement.[19,20] SIBO has long been regarded as a potential complication of celiac disease and one of the causes of nonresponsiveness to gluten withdrawal.[8,9] Rubio-Tapia and colleagues[21] analyzed intestinal aspirates from 79 patients with nonresponsive celiac disease and documented SIBO in 14 (9.3%). Those who were positive for SIBO had evidence of worse malabsorption and 67% had a coexistent disorder. In contrast, results from a study that showed no effect of rifaximin on tropical enteropathy suggest that SIBO may not be a major factor in the pathogenesis of this disorder, contrary to previous opinion.[22] SIBO has also been well documented in liver disease; Gunnarsdottir and colleagues[23] found that their cirrhotic patients with portal hypertension had a higher prevalence of SIBO, diagnosed by culture of a jejunal aspirate, than those without portal hypertension. In contrast to previous studies, which used the glucose breath test, Bauer and colleagues[4] did not find an association between SIBO, diagnosed by jejunal aspirate and the risk of developing spontaneous bacterial peritonitis. In a more recent study in which SIBO was diagnosed in half of their group of 53 cirrhotic patients, Pande and colleagues[24] found that the prevalence of SIBO was greater among those with more severe disease and was predicted by the presence

Box 1
Clinical conditions associated with SIBO

Small intestinal stasis:

Anatomic abnormalities:

- Small-intestinal diverticulosis
- Surgical (Billroth II, end-to-side anastomosis)
- Strictures (Crohn's disease, radiation, surgery)

Abnormal small-intestinal motility:

- Diabetic autonomic neuropathy
- Scleroderma
- Amyloidosis
- Hypothyroidism
- Idiopathic intestinal pseudobstruction
- Radiation enteritis
- Crohn's disease

Abnormal communication between proximal and distal gastrointestinal tract

- Gastrocolic or jejunocolic fistula
- Ileocecal valve resection

Multifactorial

- Liver disease
- IBS
- Celiac disease
- Chronic pancreatitis
- Immune deficiency (eg, AIDS, severe malnutrition)
- End-stage renal disease
- Elderly patients

of ascites and raised serum bilirubin. Jun and colleagues[25] confirmed the link with ascites in their group of patients with cirrhosis, 60% of whom had SIBO; supporting the long-held suspicion that SIBO may play a role in sepsis in this context, these investigators isolated bacterial DNA in blood from more than 30% of SIBO-positive patients. SIBO and altered intestinal permeability may, through the systemic effects of bacterial endotoxin, also play a role in the pathogenesis of what is now one of the most common liver disorders worldwide: nonalcoholic fatty liver disease.[26] In other recent reports, SIBO has been linked with rosacea,[27] interstitial cystitis,[28] and restless legs.[29] Both of the latter reports involved patients who also suffered from IBS and must therefore be treated with the same caution that one should apply to the interpretation of reports of SIBO in IBS.

However, the greatest controversy related to SIBO in the past decade and a half has been the proposal that SIBO is linked to IBS. The initial reports from Pimentel and colleagues,[30,31] using the lactulose breath test, documented SIBO in 84% of their patients with IBS. Normalization of the lactulose breath test in this group, by use of neomycin, resulted in a significant improvement in IBS symptoms. Furthermore, methane excretion, on breath testing, was highly associated with a constipation-predominant subgroup of IBS. The same group found that their patients with IBS with SIBO showed both a lower number and duration of phase III of the MMC, on antroduodenal manometry, in comparison to control subjects. Although reports of high rates of positive lactulose breath tests continue to accumulate among both children (65%)[32] and adults (45%–81%)[28,29,33,34] with IBS, with studies using glucose breath test documenting lower rates of positivity (16%),[35] significant concerns have been raised regarding the validity of this association.[36–40] In a systematic review and meta-analysis of the link between SIBO and IBS, Ford and colleagues[41] drew attention to the effect of test modality on SIBO prevalence, the average prevalence of SIBO on breath tests being 54%, in contrast to a mean prevalence of just 4% for jejunal aspirate cultures. These investigators also drew attention to the effect of diagnostic criteria, which varied considerably between studies, on study outcome.[41] To muddy the waters further it has been suggested that the apparent link between SIBO and IBS may represent the effect of the proton pump inhibitors that are prescribed so readily in this patient population.[42] The authors' personal opinion is that, although some patients with SIBO may present with IBS-type symptoms, SIBO is not a major contributor to the pathogenesis of IBS, in general. Furthermore, we believe that the modest improvement in IBS symptoms that has now been reported with some consistency in IBS with antibiotic therapy may owe more to the effects of these agents on the colonic flora rather than SIBO.

SIBO is associated with small-intestinal diverticulosis. Diverticula in the jejunum occur in 0.07% to 2% of the population and tend to be large and multiple, whereas those in the ileum are small and single. These features explain the observation that symptoms and complications, such as SIBO, have been reported in between 10% and 40% and 6% and 40% of jejunal and ileal diverticula, respectively. Jejunal diverticula are twice as frequent in men and are observed predominantly among those more than 60 years of age. Morphologic studies suggest that disorders of intestinal motility such as progressive systemic sclerosis, visceral myopathies, and neuropathies play an important role in the formation of the small-bowel diverticula.[43]

DIAGNOSIS

Aspiration and Culture

Traditionally, the direct aspiration and culture of jejunal fluid, with results expressed as CFU/mL of jejunal fluid, although invasive, has been regarded by many investigators as the gold standard for the diagnosis SIBO[44–47] using the criteria mentioned earlier. Allowing, presumably, for a higher background level of bacterial contamination in the tropics, Bhat and colleagues[48] defined SIBO among their patients in Southern India as greater than 10^7 CFU/mL. The implications of bacterial counts in jejunal aspirates, as described in several gastrointestinal disorders, which are higher than those of healthy controls but are less than 10^5 CFU/mL[49] are unclear. This dilemma was recently exemplified by the study of Posserud and colleagues[50] among patients with IBS. Although most did not have bacterial counts greater than 10^5 and the overall prevalence of SIBO, so defined, was not different from controls, bacterial counts were numerically higher in the patients with IBS and, if a lower cutoff of, for example, 10^4, had been used, the prevalence of SIBO would have been higher in the patients with IBS.[50]

Several techniques have been used to obtain bowel contents for culture, including the classic technique of jejunal intubation under fluoroscopic guidance, a variety of endoscopically guided aspiration methods,[49] mucosal brushings using a cytology brush,[51] and even mucosal biopsies.[52] It is particularly important not to extrapolate diagnostic criteria from one technique to another, as is common in endoscopically derived aspirates, in which samples are derived from the second part of the duodenum and not the jejunum, where the microbiota may differ both quantitatively and qualitatively.

Although widely quoted and applied, the basis for the classic criteria for the definition of SIBO based on aspirate and culture ($\geq 10^5$ CFU/mL of bacteria in the proximal small bowel) is uncertain. Applying the criteria of Reid and colleagues[53] for the development and application of a diagnostic test to this approach to the diagnosis of SIBO, Khoshini and colleagues[54] concluded, in their systemic review, that no gold standard exists for the diagnosis of SIBO. They suggested that the various cutoff levels proposed have not been uniformly tested or adequately validated and many are arbitrary. Cutoffs based on duodenal aspirates are even more tenuous in terms of source and validation.

These considerable issues in relation to definition, technique, and patient selection notwithstanding, aspiration-based approaches also suffer from being invasive, time-consuming, and costly. Moreover, this approach also suffers from the potential for contamination of the aspirate by oropharyngeal flora (which are mainly gram-positive) and whose presence in the aspirate has not correlated well with SIBO-related symptoms.[55] Such contamination by the oropharyngeal gram-positive flora can be addressed by oral antisepsis or by the simultaneous culture of saliva and aspirate[56] and has led some investigators to refine the definition of SIBO to more than 10^5 CFU/mL of colonic-type bacteria (ie, gram-negatives, anaerobes, and enterococci), organisms that have been linked to SIBO symptoms and whose effects in the SIBO syndrome have a plausible pathogenetic basis. A considerable body of evidence exists to link contamination of this degree and with such organisms to what might be referred to as the classic SIBO syndrome: diarrhea, steatorrhea, B_{12} deficiency, and hypoproteinemia.

The culture technique is itself beset with problems. In one study, the reproducibility of culture of jejunal contents was found to be less than 38%, compared with 92% for a breath test.[57]

Of greatest concern are recent studies based on genomic and metabolomic methods that illustrate that only about 40% of the total gut flora can be identified readily using conventional culture methods.[58] These molecular techniques may ultimately prove to be the most precise methodology for the diagnosis and definition of SIBO.

Breath Tests

Because of the pitfalls mentioned earlier with the direct aspiration of intestinal fluid, some indirect tests have been developed. These tests are now widely used as an alternative to direct aspiration, their attractiveness enhanced because they are relatively noninvasive and less costly.

The first breath test developed for the diagnosis of SIBO was the bile acid breath test,[59,60] which, by radiolabeling bile acids with ^{14}C or ^{13}C and subsequently detecting CO_2 in breath samples, exploited the ability of the flora to deconjugate bile acids.[61] The test has a reported sensitivity of between 30% and 70% and high specificity, up to 90%.[62,63] However, one of the most commonly used bile acid breath tests, the ^{14}C glycocholic acid breath test, has low specificity and sensitivity (33.3%).[64,65]

False-positive results may also come from disease or resection of the terminal ileum, the site of bile acid absorption. When ^{14}C is used, the test also carries a radiation risk, especially problematic in children, pregnant women, or women of child-bearing potential.

The ^{14}C D-xylose breath test[66,67] depends on the capacity of intestinal bacteria to metabolize ^{14}C xylose to release $^{14}CO_2$ which is absorbed and ultimately eliminated in the breath, where it can be quantified. Radioactive ^{14}C or the stable isotope ^{13}C can be used to label 1 g of xylose. Reports from many studies revealed sensitivity for the ^{14}C xylose test ranging from 14.3% to 95% and specificity from 40% to 94%.[68–72]

Hydrogen breath tests are based on the fact that carbohydrate fermentation by bacteria of the gut flora and most notably, anaerobic bacteria in the colon, is the only source of H_2 production in the body. In malabsorption, some of the ingested sugar reaches the colon and produces excess hydrogen. The same principle applies when colonic bacteria have colonized the small intestine, as in SIBO; exposure of carbohydrate to bacteria in the small intestine produces a large and premature amount of hydrogen gas. H_2 produced in this manner diffuses into the systemic circulation and is excreted via the lung in the expired air; in all, about one-fifth of the gas produced is exhaled.[73] Hydrogen breath tests are of value for the assessment of intestinal transit time; for instance, when rapid transit is present, hydrogen is produced by the colonic bacteria within a short interval of sugar ingestion.

Hydrogen breath tests may use simple sugars that should normally be absorbed in the small intestine or may involve the use of a nonabsorbable compound. The general principles of these hydrogen-based breath tests are similar.[74,75] Following a 12-hour overnight fast, and low-fiber diet for 1 day, patients are asked to exhale into a tube connected to a bag and syringe to obtain H_2 baseline values before intake of the substrate. Then the carbohydrate substrate is administered orally and sequential end-expiratory breath samples collected at timed intervals for 3 to 5 hours.

Tests based on the excretion of hydrogen in the breath, because of their low cost and relative simplicity, have become the most commonly used of all breath tests in the diagnosis of SIBO but there are problems in interpretation:

1. First is the issue of false-negative tests. Sequestration of the hydrogen produced during the fermentation process may occur in some instances consequent on the activity of 2 types of bacteria, methanogenic and sulfide-reducing, that convert hydrogen into methane and hydrogen sulfide, respectively.[76] Both compete with each other for the same substrate, hence one species tends to predominate in a given individual.[77] If the gut harbors methanogenic species, a hydrogen breath test produces a false-negative result because only methane is produced; hence the need to measure both gases.
2. Results of hydrogen breath tests can also be significantly disrupted by alterations in gut motility and, therefore, transit, such as in gastroparesis or states of intestinal hurry. The shorter the transit time, the greater the likelihood of a false-positive result.
3. False-positive results also occur among patients who suffer from carbohydrate malabsorption caused by conditions such as chronic pancreatitis or celiac disease because the sugar is available to be fermented by the colonic flora.[78–81] Difficulties of differentiation are not uncommon between malabsorption and SIBO, because SIBO itself can result in false-positive lactose hydrogen breath tests.[79] It is recommended that SIBO should first be sought before an evaluation for sugar malabsorption is performed.
4. The oral flora may contribute a confusing early peak, as does the ingestion of a high-fiber diet on the day before the test.[82]

5. Recent food ingestion may lead to an exaggeration, and smoking and exercise a suppression, of the H_2 response, and hence all should be prohibited during the test. Accordingly, the patient is requested to fast and avoid all fluids, except for water, for 12 hours before the test.

For all of these reasons, sensitivity and specificity of breath tests, in comparison to jejunal culture, as well as inter-subject variability, have been os some concern.[82,83] In the rice flour breath hydrogen test, end-alveolar breath samples are collected for hydrogen detection at baseline and at 30-minute intervals for 5 hours following the ingestion of 30 to 50 g of rice flour.[84] This test is used for the assessment of pancreatic function, as well as SIBO. Positive results are defined as an increase in fasting hydrogen level to greater than 15 particles per million (ppm) or by more than 14 ppm after rice administration.

The hydrogen breath test using xylose (25 g of D-xylose in 250 mL of tap water) as the substrate seeks to detect the passage, in instances of malabsorption, of greater quantities of oral ingested xylose to the colon to produce excessive breath H_2.[68,75] A positive xylose breath test is defined by an increase in breath hydrogen levels more than 25 ppm above baseline.

The lactulose breath hydrogen test (LHBT), based on the use of a nonabsorbable substance, lactulose, is one of the most widely used hydrogen breath tests. The increase of hydrogen level after lactulose ingestion in SIBO was first reported by Bond and Levitt.[85] The colonic flora ferments lactulose with the production of hydrogen and/or methane. After the administration of 10 g of the sugar, breath samples are taken at 15-minute intervals for 3 hours.

Methane production on lactulose ingestion, and related to the activities of methanogenic species in the gut flora, has been estimated to occur in 36% to 50% of healthy individuals.[86,87] However, the flat H_2 curve, characteristic of a methanogenic flora[88] cannot be explained simply by an abundance of the methanogenic organism, *Methanobrevibacter smithii*, which comprises only about 10% of all anaerobes in the healthy adult colon[89]; *Bacteroidetes* and *Firmicutes* (both H_2 producers) comprise more than 90% of the flora.[90] The ability of methanogens to compete for hydrogen is a more plausible explanation.[91]

The criteria for the diagnosis of SIBO, using the LHBT, have generated controversy ever since its inception, and of all tests used in the diagnosis of SIBO, the LHBT has yielded the most conflicting data.[36,55]

Some consider an increase in the basal level of H_2, in itself, as diagnostic; the action of the bacterial flora on a previous meal or on unabsorbed carbohydrate in the gut may explain these high initial levels of H_2. The double peak on the breath hydrogen expiration graph has become an established criterion for the diagnosis of SIBO by LHBT: the first peak is caused by production of the gas by the effect of bacterial overgrowth in the small bowel; the second results from the action of cecal flora on lactulose.[55]

Others have accepted either an increase in H_2 within 90 minutes and/or an absolute increase of greater than 20 ppm above the basal H_2 level within 180 minutes,[14,30,40,50,92] as diagnostic of SIBO. This definition of a positive test must take into account that the average orocecal transit time, as assessed by LHBT, is only slightly longer; therefore, many apparently healthy individuals seem to have SIBO. Rapid transit, as may occur in conditions such as IBS, compounds interpretation further, especially given the propensity of lactulose itself to accelerate transit.

In general, lactulose seems to have a lower sensitivity (17%–89%) than specificity (44%–100%).[46,84,93–95]

Next to the LHBT, the glucose hydrogen breath test (GHBT) is the most commonly used test in the diagnosis of SIBO.[74,75,96] Glucose is normally given in a dose of 50 to 75 g dissolved in water as a 10% solution and breath sampled at base line and every 15 minutes after glucose ingestion for 3 hours. Otherwise, the preparation for, and conduct of, the test follow the same guidelines as other hydrogen-based breath tests. A glucose breath test is considered positive if the basal H_2 level is more than 12 ppm or an increase of more than 12 ppm above the baseline value occurs within 2 hours. In general, the glucose breath test has been shown to be more accurate than the lactulose test and, as a result, the GHBT is the preferred test for the diagnosis of SIBO in some centers.

Which is the best breath test? Using culture as the standard, another study compared the sensitivity, specificity, positive and negative predictive values, and diagnostic accuracy of the LHBT and GHBT. The LHBT had higher specificity (86%) compared with the GHBT (80%) but lower sensitivity and accuracy.[93] However, others failed to identify any significant differences in sensitivity or specificity between the LHBT and GHBT.[50,97,98]

Other Tests

Imaging studies are of value in SIBO to identify causative factors such as jejunal diverticulosis. Small-intestinal mucosal changes in SIBO are neither specific nor diagnostic, and mucosal injury and villous atrophy are evident only in the most severely affected individuals; most biopsies are normal in SIBO.

Cholyl-PABA, a synthetic compound created by conjugating cholic acid with para-aminobenzoic acid, is catabolized into free PABA by the bacterial enzyme hydrolase. PABA can be then detected in urine. PABA provided a simple noninvasive method for detecting SIBO but could not distinguish between SIBO and other causes of malabsorption with any degree of reliability. Moreover, this test correlated well with results of the ^{14}C xylose breath test.

Urinary indican (indoxyl sulfate, a by-product of intestinal bacterial metabolism of tryptophan) levels have also been used to test for SIBO. Although the overall sensitivity of this urinary marker was promising at 80% to 90%[99,100] in early studies, no recent studies have been performed to support the validity of the test.

Various serum markers, such as bile acids, folic acid, and cobalamin have been proposed as a marker for SIBO; none has sufficient diagnostic accuracy to be of value in the detection of SIBO.

These tests, although indirect, are relatively noninvasive and have appeal for clinical practice. However, although abnormal results may support the diagnosis of SIBO, none has been adequately validated as a diagnostic test of SIBO; some have not been extensively tested in humans, and those that have are less than optimal in terms of sensitivity and specificity. More work needs to be done.

The Therapeutic Trial

Given the problems associated with all of the tests described for the diagnosis of SIBO, clinicians have turned to therapeutic trials of antibiotics as an alternative diagnostic strategy. However, appealing as the therapeutic trial may seem, it currently lacks standardization with respect to choice of antibiotic, dose, duration of therapy, or appropriate outcome measures. It is for now an entirely empiric approach.

The limitations of our currently available diagnostic methods were vividly illustrated in the study by Kerckhoffs and colleagues.[101] These investigators performed both a lactulose breath test and jejunal aspirate on 11 health controls and 15 patients predisposed to SIBO; breath testing was associated with a high false-positive rate, and using molecular methods did not increase the yield of aspirates.

Treatment

There are 3 components to the treatment of SIBO: first, treating the underlying disease; second, eradicating overgrowth; and third, addressing any associated nutritional deficiencies. The primary goal should be the treatment or correction of any underlying disease or defect, when possible. Several of the clinical conditions that are associated with SIBO, such as visceral myopathies and multiple jejunal diverticula, are not readily reversible. Medications associated with intestinal stasis such as those drugs known to inhibit intestinal motility or the inhibition of gastric acid secretion should be eliminated or substituted.

When surgical correction of the clinical condition associated with SIBO is not an option, management is based on antibiotic therapy. Its objective should not be to eradicate the bacterial flora but to alter it in a way that leads to symptomatic improvement. Although, ideally, the choice of antimicrobial agents should reflect in vitro susceptibility testing, this is usually impractical because many different bacterial species, with different antibiotic sensitivities, typically coexist. Antibiotic treatment remains, therefore, primarily empiric. Despite the volumes that have been written on the prevalence and causes of SIBO, clinicians faced with treating this condition have few studies to guide them. Effective antibiotic therapy must cover both aerobic and anaerobic enteric bacteria; different schedules have been suggested (**Box 2**). In general, a single 7- to 10-day course of antibiotic may improve symptoms for up to several months in between 46% and 90% of patients with SIBO and render breath tests negative in 20% to 75%.

In recent years, the more widespread availability of the poorly absorbed antibiotic rifaximin has led to a significant increase in the number of randomized trials of SIBO therapy. In controlled studies, rifaximin in doses of 800 per day for 4 weeks or 1200 mg per day for 7 days was effective in eradicating SIBO[102,103] and, in one trial at least, was superior to metronidazole.[102] These findings were supported by a retrospective review.[104]

Recurrence following one course of therapy remains an issue (up to 44% at 9 months after antibiotic therapy) and is more likely among older patients, those who have undergone an appendectomy and those with a history of chronic use of proton pump inhibitors.[105] Because of recurrent symptoms, some patients need either repeated (eg, the first 5–10 days out of every month) or continuous courses of

Box 2
Antibiotic therapy for SIBO

- Ciprofloxacin (250 mg twice a day)
- Norfloxacin (800 mg/d)
- Metronidazole (250 mg 3 times a day)
- Trimethoprim-sulfamethoxazole (1 double-strength twice a day)
- Doxycycline (100 mg twice a day)
- Amoxicillin-clavulanic acid (500 mg 3 times a day)
- Tetracycline (250 mg 4 times a day)
- Chloramphenicol (250 mg 4 times a day)
- Neomycin (500 mg twice a day)
- Rifaximin (800–1200 mg/d)

antibiotic therapy. For the latter, rotating antibiotic regimens are recommended to prevent the development of resistance. Decisions on management should be individualized and consider such risks of long-term antibiotic therapy as diarrhea, *Clostridium difficile* infection, intolerance, bacterial resistance, and costs. Therefore, we recommend the use of antibiotics with less toxicity and lower systemic absorption; 7-day regimes incorporating norfloxacin, amoxicillin-clavulanic acid, metronidazole or, where available, rifaximin seem to be good options. It is not necessary to repeat diagnostic tests for SIBO after antibiotic therapy if gastrointestinal symptoms respond.

Although recent studies have reported some effects for probiotic microbial supplements in the treatment and evolution of some gastrointestinal diseases such as IBD and IBS, results in SIBO have been inconclusive. The value of adding prokinetic agents such as cisapride and erythromycin is uncertain. Moreover, cisapride has been withdrawn in many countries because of cardiovascular side effects. As octreotide stimulates propagative phase 3 activity in the small intestine, low doses (50 μg per day) have been advocated for patients who do not respond to antibiotics, cannot tolerate them, or develop antibiotic-related complications. Nonabsorbable purgative solutions may improve gastrointestinal symptoms in children with short-bowel syndrome and SIBO.

Nutritional support is an important component of the management of SIBO. Dietary modifications such as a lactose-free diet, replacement of vitamin deficiencies (especially fat-soluble vitamins), and correction of deficiencies in nutrients such as calcium, magnesium, and B_{12} are necessary. Because mucosal damage may persist for some time even after complete eradication of bacterial overgrowth, nutritional support may be required for a prolonged period.

SUMMARY

There is no single valid test for SIBO, and the accuracy of all current tests remains limited. Furthermore, the concept of SIBO is under challenge; do we confine this definition to those with a malabsorption syndrome or do we accept a role for SIBO in functional gastrointestinal complaints and other ills? If we adhere to the former restrictive concept (classic SIBO), then culture of jejunal fluid remains valuable because pathologic results (defined according to conventional criteria) do seem to correlate with various clinical consequences, such as steatorrhea and anemia. If we seek to extend the concept, then we are bereft of a gold standard, and lower levels of contamination and issues like distal overgrowth come into play; this issue is unresolved. From a clinical perspective, only a full clinical response to a course of appropriate antibiotics can satisfy the clinician but here, again, effects on the colonic flora, in the proposed role for SIBO in IBS, may complicate interpretation. Modern genomic and metabolomic techniques offer promise in fully identifying alterations in the flora in disease states; we look forward to their application in the diagnosis and management of SIBO.

REFERENCES

1. Simon GL, Gorbach SL. The human intestinal microflora. Dig Dis Sci 1986;31:147–62.
2. Bouknik Y, Alain S, Attar A. Bacterial populations contaminating the upper gut in patients with small intestinal overgrowth syndrome. Am J Gastroenterol 1999;94:1327–31.
3. Toskes PP. Bacterial overgrowth of the gastrointestinal tract. Adv Intern Med 1993;38:387–407.

4. Bauer T, Steinbrückner B, Brinkmann F, et al. Small intestinal bacterial overgrowth in patients with cirrhosis: prevalence and relation with spontaneous bacterial peritonitis. Am J Gastroenterol 2001;96:2962–7.
5. Cole CR, Ziegler TR. Small bowel bacterial overgrowth: a negative factor in gut adaptation in pediatric SBS. Curr Gastroenterol Rep 2007;9:456–62.
6. Ghoshal U, Ghoshal UC, Ranjan P, et al. Spectrum and antibiotic sensitivity of bacteria contaminating the upper gut in patients with malabsorption syndrome from the tropics. BMC Gastroenterol 2003;3:9.
7. Fan X, Sellin JH. Review article: small intestinal bacterial overgrowth, bile acid malabsorption and gluten intolerance as possible causes of chronic watery diarrhoea. Aliment Pharmacol Ther 2009;29:1069–77.
8. Ghoshal UC, Ghoshal U, Misra A, et al. Partially responsive celiac disease resulting from small intestinal bacterial overgrowth and lactose intolerance. BMC Gastroenterol 2004;4:10.
9. Tursi A, Brandimarte G, Giorgetti G. High prevalence of small intestinal bacterial overgrowth in celiac patients with persistence of gastrointestinal symptoms after gluten withdrawal. Am J Gastroenterol 2003;98:839–43.
10. Funayama Y, Sasaki I, Naito H, et al. Monitoring and antibacterial treatment for postoperative bacterial overgrowth in Crohn's disease. Dis Colon Rectum 1999; 42:1072–7.
11. Castiglione F, Rispo A, Di Girolamo E, et al. Antibiotic treatment of small bowel bacterial overgrowth in patients with Crohn's disease. Aliment Pharmacol Ther 2003;18:1107–12.
12. Pimentel M, Park S, Mirocha J, et al. The effect of a nonabsorbed oral antibiotic (rifaximin) on the symptoms of the irritable bowel syndrome: a randomized trial. Ann Intern Med 2006;145:557–63.
13. Fumi AL, Trexler K. Rifaximin treatment for symptoms of irritable bowel syndrome. Ann Pharmacother 2008;42:408–12.
14. Sharara AI, Aoun E, Abdul-Baki H, et al. A randomized double-blind placebo-controlled trial of rifaximin in patients with abdominal bloating and flatulence. Am J Gastroenterol 2006;101:326–33.
15. Rana SV, Bhardwaj SB. Small intestinal bacterial overgrowth. Scand J Gastroenterol 2008;43:1030–7.
16. McEvoy A, Dutton J, James OF. Bacterial contamination of the small intestine is an important cause of occult malabsorption in the elderly. Br Med J 1983;287:789–93.
17. Vantrappen G, Janssens J, Coremans G, et al. Gastrointestinal motility disorders. Dig Dis Sci 1986;31:5S–25.
18. Khloloussy AM, Yang Y, Bonacquisti K, et al. The competence and bacteriologic effect of the telescoped intestinal valve after small bowel resection. Am Surg 1986;52:555–9.
19. Marie I, Ducrotté P, Denis P, et al. Small intestinal bacterial overgrowth in systemic sclerosis. Rheumatology 2009;48:1314–9.
20. Parodi A, Sessarego M, Greco A, et al. Small intestinal bacterial overgrowth in patients suffering from scleroderma: clinical effectiveness of its eradication. Am J Gastroenterol 2008;103:1257–62.
21. Rubio-Tapia A, Barton SH, Rosenblatt JE, et al. Prevalence of small intestine bacterial overgrowth diagnosed by quantitative culture of intestinal aspirate in celiac disease. J Clin Gastroenterol 2009;43:157–61.
22. Trehan I, Shulman RJ, Ou CN, et al. A randomized, double-blind, placebo-controlled trial of rifaximin, a nonabsorbable antibiotic, in the treatment of tropical enteropathy. Am J Gastroenterol 2009;104:2326–33.

23. Gunnarsdottir S, Sadik R, Shev S, et al. Small intestinal motility disturbances and bacterial overgrowth in patients with liver cirrhosis and portal hypertension. Am J Gastroenterol 2003;98:1362–70.
24. Pande C, Kumar A, Sarin SK. Small-intestinal bacterial overgrowth in cirrhosis is related to the severity of liver disease. Aliment Pharmacol Ther 2009;29: 1273–81.
25. Jun DW, Kim KT, Lee OY, et al. Association between small intestinal bacterial overgrowth and peripheral bacterial DNA in cirrhotic patients. Dig Dis Sci 2009 Jun 11. [Epub ahead of print].
26. Miele L, Valenza V, La Torre G, et al. Increased intestinal permeability and tight junction alterations in nonalcoholic fatty liver disease. Hepatology 2009;49: 1877–87.
27. Parodi A, Paolino S, Greco A, et al. Small intestinal bacterial overgrowth in rosacea: clinical effectiveness of its eradication. Clin Gastroenterol Hepatol 2008;6: 759–64.
28. Weinstock LB, Klutke CG, Lin HC. Small intestinal bacterial overgrowth in patients with interstitial cystitis and gastrointestinal symptoms. Dig Dis Sci 2008;53:1246–51.
29. Weinstock LB, Fern SE, Duntley SP. Restless legs syndrome in patients with irritable bowel syndrome: response to small intestinal bacterial overgrowth therapy. Dig Dis Sci 2008;53:1252–6.
30. Pimentel M, Chow EJ, Lin HC. Eradication of small intestinal bacterial overgrowth reduces symptoms of irritable bowel syndrome. Am J Gastroenterol 2000;95:3503–6.
31. Pimentel M, Chow EJ, Lin HC. Normalization of lactulose breath testing correlates with symptom improvement in irritable bowel syndrome: a double-blind, randomized, placebo-controlled study. Am J Gastroenterol 2003;98:412–9.
32. Scarpellini E, Giorgio V, Gabrielli M, et al. Prevalence of small intestinal bacterial overgrowth in children with irritable bowel syndrome: a case-control study. J Pediatr 2009;155:416–20.
33. Peralta S, Cottone C, Doveri T, et al. Small intestine bacterial overgrowth and irritable bowel syndrome-related symptoms: experience with Rifaximin. World J Gastroenterol 2009;15:2628–31.
34. Esposito I, de Leone A, Di Gregorio G, et al. Breath test for differential diagnosis between small intestinal bacterial overgrowth and irritable bowel disease: an observation on non-absorbable antibiotics. World J Gastroenterol 2007;13: 6016–21.
35. Parodi A, Dulbecco P, Savarino E, et al. Positive glucose breath testing is more prevalent in patients with IBS-like symptoms compared with controls of similar age and gender distribution. J Clin Gastroenterol 2009;43:962–6.
36. Hasler WL. Lactulose breath testing, bacterial overgrowth, and IBS: just a lot of hot air? Gastroenterology 2003;125:1898–900.
37. Quigley EM. A 51-year-old with irritable bowel syndrome: test or treat for bacterial overgrowth? Clin Gastroenterol Hepatol 2007;5:1140–3.
38. Vanner S. The lactulose breath test for diagnosing SIBO in IBS patients: another nail in the coffin. Am J Gastroenterol 2008;103:964–5.
39. Vanner S. The small intestinal bacterial overgrowth. Irritable bowel syndrome hypothesis: implications for treatment. Gut 2008;57:1315–21.
40. Bratten J, Spanier J, Jones MP. Lactulose hydrogen breath testing (LHBT) in patients with IBS and controls: differences in methane (CH4) but not hydrogen (H2). Am J Gastroenterol 2006;101:S479.

41. Ford AC, Spiegel BM, Talley NJ, et al. Small intestinal bacterial overgrowth in irritable bowel syndrome: systematic review and meta-analysis. Clin Gastroenterol Hepatol 2009;7:1279–86.
42. Spiegel BM, Chey WD, Chang L. Bacterial overgrowth and irritable bowel syndrome: unifying hypothesis or a spurious consequence of proton pump inhibitors? Am J Gastroenterol 2008;103:2972–6.
43. Krishnamurthy S, Kelly MM, Rohrmann CA, et al. Jejunal diverticulosis: a heterogeneous disorder caused by a variety of abnormalities of smooth muscle or myenteric plexus. Gastroenterology 1983;85:538–47.
44. Guarner F, Malagelada JR. Gut flora in health and disease. Lancet 2003;361: 512–9.
45. Husebye E. The pathogenesis of gastrointestinal bacterial overgrowth. Chemotherapy 2005;51(Suppl 1):1–22.
46. Riordan SM, McIver CJ, Walker BM, et al. The lactulose breath hydrogen test and small intestinal bacterial overgrowth. Am J Gastroenterol 1996;91:1795–803.
47. Riordan SM, McIver CJ, Duncombe VM, et al. Small intestinal bacterial overgrowth and the irritable bowel syndrome. Am J Gastroenterol 2001;96:2506–8.
48. Bhat P, Shantakumari S, Rajan D, et al. Bacterial flora of the gastrointestinal tract in southern Indian control subjects and patients with tropical sprue. Gastroenterology 1972;62:11–21.
49. Bardhan PK, Gyr K, Beglinger C, et al. Diagnosis of bacterial overgrowth after culturing proximal small-bowel aspirate obtained during routine upper gastrointestinal endoscopy. Scand J Gastroenterol 1992;27:253–6.
50. Posserud I, Stotzer PO, Bjornsson ES, et al. Small intestinal bacterial overgrowth in patients with irritable bowel syndrome. Gut 2007;56:802–8.
51. Leon-Barua R, Gilman RH, Rodriguez C, et al. Comparison of three methods to obtain upper small bowel contents for culture. Am J Gastroenterol 1993;88: 925–8.
52. Riordan SM, McIver CJ, Duncombe VM, et al. Bacteriologic analysis of mucosal biopsy specimens for detecting small-intestinal bacterial overgrowth. Scand J Gastroenterol 1995;30:681–5.
53. Reid MC, Lachs MS, Feinstein AR. Use of methodological standards in diagnostic test research. Getting better but still not good. JAMA 1995;274:645–51.
54. Khoshini R, Dai SC, Lezcano S, et al. A systematic review of diagnostic tests for small intestinal bacterial overgrowth. Dig Dis Sci 2008;53:1443–54.
55. Simren M, Stotzer PO. Use and abuse of hydrogen breath tests. Gut 2006;55: 297–303.
56. Hamilton I, Worsley BW, Cobden I, et al. Simultaneous culture of saliva and jejunal aspirate in the investigation of small bowel bacterial overgrowth. Gut 1982;23:847–53.
57. Quigley EMM, Quera R, Abu-Shanab A. The enteric flora in intestinal failure. In: Lagnas AN, Goulet O, Quigley EMM, Tappenden KA, editors. Intestinal failure; diagnosis, management and transplantation. Oxford: Blackwell Publishing; 2008. p. 167–83.
58. Tannock GW, Munro K, Harmsen HJ, et al. Analysis of the fecal microflora of human subjects consuming a probiotic product containing Lactobacillus rhamnosus DR20. Appl Environ Microbiol 2000;66:2578–88.
59. Fromm H, Hofmann AF. Breath test for altered bile-acid metabolism. Lancet 1971;2:621–5.
60. Sherr HP, Sasaki Y, Newman A, et al. Detection of bacterial deconjugation of bile salts by a convenient breath-analysis technic. N Engl J Med 1971;285:656–61.

61. Donaldson RM Jr. Role of enteric microorganisms in malabsorption. Fed Proc 1967;26:1426–31.
62. Donald IP, Kitchingmam G, Donald F, et al. The diagnosis of small bowel bacterial overgrowth in elderly patients. J Am Geriatr Soc 1992;40:692–6.
63. Lauterburg BH, Newcomer AD, Hofmann AF. Clinical value of the bile acid breath test. Evaluation of the Mayo Clinic experience. Mayo Clin Proc 1978; 53:227–33.
64. King CE, Toskes PP, Guilarte TR, et al. Comparison of the one-gram d-[14C] xylose breath test to the [14C]bile acid breath test in patients with small-intestine bacterial overgrowth. Dig Dis Sci 1980;25:53–8.
65. Ferguson J, Walker K, Thomson AB. Limitations in the use of 14C-glycocholate breath and stool bile acid determinations in patients with chronic diarrhea. J Clin Gastroenterol 1986;8:258–62.
66. Toskes PP, King CE, Spivey JC, et al. Xylose catabolism in the experimental rat blind loop syndrome: studies, including use of a newly developed d-[14C] xylose breath test. Gastroenterology 1978;74:691–7.
67. King CE, Toskes PP, Spivey JC, et al. Detection of small intestine bacterial overgrowth by means of a 14C-D-xylose breath test. Gastroenterology 1979;77:75–82.
68. Rumessen JJ, Gudmand-Hoyer E, Bachmann E, et al. Diagnosis of bacterial overgrowth of the small intestine. Comparison of the 14C-D-xylose breath test and jejunal cultures in 60 patients. Scand J Gastroenterol 1985;20:1267–75.
69. King CE, Toskes PP. Comparison of the 1-gram [14C]xylose, 10-gram lactulose-H2, and 80-gram glucose-H2 breath tests in patients with small intestine bacterial overgrowth. Gastroenterology 1986;91:1447–51.
70. Riordan SM, McIver CJ, Duncombe VM, et al. Factors influencing the 1-g 14C-D-xylose breath test for bacterial overgrowth. Am J Gastroenterol 1995;90: 1455–60.
71. Valdovinos MA, Camilleri M, Thomforde GM, et al. Reduced accuracy of 14C-D-xylose breath test for detecting bacterial overgrowth in gastrointestinal motility disorders. Scand J Gastroenterol 1993;28:963–8.
72. Lewis SJ, Young G, Mann M, et al. Improvement in specificity of [14C]d-xylose breath test for bacterial overgrowth. Dig Dis Sci 1997;42:1587–92.
73. Romagnuolo J, Schiller D, Bailey RJ. Using breath tests wisely in a gastroenterology practice: an evidence-based review of indications and pitfalls in interpretation. Am J Gastroenterol 2002;97:1113–26.
74. Kerlin P, Wong L. Breath hydrogen testing in bacterial overgrowth of the small intestine. Gastroenterology 1988;95:982–8.
75. Cook GC. Breath hydrogen after oral xylose in tropical malabsorption. Am J Clin Nutr 1980;33:555–60.
76. Strocchi A, Furne J, Ellis C, et al. Methanogens outcompete sulphate reducing bacteria for H2 in the human colon. Gut 1994;35:1098–101.
77. Lin HC. Small intestinal bacterial overgrowth: a framework for understanding irritable bowel syndrome. JAMA 2004;292:852–8.
78. Corazza GR, Strocchi A, Gasbarrini G. Fasting breath hydrogen in celiac disease. Gastroenterology 1987;93:53–8.
79. Pimentel M, Kong Y, Park S. Breath testing to evaluate lactose intolerance in irritable bowel syndrome correlates with lactulose testing and may not reflect true lactose malabsorption. Am J Gastroenterol 2003;98:2700–4.
80. Nucera G, Gabrielli M, Lupascu A, et al. Abnormal breath tests to lactose, fructose and sorbitol in irritable bowel syndrome may be explained by small intestinal bacterial overgrowth. Aliment Pharmacol Ther 2005;21:1391–5.

81. Thompson DG, Binfield P, De Belder A, et al. Extra intestinal influences on exhaled breath hydrogen measurements during the investigation of gastrointestinal disease. Gut 1985;26:1349–52.
82. Riordan SM, McIver CJ, Bolin TD, et al. Fasting breath hydrogen concentrations in gastric and small-intestinal bacterial overgrowth. Scand J Gastroenterol 1995; 30:252–7.
83. Corazza GR, Menozzi MG, Strocchi A, et al. The diagnosis of small bowel bacterial overgrowth. Reliability of jejunal culture and inadequacy of breath hydrogen testing. Gastroenterology 1990;98:302–9.
84. Kerlin P, Wong L, Harris B, et al. Rice flour, breath hydrogen, and malabsorption. Gastroenterology 1984;87:578–85.
85. Bond JH, Levitt MD. Use of pulmonary hydrogen (H2) measurements to quantitate carbohydrate absorption. Study of partially gastrectomized patients. J Clin Invest 1972;51:1219–25.
86. Peled Y, Weinberg D, Hallak A, et al. Factors affecting methane production in humans. Gastrointestinal diseases and alterations of colonic flora. Dig Dis Sci 1987;32:267–71.
87. McKay LF, Eastwood MA, Brydon WG. Methane excretion in man–a study of breath, flatus, and faeces. Gut 1985;26:69–74.
88. Minocha A, Rashid S. Reliability and reproducibility of breath hydrogen and methane in male diabetic subjects. Dig Dis Sci 1997;42:672–6.
89. Miller TL, Wolin MJ, Zhao HX, et al. Characteristics of methanogens isolated from bovine rumen. Appl Environ Microbiol 1986;51:201–2.
90. Eckburg PB, Bik EM, Bernstein CN, et al. Diversity of the human intestinal microbial flora. Science 2005;308:1635–8.
91. Samuel BS, Gordon JI. A humanized gnotobiotic mouse model of host-archaeal-bacterial mutualism. Proc Natl Acad Sci U S A 2006;103:10011–6.
92. Walters B, Vanner SJ. Detection of bacterial overgrowth in IBS using the lactulose H2 breath test: comparison with 14C-D-xylose and healthy controls. Am J Gastroenterol 2005;100:1566–70.
93. Ghoshal UC, Ghoshal U, Das K, et al. Utility of hydrogen breath tests in diagnosis of small intestinal bacterial overgrowth in malabsorption syndrome and its relationship with oro-cecal transit time. Indian J Gastroenterol 2006;25:6–10.
94. Rhodes JM, Middleton P, Jewell DP. The lactulose hydrogen breath test as a diagnostic test for small-bowel bacterial overgrowth. Scand J Gastroenterol 1979;14:333–6.
95. Mendoza E, Crismatt C, Matos R, et al. [Diagnosis of small intestinal bacterial overgrowth in children: the use of lactulose in the breath hydrogen test as a screening test]. Biomedica 2007;27(3):325–32 [in Spanish].
96. Metz G, Gassull MA, Drasar BS, et al. Breath-hydrogen test for small-intestinal bacterial colonisation. Lancet 1976;1:668–9.
97. Saltzman JR, Kowdley KV, Pedrosa MC, et al. Bacterial overgrowth without clinical malabsorption in elderly hypochlorhydric subjects. Gastroenterology 1994; 107:1214–5.
98. Bjorneklett A, Fausa O, Midtvedt T. Small-bowel bacterial overgrowth in the postgastrectomy syndrome. Scand J Gastroenterol 1983;18:277–87.
99. Patney NL, Mehrotra MP, Khanna HK, et al. Urinary indican as a screening index of jejunal bacterial flora in Indian adulthood cirrhosis. Indian J Med Sci 1979;33: 150–6.
100. Patney NL, Saxena SK, Mehrotra MP, et al. A correlative study of indicanuria and jejunal bacteriology in diabetes mellitus. Indian J Med Sci 1979;33:115–20.

101. Kerckhoffs AP, Visser MR, Samsom M, et al. Critical evaluation of diagnosing bacterial overgrowth in the proximal small intestine. J Clin Gastroenterol 2008; 42:1095–102.
102. Lauritano EC, Gabrielli M, Scarpellini E, et al. Antibiotic therapy in small intestinal bacterial overgrowth: rifaximin versus metronidazole. Eur Rev Med Pharmacol Sci 2009;13:111–6.
103. Majewski M, Reddymasu SC, Sostarich S, et al. Efficacy of rifaximin, a nonabsorbed oral antibiotic, in the treatment of small intestinal bacterial overgrowth. Am J Med Sci 2007;333:266–70.
104. Yang J, Lee HR, Low K, et al. Rifaximin versus other antibiotics in the primary treatment and retreatment of bacterial overgrowth in IBS. Dig Dis Sci 2008;53: 169–74.
105. Lauritano EC, Gabrielli M, Scarpellini E, et al. Small intestinal bacterial overgrowth recurrence after antibiotic therapy. Am J Gastroenterol 2008;103: 2031–5.

Pathogenic Factors Involved in the Development of Irritable Bowel Syndrome: Focus on a Microbial Role

Carolina M. Bolino, MD, Premysl Bercik, MD*

KEYWORDS

- Irritable bowel syndrome • Pathophysiology • Dysbiosis
- Gastroenteritis • Intestinal microbiota

IRRITABLE BOWEL SYNDROME DEFINITION, EPIDEMIOLOGY, CLASSIFICATION, AND IMPACT ON HEALTH CARE

Irritable bowel syndrome (IBS) is a prototype of functional gastrointestinal diseases. Disorders exist that have symptoms arising from the gastrointestinal tract in the absence of any discernible organic cause. According to Rome III diagnostic criteria, IBS is characterized by recurrent abdominal pain or discomfort for at least 3 days per month in the past 3 months associated with two or more of the following: improvement with defecation, onset associated with a change in frequency of stool, or onset associated with a change in form (appearance) of stool. Additional symptoms that are not part of the diagnostic criteria include abnormal stool frequency, abnormal stool form, straining on defecation, urgency, feeling of incomplete bowel movement, passing mucus, and bloating.[1]

IBS seems to be a rather heterogeneous disorder, or symptom complex, with multiple presentations and likely different origins.[2,3] To improve diagnosis and management, patients with IBS are classified into different groups according to their predominant symptoms. Earlier classifications (Rome II criteria) were based on a combination of symptoms, such as stool frequency and form, and the absence or

Department of Medicine, Farncombe Family Digestive Health Research Institute, Faculty of Health Sciences, McMaster University, 1200 Main Street West, Hamilton, ON L8N 3Z5, Canada
* Corresponding author. Department of Medicine, HSC-4W8-D, 1200 Main Street West, Hamilton, ON L8N 3Z5, Canada.
E-mail address: bercikp@mcmaster.ca

Infect Dis Clin N Am 24 (2010) 961–975
doi:10.1016/j.idc.2010.07.005
0891-5520/10/$ – see front matter

presence of defecation, straining, or urgency.[4] The latest Rome III criteria subtype patients exclusively according to their stool form because it better reflects transit time:

1. IBS with constipation (IBS-C): hard or lumpy stools more than 25% of the time and loose/watery stools appearing in fewer then 25% of bowel movements.
2. IBS with diarrhea (IBS-D): loose/watery stools more than 25% of the time and hard or lumpy stool appearing in fewer than 25% of bowel movements.
3. Mixed IBS (IBS-M): hard or lumpy stools more than 25% of the time and loose/watery stools in more than 25% of bowel movements.
4. Unsubtyped IBS: insufficient abnormality of stool consistency to meet criteria for IBS-C, -D, or -M.

The first three subtypes have a similar distribution, each accounting for approximately 30% of cases.[5–7]

IBS is one of the most common diseases encountered by gastroenterologists and general practitioners. Its prevalence varies considerably according to the definition used; the earlier Manning criteria were more general and less restrictive than Rome criteria.[8–10] Prevalence estimates across studies vary widely, ranging between 3% and 25%, with most studies finding prevalence close to 10%.[11,12] Recent United States data using strict criteria suggest that IBS prevalence is 7% to 10%.[13] IBS prevalence, gender distribution, and clinical spectrum seem to vary between western countries and Asia. The prevalence rates in the Asian studies have been generally lower (6.9%) independent of the criteria applied, with more heterogeneity in the estimates, possibly explained by the different nature of the population surveys (rural vs urban).[14]

IBS is more common in women. In the community, the ratio of women to men with IBS is estimated to be 2:1, and the difference is even greater in the health care–seeking population, with women leading men by up to 4:1. Female patients report greater overall IBS symptom severity, intensity of abdominal pain and bloating, and impact of symptoms on daily life, and lower health-related quality of life than male patients. The reason for this is not fully understood, but women also report more extraintestinal symptoms, such as nausea and urinary urgency. IBS symptoms in women vary according to the menstrual cycle, with increased symptoms just before and during the menses.[15]

Although IBS is not a life-threatening disease, its chronic nature can have a strong impact on a patient's quality of life, interfering with normal daily living. Leisure activities, work, travel, and social relationships are affected by IBS, often more than in patients with organic diseases.[16,17] Patients with IBS and comorbid somatic disorders report more severe IBS symptoms and lower health-related quality of life: 20% to 50% have fibromyalgia, 50% chronic fatigue syndrome, 64% temporomandibular joint disorder, and 50% chronic pelvic pain.[18]

In addition to individual patient discomfort, the costs related to IBS are substantial. A recent review showed that total direct cost estimates per patient per year ranged from $348 to $8750. In Canada, the total direct costs related to IBS for 1999 were estimated to be more than $300 million, with $1 billion in wages lost.[19] In the United States, the total costs associated with IBS include $10 billion in direct medical costs and $ 20 billon in indirect costs, such as absenteeism from work and lost work productivity.[20]

PATHOPHYSIOLOGY OF IBS

The pathophysiology of IBS is still not well understood,[21] limiting the capacity to effectively treat the disorder. Several mechanisms have been proposed, including psychological illnesses, abnormal gastrointestinal motility, visceral hyperalgesia, altered central perception of visceral events, hypothalamic–pituitary axis (HPA) dysfunction, and low-grade gut inflammation.[22]

The original hypothesis suggested that IBS was a psychosomatic disorder because of a higher prevalence of psychiatric disorders, such as anxiety and depression, in the IBS population compared with healthy individuals. This association applies to patients with IBS across the spectrum: the prevalence of psychiatric comorbidities in the community accounts for 18%, in clinics for 40% to 60%, and in referral centers it reaches up to 94%. A high degree of overlap also exists between IBS and somatization disorders.[23] Early life events, including traumatic episodes during infancy, affluent childhood socioeconomic status, and social learning of illness behavior, also have been shown to contribute to IBS in adulthood.[24]

Abnormal gastrointestinal motility also has been proposed as a cause of IBS. Manometric and electrophysiologic abnormalities were found in the colon of patients with IBS, frequently occurring in response to stressful stimulation or after meal ingestion.[25] Although IBS is considered to affect mainly the large bowel, several studies have found altered motility of the small intestine, stomach, and esophagus. The most striking feature was an occurrence of repetitive bursts or clusters of contractions, which seemed to correlate with patients' symptoms.[26] However, these motor patterns are not specific to IBS and can be found in other disorders.[27,28] Furthermore, motor disturbances vary among patient subtypes and may change in parallel with the change in patient's bowel habits.[29]

Altered intestinal transit also has been reported in patients with IBS, which may result in altered gas handling within the gut.[30,31] Despite many motor abnormalities described in these patients, dysmotility has been documented only in a proportion of patients, suggesting that it may be one of many causes of IBS.[32]

Visceral hypersensitivity and hyperalgesia, together with exaggerated viscerosomatic referral, have been described in patients with IBS.[33–37] However, similar to dysmotility, the sensory abnormalities are present only in a proportion of patients with IBS. Lower sensory thresholds have been shown to correlate with symptom intensity,[17,38] but this finding was not confirmed by other studies.[39] Visceral hypersensitivity seems to be related to the symptom of bloating, but not to that of abdominal distension.[40] Age, central nervous system activity, psychological stress, and food intake are factors that influence the measurement of a sensory threshold. However, no gender differences in visceral perception have been described.[41] Patients with IBS generally do not exhibit somatic hypersensitivity to somatic stimulation; however, some evidence shows that patients with IBS and fibromyalgia have concomitant somatic hyperalgesia occurring at lumbosacral levels.[42,43] The cause and mechanisms of visceral hypersensitivity in patients with IBS are unknown. Several mechanisms have been proposed, including peripheral sensitization of intestinal nerve endings,[44,45] hyperexcitability of spinal dorsal horn neurons,[46] and altered central processing of visceral afferent information.[47,48]

Functional neuroimaging studies have shown evidence of altered regional brain activation responses during visceral and somatic stimuli in patients with IBS, which have been associated with perceptual differences.[49,50] Altered brain responses include activation of regions concerned with attentional processes and response selection, corticolimbic regions concerned with emotions, and subcortical regions associated with arousal and autonomic responses.[51–55] Several studies have also shown that patients with IBS have alterations in central autonomic regulation.[56,57]

Studies in animal models showed that mucosal inflammation alters gut sensory-motor function[58,59] and that deeper layers of the gut wall, including muscle and nerves, actively participate in the inflammatory response to luminal stimuli.[60] Increasing evidence shows that inflammation has a role in at least a subset of patients with functional bowel disorders. Studies in patients with IBS with no history of gastroenteritis have shown that biopsy specimens contained increased numbers of neutrophils and mast cells in the colonic mucosa,[61] and chronic inflammatory infiltrate with neuronal degeneration in the myenteric plexus of the jejunum.[62] Infiltration and activation of mast cells, found in the intestinal mucosa in proximity to enteric nerves, with consequent release of bioactive substances, have been also documented in patients with IBS.[63–65] Other experiments have shown that biopsy culture supernatants from patients with IBS have the capacity to activate enteric nerves, likely through mast cell–dependent mechanisms.[66–68] Also, increased rectal lymphocytes, altered mucosal enteroendocrine cells, and gut permeability have been described in patients with postinfective IBS.[69–71] Recent studies suggest that immune alterations are not confined to the gut level, because increased levels of circulating inflammatory cytokines, T-cell activation, and cytokine gene polymorphism were found in patients with IBS.[72–75] These observations provide insight into the expression of chronic gut disorders, including inflammatory bowel disease and IBS, and may reflect distinct manifestations of a broad spectrum of inflammation in the gastrointestinal tract.[76]

One of the possible mechanisms leading to low-grade inflammation of the gut is psychological and physical stress. Studies in animal models showed that acute stress alters intestinal permeability through mechanisms involving corticotropin-releasing hormone.[77] Chronic water-avoidance stress induces low-grade inflammation and can lead to visceral hyperalgesia.[78] Enhanced stress responsiveness has been implicated as a potential mechanism contributing to the pathophysiology of IBS, because stress also causes a reactivation of previous enteric inflammation and enhances the response to subsequent inflammatory stimuli.[79] Good evidence shows that patients with IBS have a dysregulated HPA axis under basal conditions, consistent with an enhanced central response system. In response to a visceral stressor, there is a significant positive correlation of basal cortisol levels and anxiety symptoms scores.[80,81] The role of the corticotropin-releasing factor (CRF) as a possible mediator in IBS has been supported by experiments showing that central CRF administration mimics acute stress-induced colonic responses and enhances colorectal distension-induced visceral pain, whereas the peripheral CRF alters neuromotor gut function.[82]

Serotonin (5-hydroxtryptamine, 5-HT), a recognized key neurotransmitter secreted in copious amounts from gut enteroendocrine cells, has a role in intestinal secretory, sensory, and motor gut function.[83] Mounting evidence shows that abnormalities in its metabolism may be associated with functional bowel diseases.[84] 5-HT transporter (SERT)–deficient mice display abnormal gut motility and anxiety-like behavior.[85,86] Clinical studies showed that patients with constipation-predominant IBS have lower postprandial levels of plasma 5-HT, associated with delayed intestinal transit,[87] whereas the opposite was shown in patients with diarrhea-predominant IBS.[88] Altered 5-HT metabolism may be a consequence of up-regulated immune system in the gut, because cytokines were shown to alter SERT.[89,90] Genetic influences may be also important because SERT polymorphisms have been reported in patients with IBS,[91–93] although the association between genetic polymorphisms and the clinical pattern of IBS remains controversial.[94]

Several lines of evidence suggest that symptoms in a proportion of patients with IBS can be caused by food allergy or generalized immune hypersensitivity.[95] Recently, more attention has been given to gluten sensitivity, which can present with IBS or dyspepsia-like symptoms in the absence of overt enteropathy or positive TTG antibodies.[96–98] The symptoms in these patients seem to improve after gluten is excluded from the diet.

THE ROLE OF INFECTIOUS GASTROENTERITIS AND INTESTINAL MICROBIOTA IN IBS

Epidemiologic studies have shown that gastrointestinal infection is the strongest environmental risk factor for the development of IBS.[99,100] Although most subjects with gastroenteritis recover completely after eviction of the infectious agent, a small but significant proportion of subjects (7%–31%) develop postinfectious (PI) IBS, dyspepsia, or both. A recent systematic review and meta-analysis identified that the pooled incidence for IBS development after infectious gastroenteritis was 10%.[101] PI-IBS has mainly been reported in Western countries,[69,102–104] but recent studies have reported that PI-IBS also occurs in Eastern countries with a prevalence similar to that found in the West.[105–107] *Salmonella*, *Shigella*, and *Campylobacter* are among the most frequently isolated infectious agents, but viral infection has also been documented as a trigger of IBS.[104] Several risk factors increase the risk of PI-IBS development, including prolonged duration of the initial illness; toxicity of infecting bacterial strain; smoking; degree of mucosal inflammation; female gender; presence of psychological disorders, such as depression and anxiety; and treatment with antibiotics during the acute gastroenteritis episode.[100,108–110] Most patients with PI-IBS (63%) develop diarrhea, approximately 24% have an "alternate" subtype, and 13% report constipation. Follow-up studies of patients with PI-IBS suggest that symptoms may persist for up to 6 years but will gradually improve in a substantial proportion of patients.[111–113]

The underlying mechanisms of PI-IBS have not been clearly identified, but persistence of mucosal inflammation in the colon suggests that IBS is the result of inefficient down-regulation of inflammatory response to infection. Several studies have documented persistent immune activation, including increased intraepithelial lymphocytes and up-regulated cytokines in the rectal mucosa in patients with PI-IBS.[69,70,72,114] Low-grade intestinal inflammation and enterochromaffin cell hyperplasia PI-IBS are also accompanied by increased intestinal permeability, which likely leads to an increased antigenic load and further activation of the immune system 68.

Intestinal dysbiosis induced by infection also has been proposed to produce low-grade inflammation and chronic gut dysfunction. Small intestinal bacterial overgrowth (SIBO) has been documented in a proportion of patients with IBS (10%–84%)[115,116] who had marked symptom improvement after antibiotic treatment.[117] However, other studies were unable to confirm these finding, and the importance of SIBO as an etiologic factor of IBS remains controversial.[118–121]

The human gastrointestinal tract is colonized from birth by a complex and diverse collection of microbial species. The constituents of this microbiota are known to influence several biochemical, physiologic, and immunologic characteristics of the hosts, thus contributing to the overall health status.[122] The microbiota serves the host by protecting against pathogens, harvesting nutrients from the diet, metabolizing certain drugs and carcinogens, and influencing the absorption and distribution of the body fat.[123] The gastrointestinal microbiota can be divided into two distinct ecosystems: luminal bacteria and mucosa-associated bacteria.[124,125] Each of these ecosystems has a distinct microenvironment and both have the potential to play a roles in the symptomatology of IBS. The luminal microbiota, through its metabolic capacity, may play a crucial role in gastrointestinal homeostasis, whereas the mucosa-associated microbiota has the potential to influence the host through immune–microbial interactions.[126–128] A recent study found higher concentrations of acetic and propionic acids in fecal samples of patients with IBS.[129] These patients also presented with worse IBS symptoms and quality of life.

It is generally accepted that the intestinal microbiota is unique in each individual and remains fairly stable under normal circumstances.[130,131] However, some studies have shown a marked variation in the complexity and stability of *Bifidobacteria* and *Lactobacillus* populations over a 1-year period[132] and significant alterations in the microbiota composition from environmental factors.[133,134] Antibiotics are known to affect the gut microbiota, with possible long-lasting effects.[135] For instance, a 1-week course of clindamycin caused changes in the *Bacteroides* community detectable for up to 2 years.[136]

Accumulating evidence shows that patients with IBS have a higher temporal instability of the bacterial populations and that the microbiota composition is different compared with healthy controls.[137–140] Initial molecular-based studies found lower levels of coliform bacteria, *Lactobacilli*, and *Bifidobacteria* species with higher numbers of Clostridia and *Enterobacteriaceae* in the feces of patients with IBS compared with controls.[141]

A recent study investigating 300 bacterial species using quantitative real-time polymerase chain reaction assays showed lower amounts of *Lactobacillus* species in samples from patients with diarrhea-predominant IBS, whereas patients with constipation-predominant IBS had increased amounts of *Veillonella* species.[142] In another study using denaturing gradient gel electrophoresis, amounts of *Clostridium coccoides–Eubacterium rectale* were found to be significantly lower in patients with constipation-predominant IBS than in control subjects, while tending to be higher in patients with diarrhea-predominant IBS.[143]

The same study also showed that the bacterial population had a higher temporal instability in patients with IBS than in healthy controls. The predominant bacteria adherent to the intestinal mucosa in patients with IBS (the *Clostridium coccoides–Eubacterium rectale* group) accounted for 48% of the total adherent bacteria, compared with 32% in healthy controls, showing a difference in the composition of the adherent microbiota between patients with IBS and healthy controls.[144] The qualitative changes in the colonic flora could lead to the proliferation of species that produce more gas and short-chain fatty acids, and that are more avid in the deconjugation of bile acids. The latter could, in turn, lead to clinically significant changes in water and electrolyte transport in the colon, and affect colonic motility or sensitivity. Thus, changes in microbiota composition may affect several aspects of intestinal physiology, resulting in altered motor-sensory function of the gut. These abnormalities could further perpetuate changes in the microbiota and subsequently cause low-grade inflammation contributing to symptom generation.

An improved understanding of host–microbiota interactions in IBS is important to gain insight on its pathogenesis and to enable therapeutic modulation through the rational use of antibiotics, probiotics, and prebiotics. Antibiotics such as rifaximin might be used to treat SIBO present in some patients with IBS.[115–117] Probiotics can introduce microbial components with known beneficial functions for the human host. Since the first study in an animal model of PI-IBS, which showed a beneficial effect of specific probiotic bacteria on PI muscle hypercontractility,[145] many other studies have documented improvement in visceral sensitivity, intestinal motility, permeability, and immune activation using various probiotic strains.[146–150] Most of the clinical trials with probiotics have shown improvement in IBS symptoms,[75,151,152] but individual clinical trials are difficult to compare because their design and methodology, and especially the probiotics used differ significantly. However, a recent systematic review concluded that probiotics seem to be efficacious in treating

IBS, although the magnitude of benefit and the most effective bacteria are still uncertain.[153]

SUMMARY

IBS is a multifactorial disorder. It is a symptom complex characterized by recurrent abdominal pain or discomfort, and accompanied by abnormal bowel habits, in the absence of any discernible organic abnormality. IBS is a prototype of functional bowel diseases and affects up to 10% of the general population, with significant socioeconomic impact. Its origin remains unclear, partly because multiple pathophysiologic mechanisms are likely to be involved. Psychosomatic disorders and stress, intestinal dysmotility, visceral hyperalgesia, abnormal brain processing of luminal stimuli, and chronic low-grade inflammation have all been suggested to play a role in the development of IBS. A significant proportion of patients develop IBS symptoms after an episode of gastrointestinal infection. In addition to gastrointestinal pathogens, recent evidence suggests that patients with IBS have abnormal composition and higher temporal instability of their intestinal microbiota. Because the intestinal microbiota is an important determinant of normal gut function and immunity, this instability may constitute an additional mechanism that leads to symptom generation and IBS. More importantly, a role for altered microbiota composition in IBS raises the possibility of therapeutic interventions through selective antibiotic or probiotic administration. The new concept of functional bowel diseases incorporates the bidirectional communication between the gut and the central nervous system (gut–brain axis), which may explain the multiple facets of IBS by linking emotional and cognitive centers of the brain with peripheral functioning of the gastrointestinal tract and vice versa.

REFERENCES

1. Longstreth GF, Thompson WG, Chey WD, et al. Functional bowel disorders. Gastroenterology 2006;130(5):1480–91.
2. Mearin F. IBS: New Rome III criteria. Med Clin (Barc) 2007;128(9):335–43.
3. Gwee KA. Irritable bowel syndrome and the Rome III criteria: for better or for worse? Eur J Gastroenterol Hepatol 2007;19(6):441–7.
4. Longstreth GF. IBS: definition and classification of IBS: current consensus and controversies. Gastroenterol Clin North Am 2005;34:173–87.
5. Ersryd A, Posserud I, Abrahamsson H, et al. Subtyping the IBS by predominant habit: Rome II vs Rome III. Aliment Pharmacol Ther 2007;26(6):953–61.
6. Guilera M, Balboa A, Mearin F. Bowel habits subtypes and temporal patterns in IBS: systematic review. Am J Gastroenterol 2005;100(5):1174–84.
7. Dorn SD, Morris CB, Hu Y, et al. IBS subtypes defined by Rome II and Rome III criteria are similar. J Clin Gastroenterol 2009;43(3):214–20.
8. Manning AP, Thompson WG, Heaton KW, et al. Towards positive diagnosis of the irritable bowel. Br Med J 1978;2(6138):653–4.
9. Thompson WG, Dotevall DA, Drossman DA, et al. Irritable bowel syndrome: guidelines for the diagnosis. Gastroenterol Int 1989;2(2):92–5.
10. Drossman DA, Corazziari E, Talley NJ, et al. The functional gastrointestinal disorders. 2nd edition. McLean (VA): Degnon; 2000.
11. Spiller R, Aziz Q, Creed F, et al. Guidelines on IBS: mechanisms and practical management. Gut 2007;56(12):1770–98.
12. Marshall JK. Post-infectious irritable bowel syndrome following water contamination. Kidney Int Suppl 2009;112:S42–3.

13. Spiegel BM. The burden of IBS: looking at metrics. Curr Gastroenterol Rep 2009;11(4):265–9.
14. Cremonini F, Talley NJ. Irritable bowel syndrome: epidemiology, natural history, health care seeking and emerging risk factors. Gastroenterol Clin North Am 2005;34(2):189–204.
15. Videlock EJ, Chang L. IBS: current approach to symptoms, evaluation and treatment. Gastroenterol Clin North Am 2007;36(3):665–85.
16. Amouretti M, Le Pen C, Gaudin AF, et al. Impact of irritable bowel syndrome (IBS) on health-related quality of life (HRQOL). Gastroenterol Clin Biol 2006; 30(2):241–6.
17. Drossman DA, Morris CB, Schneck S, et al. International survey of patients with IBS symptom features and their severity, health status, treatments and risk taking to achieve clinical benefit. J Clin Gastroenterol 2009;43(6):541–50.
18. Williams RE, Hartmann KE, Sandler RS, et al. Prevalence and characteristics of irritable bowel syndrome among women with chronic pelvis pain. Obstet Gynecol 2004;104(3):452–8.
19. Balshaw R, Khorasheh S, Barbeau M. Longitudinal Outcomes of GI symptoms in Canada (LOGIC): key factors for an effective patient retention in observational studies. Can J Clin Pharmacol 2009;16(1):el40–50.
20. Dean BB, Aguilar D, Barghout V, et al. Impairment in work productivity and health-related QoL in patients with IBS. Am J Manag Care 2005;11(Suppl 1): S17–26.
21. Gasbarrini A, Lauritano EC, Garcovich M, et al. New insights into the pathophysiology of IBS: intestinal microflora, gas production and gut motility. Eur Rev Med Pharmacol Sci 2008;12(Suppl 1):111–7.
22. Quigley EM. Disturbances of motility and visceral hypersensitivity in irritable bowel syndrome: biological markers or epiphenomenon. Gastroenterol Clin North Am 2005;34:221–33.
23. Miller V, Hopkins L, Whorwell PJ. Suicidal ideation in patients with irritable bowel syndrome. Clin Gastroenterol Hepatol 2004;2(12):1064–8.
24. Chitkara DK, van Tilburg MA, Blois-Martin N, et al. Early life risk factors that contribute to IBS in adults: a systematic review. Am J Gastroenterol 2008; 103(3):765–74.
25. Drossman DA, Camilleri M, Mayer EA, et al. AGA technical review on irritable bowel syndrome. Gastroenterology 2002;123(6):2108–31.
26. Quigley EM. Disturbances in small bowel motility. Baillieres Best Pract Res Clin Gastroenterol 1999;13(3):385–95.
27. McKee DP, Quigley EM. Intestinal motility in irritable bowel syndrome: is IBS a motility disorder? Part 1: definition of IBS and colonic motility. Dig Dis Sci 1993;38(10):1761–72.
28. McKee DP, Quigley EM. Intestinal motility in irritable bowel syndrome: is IBS a motility disorder? Part 2: motility of the small bowel, esophagus, stomach and gall bladder. Dig Dis Sci 1993;38(10):1773–82.
29. Hungin AP, Whorwell PJ, Tack J, et al. The prevalence, patterns and impact of irritable bowel syndrome: an international survey of 40,000 subjects. Aliment Pharmacol Ther 2003;17:643–50.
30. Serra J, Azpiroz F, Malagelada JR. Mechanisms of intestinal gas retention in humans: impaired propulsion versus obstructed evacuation. Am J Physiol Gastrointest Liver Physiol 2001;281(1):G138–43.
31. Simrén M. Bloating and abdominal distention: not so poorly understood anymore. Gastroenterology 2009;136:1487–505.

32. Brandt LJ, Chey WD, Foxx-Orenstein AE, et al. An evidence-based systematic review on the management of irritable bowel syndrome American college of gastroenterology task force on IBS. Am J Gastroenterol 2009;104(Suppl 1): S1–35.
33. Mertz H, Naliboff B, Munakata J, et al. Altered rectal perception is a biological marker of patients with irritable bowel syndrome. Gastroenterology 1995;109: 40–52.
34. Schmulson M, Chang L, Malakoff B, et al. Correlation of symptom criteria with perception thresholds during rectosigmoid distension in irritable bowel syndrome patients. Am J Gastroenterol 2000;95:152–6.
35. Bouin M, Meunier P, Riberdy-Poitras M, et al. Pain hypersensitivity in patients with functional gastrointestinal disorders: a gastrointestinal specific defect or a general systemic condition. Dig Dis Sci 2001;46:2542–8.
36. Accarino AM, Azpiroz F, Malagelada JR. Mechanosensitive intestinal afferents in irritable bowel syndrome. Gastroenterology 1995;108(3):636–43.
37. Simrén M, Abrahamsson H, Björnsson ES. An exaggerated sensory component of the gastro colonic response in patients with irritable bowel syndrome. Gut 2001;48(1):20–7.
38. van der Veek PP, Van Rood YR, Masclee AA. Symptom severity but not psychopathology predicts visceral hypersensitivity in irritable bowel syndrome. Clin Gastroenterol Hepatol 2008;6(3):321–8.
39. Sabate JM, Veyrac M, Mion F, et al. Relationship between rectal sensitivity, symptoms intensity and quality of life in patients with irritable bowel syndrome. Aliment Pharmacol Ther 2008;28(4):484–90.
40. Agrawal A, Houghton LA, Lea R, et al. Bloating and distention in irritable bowel syndrome: the role of visceral sensation. Gastroenterology 2008;134(7):1882–9.
41. Kim HS, Rhee PL, Park J, et al. Gender-related differences in visceral perception in health and irritable bowel syndrome. J Gastroenterol Hepatol 2006;21(2):468–73.
42. Verne GN, Robinson ME, Price DD. Hypersensitivity to visceral and cutaneous pain in irritable bowel syndrome. Pain 2001;93(1):7–14.
43. Chang L, Mayer EA, Johnson T, et al. Differences in somatic perception in patients with irritable bowel syndrome with and without fibromyalgia. Pain 2000;84(2-3):297–307.
44. Delvaux M. Role of visceral sensitivity in the pathophysiology of irritable bowel syndrome. Gut 2002;51(Suppl 1):i67–71.
45. Kwan CL, Diamant NE, Mikula K, et al. Characteristics of rectal perception are altered in irritable bowel syndrome. Pain 2005;113(1–2):160–71.
46. Lembo T, Munakata J, Mertz H, et al. Evidence for the hypersensitivity of lumbar splanchnic afferents in irritable bowel syndrome. Gastroenterology 1994;107(6): 1686–96.
47. Drewes AM, Petersen P, Rössel P, et al. Sensitivity and distensibility of the rectum and sigmoid colon in patients with irritable bowel syndrome. Scand J Gastroenterol 2001;36(8):827–32.
48. Naliboff BD, Munakata J, Fullerton S, et al. Evidence of two distinct perceptual alterations in irritable bowel syndrome. Gut 1997;41(4):505–12.
49. Rapps N, van Oudenhove L, Enck P, et al. Brain imaging of visceral functions in healthy volunteers and IBS patients. J Psychosom Res 2008;64(6):599–604.
50. Berman SM, Naliboff BD, Suyenobu B, et al. Reduced brainstem inhibition during anticipated pelvic visceral pain correlates with enhanced brain response to visceral stimulus in women with irritable bowel syndrome. J Neurosci 2008; 28(2):349–59.

51. Mertz H, Morgan V, Tanner G, et al. Regional cerebral activation in irritable bowel syndrome with painful and nonpainful stimuli. Gastroenterology 2000;118(5): 842–8.
52. Naliboff BD, Derbyshire SW, Munakata J, et al. Cerebral activation in patients with irritable bowel syndrome and control subjects during rectosigmoid stimulation. Psychosom Med 2001;63(3):365–75.
53. Naliboff BD, Berman S, Suyenobu B, et al. Longitudinal change in perceptual and brain activation response to visceral stimuli in irritable bowel syndrome patients. Gastroenterology 2006;131(2):352–65.
54. Wilder-Smith CH, Schindler D, Lovblad K, et al. Brain functional magnetic resonance imaging of rectal pain and activation of endogenous inhibitory mechanisms in irritable bowel syndrome patient subgroups and healthy controls. Gut 2004;53(11):1595–601.
55. Lawal A, Kern M, Sidhu H, et al. Novel evidence for hypersensitivity of visceral sensory neural circuitry in irritable bowel syndrome patients. Gastroenterology 2006;130(1):26–33.
56. Gupta V, Sheffield D, Verne GN. Evidence for autonomic dysregulation in the irritable bowel syndrome. Dig Dis Sci 2002;47(8):1716–22.
57. Spaziani R, Bayati A, Redmond K, et al. Vagal dysfunction in irritable bowel syndrome assessed by rectal distension and baroreceptor sensitivity. Neurogastroenterol Motil 2008;20(4):336–42.
58. Collins SM, McHugh K, Jacobson K, et al. Previous inflammation alters the response of the rat colon to stress. Gastroenterology 1996;111(6):1509–15.
59. Bercík P, Wang L, Verdú EF, et al. Visceral hyperalgesia and intestinal dysmotility in a mouse model of post infective gut dysfunction. Gastroenterology 2004; 127(1):179–87.
60. Collins SM. The immunomodulation of enteric neuromuscular function: implications for motility and inflammatory disorders. Gastroenterology 1996;111(6): 1683–99.
61. Chadwick VS, Chen W, Shu D, et al. Activation of the mucosal immune system in irritable bowel syndrome. Gastroenterology 2002;122(7):1778–83.
62. Törnblom H, Lindberg G, Nyberg B, et al. Full-thickness biopsy of the jejunum reveals inflammation and enteric neuropathy in irritable bowel syndrome. Gastroenterology 2002;123(6):1972–9.
63. Guilarte M, Santos J, de Torres I, et al. Diarrhea-predominant IBS patients show mast cell activation and hyperplasia in the jejunum. Gut 2007;56(2):203–9.
64. Ohman L, Isaksson S, Lindmark AC, et al. T-cell activation in patients with irritable bowel syndrome. Am J Gastroenterol 2009;104(5):1205–12.
65. Barbara G, Stanghellini V, De Giorgio R, et al. Activated mast cells in proximity to colonic nerves correlate with abdominal pain in irritable bowel syndrome. Gastroenterology 2004;126(3):693–702.
66. Cenac N, Andrews CN, Holzhausen M, et al. Role for protease activity in visceral pain in irritable bowel syndrome. J Clin Invest 2007;117(3):636–47.
67. Barbara G, Wang B, Stanghellini V, et al. Mast cell-dependent excitation of visceral-nociceptive sensory neurons in irritable bowel syndrome. Gastroenterology 2007;132(1):26–37.
68. Buhner S, Li Q, Vignali S, et al. Activation of human enteric neurons by supernatants of colonic biopsy specimens from patients with irritable bowel syndrome. Gastroenterology 2009;137(4):1425–34.
69. Spiller RC, Jenkins D, Thornley JP, et al. Increased rectal mucosal enteroendocrine cells, T lymphocytes, and increased gut permeability following acute

Campylobacter enteritis and in post-dysenteric irritable bowel syndrome. Gut 2000;47(6):804–11.
70. Dunlop SP, Jenkins D, Spiller RC. Distinctive clinical, psychological, and histological features of post infective irritable bowel syndrome. Am J Gastroenterol 2003;98(7):1578–83.
71. Dunlop SP, Hebden J, Campbell E, et al. Abnormal intestinal permeability in subgroups of diarrhea predominant irritable bowel syndromes. Am J Gastroenterol 2006;101(6):1288–94.
72. van der Veek PP, van den Berg M, de Kroon YE, et al. Role of tumor necrosis factor-alpha and interleukin-10 gene polymorphisms in irritable bowel syndrome. Am J Gastroenterol 2005;100(11):2510–6.
73. Dinan TG, Quigley EM, Ahmed SM, et al. Hypothalamic-pituitary-gut axis dysregulation in irritable bowel syndrome: plasma cytokines as a potential biomarker? Gastroenterology 2006;130(2):304–11.
74. Liebregts T, Adam B, Bredack C, et al. Immune activation in patients with irritable bowel syndrome. Gastroenterology 2007;132(3):913–20.
75. O'Mahony L, McCarthy J, Kelly P, et al. Lactobacillus and bifidobacterium in irritable bowel syndrome: symptom responses and relationship to cytokine profiles. Gastroenterology 2005;128(3):541–51.
76. Bercik P, Verdu EF, Collins SM. Is irritable bowel syndrome a low-grade inflammatory bowel disease? Gastroenterol Clin North Am 2005;34(2):235–45, vi–vii.
77. Saunders PR, Santos J, Hanssen NP, et al. Physical and psychological stress in rats enhances colonic epithelial permeability via peripheral CRH. Dig Dis Sci 2002;47(1):208–15.
78. Bradesi S, Schwetz I, Ennes HS, et al. Repeated exposure to water avoidance stress in rats: a new model for sustained visceral hyperalgesia. Am J Physiol Gastrointest Liver Physiol 2005;289(1):G42–53.
79. Collins SM. Stress and the gastrointestinal tract IV. Modulation of intestinal inflammation by stress: basic mechanisms and clinical relevance. Am J Physiol Gastrointest Liver Physiol 2001;280(3):G315–8.
80. Chang L, Sundaresh S, Elliott J, et al. Dysregulation of the hypothalamic-pituitary- adrenal (HPA) axis in IBSA. Neurogastroenterol Motil 2009;21(2): 149–59.
81. Mawdsley JE, Rampton DS. Psychological stress in IBD: new insights into pathogenic and therapeutic implications. Gut 2005;54(10):1481–91.
82. Martinez V, Taché Y. CRF1 receptors as a therapeutic target for irritable bowel syndrome. Curr Pharm Des 2006;12(31):4071–88.
83. Gershon MD. Review article: roles played by 5-hydroxytryptamine in the physiology of the bowel. Aliment Pharmacol Ther 1999;13(Suppl 2):15–30.
84. Garvin B, Wiley JW. The role of serotonin in irritable bowel syndrome: implications for management. Curr Gastroenterol Rep 2008;10(4):363–8.
85. Chen JJ, Li Z, Pan H, et al. Maintenance of serotonin in the intestinal mucosa and ganglia of mice that lack the high-affinity serotonin transporter: abnormal intestinal motility and the expression of cation transporters. J Neurosci 2001; 21(16):6348–61.
86. Liu MT, Rayport S, Jiang Y, et al. Expression and function of 5-HT3 receptors in the enteric neurons of mice lacking the serotonin transporter. Am J Phys 2002; 283:G1398–411.
87. Dunlop SP, Coleman NS, Blackshaw E, et al. Abnormalities of 5-Hydroxytryptamine metabolism in irritable bowel syndrome. Clin Gastroenterol Hepatol 2005; 3(4):349–57.

88. Bearcroft CP, Perrett D, Farthing MJ. Postprandial plasma 5- hydroxytriptamine in diarrhea predominant irritable bowel syndrome: a pilot study. Gut 1998;42(1): 42–6.
89. Wheatcroft J, Wakelin D, Smith A, et al. Enterochromaffin cell hyperplasia and decreased serotonin transporter in a mouse model of postinfectious bowel dysfunction. Neurogastroenterol Motil 2005;17(6):863–70.
90. Mössner R, Daniel S, Schmitt A, et al. Modulation of serotonin transporter function by interleukin-4. Life Sci 2001;68(8):873–80.
91. Pata C, Erdal ME, Derici E, et al. Serotonin transporter gene polymorphism in irritable bowel syndrome. Am J Gastroenterol 2002;97(7):1780–4.
92. Kim HJ, Camilleri M, Carlson PJ, et al. Association of distinct 2A adrenoceptor and serotonin-transporter polymorphisms associated with constipation and somatic symptoms in functional gastrointestinal disorders. Gut 2004;53(6): 829–37.
93. Yeo A, Boyd P, Lumsden S, et al. Association between a functional polymorphism in the serotonin transporter gene and diarrhea predominant irritable bowel syndrome in women. Gut 2004;53(10):1452–8.
94. Park MI, Camilleri M. Genetics and genotypes in irritable bowel syndrome: implications for diagnosis and treatment. Gastroenterol Clin North Am 2005;34(2): 305–17.
95. Park MI, Camilleri M. Is there a role of food allergy in irritable bowel syndrome and functional dyspepsia? A systematic review. Neurogastroenterol Motil 2006;18(8):595–607.
96. Wahnschaffe U, Ullrich R, Riecken EO, et al. Celiac disease-like abnormalities in a subgroup of patients with irritable bowel syndrome. Gastroenterology 2001; 121(6):1329–38.
97. Wahnschaffe U, Schulzke JD, Zeitz M, et al. Predictors of clinical response to gluten-free diet in patients diagnosed with diarrhea-predominant irritable bowel syndrome. Clin Gastroenterol Hepatol 2007;5(7):844–50.
98. Verdu EF, Armstrong D, Murray JA. Between celiac disease and irritable bowel syndrome: the "no man's land" of gluten sensitivity. Am J Gastroenterol 2009; 104(6):1587–94.
99. Rodríguez LA, Ruigómez A. Increased risk of irritable bowel syndrome after bacterial gastroenteritis: cohort study. BMJ 1999;318(7183):565–6.
100. Ruigómez A, García Rodríguez LA, Panés J. Risk of irritable bowel syndrome after an episode of bacterial gastroenteritis in general practice: influence of comorbidities. Clin Gastroenterol Hepatol 2007;5(4):465–9.
101. Thabane M, Kottachchi DT, Marshall JK. Systematic review and meta-analysis: the incidence and prognosis of post-infectious irritable bowel syndrome. Aliment Pharmacol Ther 2007;26(4):535–44.
102. Spiller RC. Role of infection in irritable bowel syndrome. J Gastroenterol 2007; 42(Suppl 17):41–7.
103. Neal KR, Hebden J, Spiller R. Prevalence of gastrointestinal symptoms six months after bacterial gastroenteritis and risk factors for development of the irritable bowel syndrome: postal survey of patients. BMJ 1997;314(7083): 779–82.
104. Marshall JK, Thabane M, Borgaonkar MR, et al. Postinfectious irritable bowel syndrome after a food-borne outbreak of acute gastroenteritis attributed to a viral pathogen. Clin Gastroenterol Hepatol 2007;5(4):457–60.
105. Ji S, Park H, Lee D, et al. Post-infectious irritable bowel syndrome in patients with Shigella infection. J Gastroenterol Hepatol 2005;20(3):381–6.

106. Wang LH, Fang XC, Pan GZ. Bacillary dysentery as a causative factor of irritable bowel syndrome and its pathogenesis. Gut 2004;53(8):1096–101.
107. Mearin F, Pérez-Oliveras M, Perelló A, et al. Dyspepsia and irritable bowel syndrome after a Salmonella gastroenteritis outbreak: one-year follow-up cohort study. Gastroenterology 2005;129(1):98–104.
108. Spiller R, Garsed K. Infection, inflammation, and the irritable bowel syndrome. Dig Liver Dis 2009;41(12):844–9.
109. Thabane M, Marshall JK. Post-infectious irritable bowel syndrome. World J Gastroenterol 2009;15(29):3591–6.
110. Barbara G, Cremon C, Pallotti F, et al. Postinfectious irritable bowel syndrome. J Pediatr Gastroenterol Nutr 2009;48(Suppl 2):S95–7.
111. Neal KR, Barker L, Spiller RC. Prognosis in post-infective irritable bowel syndrome: a six year follow up study. Gut 2002;51(3):410–3.
112. Törnblom H, Holmvall P, Svenungsson B, et al. Gastrointestinal symptoms after infectious diarrhea: a five-year follow-up in a Swedish cohort of adults. Clin Gastroenterol Hepatol 2007;5(4):461–4.
113. Jung IS, Kim HS, Park H, et al. The clinical course of postinfectious irritable bowel syndrome: a five-year follow-up study. J Clin Gastroenterol 2009;43(6):534–40.
114. Gwee KA, Collins SM, Read NW, et al. Increased rectal mucosal expression of interleukin 1beta in recently acquired post-infectious irritable bowel syndrome. Gut 2003;52(4):523–6.
115. Pimentel M, Chow EJ, Lin HC. Eradication of small intestinal bacterial overgrowth reduces symptoms of irritable bowel syndrome. Am J Gastroenterol 2000;95(12):3503–6.
116. Pimentel M, Chow EJ, Lin HC. Normalization of lactulose breath testing correlates with symptom improvement in irritable bowel syndrome. A double-blind, randomized, placebo-controlled study. Am J Gastroenterol 2003;98(2):412–9.
117. Pimentel M, Park S, Mirocha J, et al. The effect of a nonabsorbed oral antibiotic (rifaximin) on the symptoms of the irritable bowel syndrome. Ann Intern Med 2006;145(8):557–63.
118. Posserud I, Stotzer PO, Björnsson ES, et al. Small intestinal bacterial overgrowth in patients with irritable bowel syndrome. Gut 2007;56(6):802–8.
119. Grover M, Kanazawa M, Palsson OS, et al. Small intestinal bacterial overgrowth in irritable bowel syndrome: association with colon motility, bowel symptoms, and psychological distress. Neurogastroenterol Motil 2008;20(9):998–1008.
120. Walters B, Vanner SJ. Detection of bacterial overgrowth in IBS using the lactulose H2 breath test: comparison with 14C-D-xylose and healthy controls. Am J Gastroenterol 2005;100(7):1566–70.
121. Ford AC, Spiegel BM, Talley NJ, et al. Small intestinal bacterial overgrowth in irritable bowel syndrome: systematic review and meta-analysis. Clin Gastroenterol Hepatol 2009;7(12):1279–86.
122. Montalto M, D'Onofrio F, Gallo A, et al. Intestinal microbiota and its functions. Dig Liver Dis Suppl 2009;3(2):30–4.
123. Bäckhed F, Ley RE, Sonnenburg JL, et al. Host-bacterial mutualism in the human intestine. Science 2005;307(5717):1915–20.
124. Zoetendal EG, von Wright A, Vilpponen-Salmela T, et al. Mucosa-associated bacteria in the human gastrointestinal tract are uniformly distributed along the colon and differ from the community recovered from feces. Appl Environ Microbiol 2002;68(7):3401–7.

125. Delgado S, Suárez A, Mayo B. Identification of dominant bacteria in feces and colonic mucosa from healthy Spanish adults by culturing and by 16S rDNA sequence analysis. Dig Dis Sci 2006;51(4):744–51.
126. Collins SM, Denou E, Verdu EF, et al. The putative role of the intestinal microbiota in the irritable bowel syndrome. Dig Liver Dis 2009;41(12):850–3.
127. Ojetti V, Gigante G, Ainora ME, et al. Microflora imbalance and gastrointestinal diseases. Dig Liver Dis Suppl 2009;3(2):35–9.
128. Parkes GC, Brostoff J, Whelan K, et al. Gastrointestinal microbiota in irritable bowel syndrome: their role in its pathogenesis and treatment. Am J Gastroenterol 2008;103(6):1557–67.
129. Tana C, Umesaki Y, Imaoka A, et al. Altered profiles of intestinal microbiota and organic acids may be the origin of symptoms in irritable bowel syndrome. Neurogastroenterol Motil 2010;22:512–9, e115.
130. Zoetendal E, Akkermans AD, DeVos WM. Temperature gradient gel electrophoresis analysis of 16S rRNA from human fecal samples reveals stable and host-specific communities of active bacteria. Appl Environ Microbiol 1998;64(10): 3854–9.
131. Tannock GW, Munro K, Harmsen HJ, et al. Analysis of the fecal microflora of human subjects consuming a probiotic containing Lactobacillus rhamnosus DR20. Appl Environ Microbiol 2000;66(6):2578–88.
132. McCartney AL, Wang W, Tannock GW. Molecular analysis of the composition of the bifidobacterial and lactobacillus microflora of humans. Appl Environ Microbiol 1996;62(12):4608–13.
133. Bartosch S, Fite A, Macfarlane GT. Characterization of bacterial communities in feces from healthy elderly volunteers and hospitalized elderly patients by using real-time PCR and effects of antibiotic treatment on the fecal microbiota. Appl Environ Microbiol 2004;70(6):3575–81.
134. Kleessen B, Schroedl W, Stueck M, et al. Microbial and immunological responses relative to high-altitude exposure in mountaineers. Med Sci Sports Exerc 2005;37(8):1313–8.
135. Jernberg C, Löfmark S, Edlund C, et al. Long-term ecological impacts of antibiotic administration on the human intestinal microbiota. ISME J 2007;1(1): 56–66.
136. Löfmark S, Jernberg C, Jansson JK, et al. Clindamycin-induced enrichment and long-term persistence of resistant Bacteroides spp. and resistance genes. J Antimicrob Chemother 2006;58(6):1160–7.
137. Mättö J, Maunuksela L, Kajander K, et al. Composition and temporal stability of gastrointestinal microbiota in irritable bowel syndrome—a longitudinal study in IBS and control subjects. FEMS Immunol Med Microbiol 2005;43(2):213–22.
138. Codling C, O'Mahony L, Shanahan F, et al. A molecular analysis of fecal and mucosal bacterial communities in irritable bowel syndrome. Dig Dis Sci 2010; 55(2):392–7.
139. Kassinen A, Krogius-Kurikka L, Mäkivuokko H, et al. The fecal microbiota of irritable bowel syndrome patients differs significantly from that of healthy subjects. Gastroenterology 2007;133(1):24–33.
140. Krogius-Kurikka L, Lyra A, Malinen E, et al. Microbial community analysis reveals high level phylogenetic alterations in the overall gastrointestinal microbiota of diarrhoea-predominant irritable bowel syndrome sufferers. BMC Gastroenterol 2009;9:95.
141. Si JM, Yu YC, Fan YJ, et al. Intestinal microecology and quality of life in irritable bowel syndrome patients. World J Gastroenterol 2004;10(12):1802–5.

142. Malinen E, Rinttilä T, Kajander K, et al. Analysis of the fecal microbiota of irritable bowel syndrome patients and healthy controls with PCR- real time. Am J Gastroenterol 2005;100(2):373–82.
143. Maukonen J, Satokari R, Mättö J, et al. Prevalence and temporal stability of selected clostridial groups in irritable bowel syndrome in relation to predominant faecal bacteria. J Med Microbiol 2006;55(Pt 5):625–33.
144. Ringel Y, Carroll IM. Alterations in the intestinal microbiota and functional bowel symptoms. Gastrointest Endosc Clin N Am 2009;19(1):141–50, vii.
145. Verdú EF, Bercík P, Bergonzelli GE, et al. Lactobacillus paracasei normalizes muscle hypercontractility in a murine model of post infective gut dysfunction. Gastroenterology 2004;127(3):826–37.
146. Liebregts T, Adam B, Bertel A, et al. Effect of E. coli Nissle 1917 on post-inflammatory visceral sensory function in a rat model. Neurogastroenterol Motil 2005; 17(3):410–4.
147. Ukena SN, Singh A, Dringenberg U, et al. Probiotic Escherichia coli Nissle 1917 inhibits leaky gut by enhancing mucosal integrity. PLoS One 2007;2(12):e1308.
148. Martin FP, Verdu EF, Wang Y, et al. Transgenomic metabolic interactions in a mouse disease model: interactions of Trichinella spiralis infection with dietary Lactobacillus paracasei supplementation. J Proteome Res 2006;5(9):2185–93.
149. Mennigen R, Nolte K, Rijcken E, et al. Probiotic mixture VSL#3 protects the epithelial barrier by maintaining tight junction protein expression and preventing apoptosis in a murine model of colitis. Am J Physiol Gastrointest Liver Physiol 2009;296(5):G1140–9.
150. Kim N, Kunisawa J, Kweon MN, et al. Oral feeding of Bifidobacterium bifidum (BGN4) prevents CD4(+) CD45RB(high) T cell-mediated inflammatory bowel disease by inhibition of disordered T cell activation. Clin Immunol 2007;123(1): 30–9.
151. Niedzielin K, Kordecki H, Birkenfeld B. A controlled, double-blind, randomized study on the efficacy of Lactobacillus plantarum 299V in patients with irritable bowel syndrome. Eur J Gastroenterol Hepatol 2001;13(10):1143–7.
152. Whorwell PJ, Altringer L, Morel J, et al. Efficacy of an encapsulated probiotic Bifidobacterium infantis 35624 in women with irritable bowel syndrome. Am J Gastroenterol 2006;101(7):1581–90.
153. Moayyedi P, Ford AC, Talley NJ, et al. The efficacy of probiotics in the therapy of irritable bowel syndrome: a systematic review. Gut 2010;59:325–32.

Influences of Intestinal Bacteria in Human Inflammatory Bowel Disease

Rachel Vanderploeg, BSc[a], Remo Panaccione, MD, FRCP(C)[b], Subrata Ghosh, MD, FRCP(C), FRCP(E)[c], Kevin Rioux, MD, PhD, FRCP(C)[d,*]

KEYWORDS

- Inflammatory bowel disease • Microbiota • Bacteria
- Dysbiosis • Adherent-invasive *E coli*
- *Mycobacterium avium paratuberculosis*

Inflammatory bowel disease (IBD) comprises at least 2 common clinical phenotypes termed Crohn's disease (CD) and ulcerative colitis (UC). These conditions are chronic inflammatory disorders that have a predilection for the distal intestinal tract, a site that coincides with the region of densest microbial colonization in the human body. The diseases are characterized by abdominal pain, diarrhea, and intestinal bleeding; symptoms that closely mimic those of a variety of specific acute and chronic gastrointestinal infections. The cause of these troublesome diseases is unknown, and the prevalence in certain populations in the last 50 years has dramatically risen, pointing, at least in part, to environmental microbial influences.

From the very moment of birth, the intestinal tract becomes colonized by a wide variety of environmental microbes, which evolve in a stochastic fashion during early life to what are believed to be relatively stable communities of symbiont gut organisms.[1] Early on, intestinal bacteria are known to play a vital role in educating both local and systemic immunity, and defenses are challenged time to time by more aggressive

[a] Gastrointestinal Research Group, Faculty of Medicine, University of Calgary, Room 1764 Health Sciences Centre, 3330 Hospital Drive NW, Calgary, Alberta, Canada T2N 4N1
[b] Department of Medicine, Division of Gastroenterology, Faculty of Medicine, University of Calgary, Room 6D28 TRW Building, 3280 Hospital Drive NW, Calgary, Alberta, Canada T2N 4Z6
[c] Department of Medicine, Division of Gastroenterology, Faculty of Medicine, University of Calgary, Room 6D31 TRW Building, 3280 Hospital Drive NW, Calgary, Alberta, Canada T2N 4Z6
[d] Department of Medicine, Division of Gastroenterology, Department of Microbiology and Infectious Diseases, Faculty of Medicine, University of Calgary, Room 1705 Health Sciences Centre, 3330 Hospital Drive NW, Calgary, Alberta, Canada, T2N 4N1
* Corresponding author. 1705 Health Sciences Centre, 3330 Hospital Drive North West, Calgary, Alberta, Canada T2N 4N1.
E-mail address: kprioux@ucalgary.ca

Infect Dis Clin N Am 24 (2010) 977–993
doi:10.1016/j.idc.2010.07.008 id.theclinics.com
0891-5520/10/$ – see front matter

or pathogenic microbes. Aberrations in immunity are an obvious prerequisite for IBD, and it is believed that maladaptive "lessons" during microbial education of host immunity play a role in IBD. The mature communities of commensal and nonpathogenic gut bacteria have important influences on day-to-day host intestinal mucosal barrier integrity, host metabolism, and nutrition. Failed assembly in terms of composition and/or functional abilities of gut bacterial communities is termed dysbiosis, and has also been linked to IBD.[2] Alternatively, there remains a compelling idea that IBD may be the sequelae of chronic infection with one or a small group of unrecognized intestinal pathogens.

The goal of this article is to summarize known microbial associations with human IBD. The rapidly unfolding field of IBD metagenomics is surveyed, highlighting the impressive advances that have occurred in the last decade while critiquing methodology and approach. Adherent-invasive strains of *Escherichia coli* (AIEC) and *Mycobacterium avium* subspecies *paratuberculosis* (MAP) have been singled out as suspects in IBD etiology and are discussed in some detail. There is a recent but preliminary description of *Campylobacter concisus* as a new candidate pathogen in CD.[3] It is clear that much remains unknown in this field, and this article concludes by offering some ideas on research priorities and speculation on which avenues of investigation are likely to be most rewarding.

DYSBIOSIS

Eli Metchnikoff formulated a concept of orthobiosis, referring to a balance and collectively beneficial influence of the indigenous microbiome on human health.[4] Dysbiosis, then, refers to an imbalance between microbes with potentially aggressive or detrimental influences and those with benign or helpful effects on the host organism.[2] In the absence of a single microbial cause of IBD, many have postulated that dysbiosis underlies the development of these chronic inflammatory conditions. Early studies using classical descriptive and quantitative bacterial culture established this concept. For example, in 1988 Van de Merwe and colleagues[5] showed that the fecal flora of CD patients contained more cultivable anaerobic gram-positive coccoid rods and gram-negative rods than healthy subjects. Similarly, fecal samples from CD patients were found to be enriched with *Escherichia coli* but depleted of lactobacillus and bifidobacteria species compared with healthy controls.[6] A specific reduction in fecal bifidobacteria has also been described in UC patients by quantitative culture, and was accompanied by substantial increase in group D streptococci.[7] The discovery of deficiencies in putatively beneficial gut bacteria in IBD patients has spawned an entire industry of remedial products in IBD such as pre-, pro-, post- and syn-biotics aimed at ameliorating microbial imbalances.[8] However, it is difficult to know whether dysbiosis is a necessary precondition of the various forms of IBD or is a consequence of mucosal injury, therapies (eg, antibiotics and immunosuppressants), or dietary adaptations. Most studies of the microbiota in IBD have examined patients with established disease and any readout in this circumstance may be a secondary finding rather than a clue to causality.

Molecular techniques have revolutionized the study of diverse microbial ecosystems in the last decade, and a multitude of recent studies using such methodologies have further documented aberrations in the intestinal microbiota of IBD.[9–31] The salient points of study design and major findings of this growing body of literature are summarized in **Table 1**. It is immediately apparent that most studies have employed relatively small numbers of patients from diverse IBD populations and disparate specimens (eg, feces, mucosal biopsies, surgical specimens). Less apparent, but of major importance, has been the nearly universal lack of control over medication and dietary influences in these studies.

It is difficult to make any strong unifying conclusions about dysbiosis in IBD from such molecular studies taken collectively. In general, however, it is reasonable to conclude that IBD is associated with a reduction in intestinal microbial diversity, reflecting changes in bacterial, fungal, and archaeal phylotypes and abundance (see **Table 1**). This common finding in IBD may not be specific to the disease state, as reduced microbial diversity has also been observed in acute infectious[32] or postradiation diarrhea,[33] as well as chronic diarrheal conditions.[34,35] As a more fundamental principle, ecological stress in any complex multispecies bacterial community (eg, soil, water, human intestine) causes reduced diversity.[36] Another common thread emerging from metagenomic studies is the increased representation of members of Enterobacteriaceae among patients with IBD (see **Table 1**) and, in particular, the identification of numerous strains of *E coli* that are invasive at mucosal surfaces, discussed later in greater detail.

One of the most robust molecular studies of the IBD microbiota was reported by Frank and colleagues[23] in 2007, and employed surgical specimens of inflamed and noninflamed intestinal tissue from CD and UC patients. Small subunit RNA gene clone libraries representing the tissue-associated microbiota were constructed and compared with the microbiota of noninflamed control subjects (mainly those undergoing resection for intestinal malignancy). Principal component analysis based on the presence or absence of identified phylotypes revealed a stereotypical "IBD-specific" microbiota in certain cases of IBD (both UC and CD), which was distinct from non-IBD controls. However, most IBD cases in this study actually clustered together with the non-IBD controls, suggesting that dysbiosis may be neither precondition nor consequence in many patients with IBD. In the IBD-specific group, there was depletion of Bacteroidetes and groups IV and XIVa Clostridia (Lachnospiraceae), and enrichment of a variety of Actinobacteria and Proteobacteria, which were the dominant factors driving distinction of the IBD subset from the remaining cases. The IBD subset correlated with 2 clinical markers of more aggressive disease—younger age at time of surgery and abscess formation—and therefore the microbiologic phenomena observed in this group could still plausibly relate to pharmacologic or nutritional influences that were not fully assessed in this study, or reflect more severe disease. Nonetheless, this study highlighted the concept that metagenomic data help characterize IBD and could inform treatment decisions and prognosis.

A unique study was recently reported by Dicksved and colleagues[29] comparing the intestinal microbiotas of identical twins concordant or discordant for CD. This approach eliminated host genetic determinants of intestinal microbiota to enable a clearer picture of disease-associated and antecedent microbial influences in CD. Six monozygotic twin pairs discordant for CD and 4 twin pairs concordant for the disease were compared with ten healthy twin pairs. Fecal microbiotas were assessed by polymerase chain reaction (PCR) targeting the 16S rRNA gene followed by terminal restriction fragment length polymorphism profiling. As shown by numerous others, total bacterial diversity was decreased among patients with CD. When analyzed within twin sets, healthy twin pairs and twin pairs concordant for CD tended to have closely matched bacterial community profiles. Within twin pairs discordant for CD, however, only the fecal microbiota of affected individuals was distinct from that of the matched healthy twin, suggesting that the observed dysbiosis was consequence of the CD or its treatment. When comparisons were made between the healthy twin in discordant sets and those in healthy twin sibling sets, there was no evidence of specific microbial

Table 1
Summary of dysbiosis in IBD: studies using molecular methodologies

Study	Patients	Methods	Summary of Main Findings
Seksik et al[9]	CD remission (n = 9) CD active (n = 8) CTRL (n = 16)	Fecal specimens 16S rDNA dot blot hybridization and TGGE	Enterobacteriaceae increased in all CD patients; Distinct microbiota in remission and active CD; *C coccoides* subgroup decreased in active disease; Bacteroides and Bifidobacteria decreased in quiescent disease
Bullock et al[10]	UC active (n = 6) UC remission (n = 6)	Dispersed fecal bacteria FISH microscopy *Lactobacillus*-specific DGGE	Depletion of Lactobacilli in patients with active disease pointing to specific means of probiotic therapy in UC
Mangin et al[11]	CD (n = 4) CTRL (n = 4)	Fecal samples, surgical and/or mucosal biopsy specimens 16S rDNA clone library	*Bacteroides vulgatus* enriched in CD patients; *E coli* was a dominant phylotype only in CD patients; numerous bacterial phylotypes seen in CD that are not commonly part of dominant microbiota in healthy individuals; this study accounted for CARD15 mutations and medication use
Prindiville et al[12]	CD and CTRL (n = 25 subjects total)	Endoscopic biopsies and surgical 16S rDNA clone library	Samples taken from early CD lesions (aphthous ulcers); no known pathogenic phylotypes identified; CD patients had increased numbers of facultative bacteria
Mylonaki et al[13]	IBD active or remission UC (n = 33) CD colonic (n = 6) CTRL (n = 14)	Rectal biopsies FISH microscopy to determine epithelium-associated microbiota	Epithelium-associated and lamina propria *E coli* were higher in both CD and UC versus CTRL; Clostridia were higher in active UC versus inactive disease; Bifidobacteria were lower in all patients with UC compared with controls
Lepage et al[14]	CD (n = 20) UC (n = 11) CTRL (n = 4)	Mucosal biopsies in all patients; Feces in subset of 7 subjects; 16S rDNA TGGE	Validates means of sample collection, showing that biopsy-associated microbiota within an individual is 95% similar between various segments of distal gut (ileum, right colon, left colon, rectum), but there are differences between fecal and biopsy-associated microbiota (<92% similar within an individual).
Manichanh et al[15]	CD remission (n = 6) CTRL (n = 6)	Fecal specimens Metagenomic library construction 16S rDNA macroarray FISH analysis of *Bacteroides* and *C coccoides/leptum* subgroups	Markedly reduced diversity of fecal microbiota in CD, particularly driven by reduced diversity within phylum Firmicutes and abundance of *Clostridium leptum* subgroup; overrepresentation of Porphyromonadaceae in CD patients

Bibiloni et al[16]	CD (n = 20) UC (n = 15)	Mucosal biopsies 16S rDNA clone libraries PCR-DGGE, qPCR	These were newly diagnosed and untreated patients. Biopsy-associated microbiota in UC was different from CD, and greater bacterial abundance in UC patients. There was no difference in dominant microbiota between inflamed and noninflamed sites within an individual
Sokol et al[17]	UC active (n = 9) CTRL (n = 9)	16S rDNA gene TGGE profiling	Unique assessment of "present" and "active" microbiota using 16S rRNA gene PCR and RT-PCR. In UC patients, there was lower diversity of the active microbiota, but it was notably enriched in *E coli*
Scanlan et al[18]	CD remission on probiotic/steroid (n = 11) or relapse (n = 5); CTRL (n = 18)	Fecal specimens 16S rDNA PCR-DGGE	Decreased fecal bacterial biodiversity among patients with CD in remission. Notable demonstration of the relative instability of the fecal microbiota in quiescent CD over 3 months, highlighting a methodological limitation of assessing fecal microbiota at a single point in time in studies of IBD. Some suggestion that greater instability may predict relapse but no specific microbial group implicated
Gophna et al[19]	CD (n = 6) UC (n = 5) CTRL (n = 5)	Mucosal biopsies 16S rDNA clone library	Dysbiosis in CD but not UC with enrichment of Proteobacteria and Bacteroidetes, but depletion of Clostridia. Microbiotas from inflamed and noninflamed site were similar within individuals with CD
Martinez-Medina et al[20]	CD (n = 19) UC (n = 2) CTRL (n = 15)	Mucosal biopsies 16S rDNA PCR-DGGE	Microbiota of CD patients distinct from UC and healthy subjects. Higher interindividual variability of microbiota among CD patients. CD enriched in *E coli* and certain species of Clostridia but deficient in *Faecalibacterium*
Sokol et al[21]	UC (n = 10)	Mucosal biopsies 16S rDNA PCR-TGGE	Biopsy-associated microbiota of inflamed and noninflamed tissue was 95% similar within an individual; There was no stereotypical microbiota that characterized UC patients
Vasquez et al[22]	CD (n = 22)	Surgical specimens ileum 16S rDNA FISH/TGGE	No significant differences in mucosa-associated bacterial populations between inflamed and adjacent noninflamed ileum; arguing against concept of localized dysbiosis
Frank et al[23]	CD (n = 35) UC (n = 55) CTRL (n = 34)	Surgical specimens Broad-range PCR; qPCR	Microbiota of most IBD patients clustered with non-IBD controls but there was a distinct subset of IBD patients (both UC and CD) that clustered together on basis of depletion of Firmicutes and Bacteroidetes. *Mycobacterium avium paratuberculosis* or other specific pathogens were not detected in any patient
Baumgart et al[24]	CD ileal (n = 13) CD colonic (n = 8) CTRL (n = 7)	Mucosal biopsies 16S rDNA clone library qPCR; FISH	*E coli* enriched but Clostridiales depleted in inflamed terminal ileum but not colonic CD. These *E coli* had invasive properties in vitro and shared genetic elements that define invasiveness among members of Enterobacteriaceae

(*continued on next page*)

Table 1
(continued)

Study	Patients	Methods	Summary of Main Findings
Scanlan et al[25]	CD (n = 27) UC (n = 29) CTRL (n = 44)	Fecal specimens PCR detection of methyl-coenzyme M reductase (*mcrA*) gene	Depletion of methanogens in UC and CD
Ott et al[26]	CD (n = 31) UC (n = 26) CTRL (n = 47)	Fecal and mucosal biopsy 18S rDNA DGGE	Fungi only represent about 0.02% of fecal or mucosal microbiota and composition of intestinal fungal communities in IBD is distinct from controls. There was higher fungal diversity in CD, but no disease-specific fungi were identified
Swidsinski et al[27]	CD (n = 82) UC (n = 105) CTRL (n = 32)	Paraffin-embedded punched fecal cylinders FISH microscopy to visualize bacteria and leukocytes	Dichotomous differences in number of fecal *Faecalibacterium prausnitzii* and leukocytes in the fecal-mucus transition zone in CD (low/low) and UC (high/high)
Martinez et al[28]	UC remission (n = 33) CTRL (n = 8)	Fecal specimens 16S rDNA PCR-DGGE	Lower fecal bacterial diversity among UC patients in remission. Whereas control microbiota showed long-term stability, progressive decline in similarity of UC from baseline over 1 year, suggesting lower fecal biodiversity, reduces resiliency of UC microbiota to environmental influences
Dicksved et al[29]	Monozygotic twin pairs CD (n = 6 discordant, n = 4 concordant) Healthy identical twin pairs (n = 8)	Fecal specimens 16S rDNA TRFLP	Decreased fecal bacterial diversity in CD. Specific imbalances induced in various species of Bacteroides that were selectively studied. Greater dissimilarity in microbiota in twin pairs discordant for CD than healthy controls of those concordant for CD. Study could not determine specific pattern of genetically and environmentally determined microbiota that predates development of CD
Nishikawa et al[30]	UC (n = 9) CTRL (n = 11)	Rectal biopsies 16S rDNA TRFLP	Reduced bacterial diversity in UC, mainly loss of commensal *C coccoides* subgroup organisms
Schwiertz et al[31]	Children/Adolescents CD (n = 40) UC (n = 29) CTRL (n = 25)	Fecal samples, qPCR	Decreased *F prausnitzii* and bifidobacteria in patients with active and inactive CD; increased *E coli* in active CD. No major differences in UC except for decreased bifidobacteria in active disease

Abbreviations: CD, Crohn's disease; CTRL, control subjects; DGGE, denaturing gradient gel electrophoresis; FISH, fluorescent in situ hybridization; PCR, polymerase chain reaction; qPCR, quantitative real-time PCR; TGGE, temperature gradient gel electrophoresis; TRFLP, terminal restriction fragment length polymorphism; UC, ulcerative colitis.

imbalances as a precondition of disease in genetically susceptible individuals, although the power of such comparisons within this small study was understandably limited.

Phylum Firmicutes is a major constituent of the human gut microbiota, and decreased diversity, particularly among the *Clostridium leptum* subgroup, is a major factor in the dysbiotic state that occurs in IBD. Reduced richness and abundance has been noted in *C leptum* phylotypes in patients with CD.[15,37] *Faecalibacterium prausnitzii* is a dominant member of the *C leptum* subgroup residing in close association with the gut mucosa, and seems to be specifically depleted in IBD, as shown by several investigators.[20,23,37] In patients undergoing intestinal resection for CD, reduced density of mucosa-associated *F prausnitzii* in the surgical specimen was a predictor of postoperative recurrence.[38] *F prausnitzii* has specific anti-inflammatory activities mediated by soluble factors that increase interleukin (IL)-10 production and inhibit nuclear factor (NF)-kB activation. Depletion of *F prausnitzii* and loss of its protective actions at the intestinal mucosa may be a predisposing factor in the development of chronic IBD. *F prausnitzii* is a rational candidate for probiotic development and testing in IBD.

STUDY OF THE MICROBIOME IN IBD: CHALLENGES AND OPPORTUNITIES

Conventional culture-based methods are limited when it comes to studying gut bacterial communities because of their fastidious nutrient and anaerobic requirements, and complex in situ interactions with the host and neighboring microbial colonizers that support bacterial growth and persistence. Although molecular approaches have largely replaced bacterial culture in the study of IBD microbiology in the past 10 years, cultivation methods should be maintained as complementary in studies of bacterial diversity and to detect organisms that molecular techniques fail to detect.[39] Indeed, there are numerous technical limitations of metagenomic methodologies (**Box 1**).

Box 1
Technical challenges and methodological issues surrounding metagenomic investigations in human IBD

Technical

Bias due to varying efficiency of bacterial nucleic acid extraction

Inherent PCR biases leading to underrepresentation or failed detection of minor phylotypes

16S rRNA gene does not accurately reflect bacterial abundance (varying copy numbers)

DNA-based techniques do not distinguish bacteria as dead or alive, autochthonous or allochthonous

Metagenomic studies in IBD have not yet assessed functional aspects of microbiome

Methodological

Patient selection (stage of disease, phenotype)

Genotype of patients in face of ever-growing number of IBD-associated genes

Confounding influence of drug treatment and diet

Contamination during sample collection

Effect of fasting and precolonoscopy bowel cleansing on relevant microbiota

Validity of mucosal biopsies as representation of "mucosa-associated" microbiota

Moving target: temporal instability of IBD microbiota

Furthermore, there are distinct methodological challenges to accurately defining the human intestinal microbiome in IBD in terms of which patients to study (eg, genotype, phenotype, stage of disease, and confounding influences of drug treatment and diet), which samples to collect (eg, fecal, endoscopic mucosal biopsy, surgical) and how to avoid contamination with irrelevant microbes during sample collection (eg, gut luminal or endoscope channel contamination of mucosal biopsies).

Further difficulties inherent to the search for microbial triggers of IBD are illustrated in **Fig. 1**. It is possible that certain subsets of IBD have a distinct, single microbial cause and that this microbe persists and perpetuates disease but has escaped recognition or discovery by available means (see **Fig. 1**A). However, it is equally plausible that a pathogen could incite the disease and be cleared by the time the disease has evolved to be clinically recognizable, in which case failed restoration of gut homeostasis is the perpetuating factor, and the inciting organism is no longer detectable (see **Fig. 1**B). If dysbiosis were at play, the primary state of imbalance that spawns the disease may be very different from the dysbiosis that many studies describe and could, to some degree, be a secondary phenomenon.

IBD likely has a long preclinical phase making the earliest immunologic and microbiologic events in the genesis of disease remote from the time of diagnosis. Study of CD after ileocolonic resection is effectively a model of the early events in CD pathogenesis. Postoperative recurrence of CD occurs in a substantial percentage of patients at the surgical anastomosis within 1 year of operative cure. Neut and colleagues[40] studied the microbiota of ileocolectomy specimens and subsequent

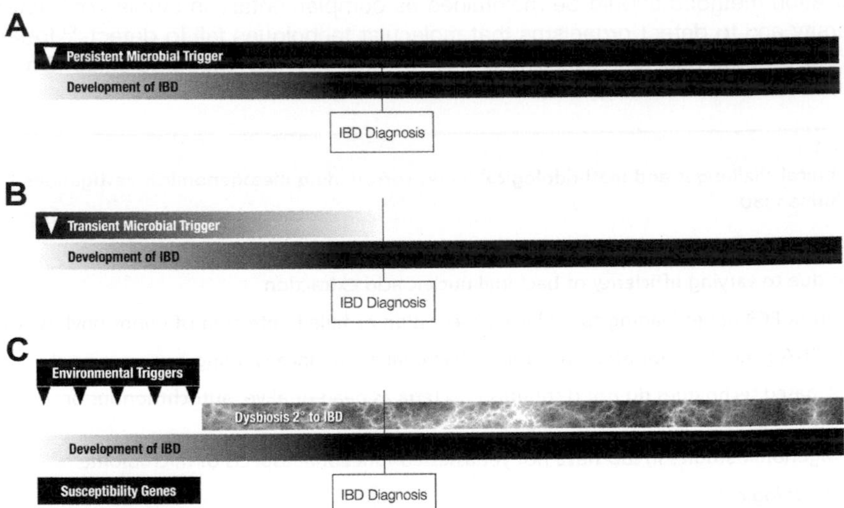

Fig. 1. Hypothetical scenarios for early events in IBD pathogenesis, highlighting the inherent challenges of identifying specific microbial triggers of IBD. (*A*) If certain subsets of IBD exist that are triggered by specific microbial pathogens that persist after development of IBD, recognition of such causative agents should be possible but at this point may simply be obscured by technical or methodological limitations. (*B*) Specific early microbial events in IBD pathogenesis may only be transient but essential triggers of a then self-perpetuating process, and are no longer present by the time that clinical disease occurs. (*C*) Environmental and immunogenetic factors are the dominant cause of IBD and microbial factors may be irrelevant, relegating much of the existing data on the microbiology of IBD to epiphenomena.

endoscopic biopsies in patients with CD. These investigators found that *E coli*, bacteroides, and fusobacteria were found in greater numbers in resected bowel from CD patients than controls (patients undergoing similar surgery for colon cancer) and correlated with early recurrence of CD.

Finally, one must consider the possibility that microbes have no role in IBD at all and that culprit environmental and immunologic triggers conspire to produce a disease in which dysbiosis is simply a reactive process (see **Fig. 1**C). Rather than an etiologic agent, the role of bacteria in IBD may be limited to one of a complicating factor, causing abscess and fistulization in perforating phenotypes of CD.

MYCOBACTERIUM AVIUM SUBSPECIES *PARATUBERCULOSIS*

As far as putative microbial causes of IBD, none has captured greater attention than MAP. MAP is the cause of Johne's disease in cattle, a chronic granulomatous enteritis that is clinically and pathologically reminiscent of Crohn's enteritis in humans. The identification of MAP in patients with CD implicates MAP as an etiologic agent. Systematic reviews and meta-analyses of recent studies employing valid design and methodology confirm the consistency and magnitude of this association.[41] Most studies do not show an association of MAP with UC, suggesting that the presence of MAP is not simply an epiphenomenon whereby an environmental mycobacterium takes hold at ulcerated and inflamed mucosa in a nonspecific fashion. It has been suggested that the source of MAP in humans may be environmental or zoonotic. Of particular concern are reports of the presence of MAP DNA or even viable MAP in milk at the retail level.[42]

Some investigators presently contend that MAP is causally related to CD, even citing that Koch's postulates have been fulfilled,[43] and clinical trials[41] and case series[44] have demonstrated long-term clinical, endoscopic, and histologic remission in select CD patients given anti-MAP therapies. Critics of these findings cite methodological issues that cast questions on the association between MAP and CD and that, even if this were a true association, causality remains unproven. As such, much controversy and debate continues in this field. Many have pointed to well-designed clinical trials of antimycobacterial therapy in CD as important in settling this debate.[45,46]

A large, randomized, controlled trial (RCT) using combination antibiotics with demonstrated efficacy against MAP (clarithromycin, clofazimine, and rifabutin) was in fact performed by the Australian Antibiotics in Crohn's Disease Study Group and reported by Selby and colleagues.[47] In this study, although antibiotics did produce a clinically meaningful increase in steroid-induced remission, there was no significant effect on maintenance of remission. The intent of long-term anti-MAP antibiotics was to eradicate MAP and to determine whether CD is causally related or at least dependent in some fashion on infection with MAP. However, the design of the trial would not have allowed for any meaningful conclusions to be drawn in this regard, mainly because patients selected for study were not assessed for the presence of MAP at study entry. A "test-and-treat" approach would have added an important strength to their design and statistical power to their conclusions.

Considerable work continues on MAP, mainly in the arena of veterinary medicine and infectious disease. Johne's disease has a major economic impact on the ranching and dairy industries in many countries, and there has been a proliferation of literature in the last 5 years on basic mycobacterial pathogenesis in Johne's disease. Better understanding of how MAP triggers chronic enteritis in cattle, and studies in highly selected subsets of "MAP-associated" CD in which known IBD genes are taken in to account, will hopefully provide some greater clarity in the field of IBD, which remains charged with controversy and skepticism.

ADHERENT-INVASIVE STRAINS OF *ESCHERICHIA COLI*

E coli is the main aerobe in the normal human intestinal microbiota. As shown in **Table 1**, increased abundance of *E coli* has been a remarkably consistent finding in IBD patients. Biopsy samples taken from IBD patients were found to contain 3 to 4 log units more Enterobacteriaceae compared with biopsies taken from healthy control patients.[48] In particular, CD patients have high numbers of *E coli* associated with early CD lesions. In one study, 100% of biopsy specimens from early CD lesions (postoperative recurrence) contained *E coli* compared with 65% of specimens obtained from chronic lesions (ileal resection).[49] These data suggest that *E coli* may play a role in the initiation of inflammation that is characteristic of CD. A separate study revealed that 99% of all invasive bacteria recovered from CD biopsies were *E coli* strains.[50] Of the 4 main phylogenetic groups of *E coli*, groups B2 and D are more pathogenic.[48] *E coli* strains recovered from IBD patients are predominantly of these 2 phylotypes.[51]

LF82 is a reference strain of invasive *E coli* recovered from a CD chronic lesion that is capable of invading intestinal epithelial cells.[52] LF82 belongs to the *E coli* serotype O83:H1.[53] LF82 does not possess the genes for intimin (EPEC), invasion effector IpaC (EIEC), Tia (EHEC),[53] or other virulence factors found in EAEC and ETEC.[49,54] For these reasons, LF82 and other invasive CD-associated *E coli* strains have been grouped together under the name adherent-invasive *E coli* (AIEC). AIEC strains are unique in that they have a specific phenotype. These bacteria can adhere to and invade intestinal epithelial cells, survive and replicate in macrophages without causing cell death, and induce the secretion of tumor necrosis factor (TNF)-α.

Adherence

AIEC strains express type 1 pili. These pili bind to eukaryotic cell mannose receptors. The presence of free mannose inhibits this binding. Some studies found that AIEC strains associated with the ileal mucosa of CD patients are still able to adhere to eukaryotic cells in the presence of D-mannose,[49] suggesting that other adhesins are also involved. The same study found that 73% of *E coli* strains isolated from CD patients possess an adhesin that is not identifiable by molecular techniques. A different study found that the presence of D-mannose blocked adherence of LF82 along with 4 other AIEC strains, suggesting that type 1 pili binds to glycosylated host receptors.[52] FimH is the adhesive subunit of the type 1 pilus. AIEC were found to have 4 amino acid substitutions in the *fim*H sequence.[55] These variant type 1 pili have FimH homologies to 2 virulent *E coli* strains: avian MT78 and a K-1 strain, IHE3034.[56,57]

CD-associated AIEC strains are capable of adhering to ileal enterocytes recovered from CD patients, but not from control patient enterocytes.[52] CD patients exhibit a high level of glycosylated CEACAM5 (carcinoembryonic antigen–related cell adhesion molecule) and CEACAM6 molecules throughout the ileum, although only antibodies against CEACAM6 prevent AIEC from adhering to CD enterocytes.[52] The amino acid changes in AIEC's *fim*H sequence may facilitate binding to CEACAM6.[55] The expression of CEACAM6 can be increased by TNF-α, interferon-γ, and AIEC infection. What remains to be known is whether AIEC induces the expression of CEACAM6 or whether increased expression of CEACAM6 induces the colonization of AIEC. It has been proposed that patients with a basal level of CEACAM6 expression may be predisposed to CD and that CEACAM6 expression could be used as a diagnostic marker.[52]

CD patients have very high concentrations of biofilm-forming bacteria associated with the gut mucosa.[58] AIEC strains have stronger biofilm formation abilities than other *E coli* strains isolated from the gastrointestinal tract.[51] It has been hypothesized that the machinery that makes AIEC pathogenic, such as flagellum and type 1 pili, are also involved in biofilm formation.[51] Recently AIEC's OmpC, regulated by the EnvX/OmpR pathway, has been shown to play a role in the bacterium's ability to adhere to and invade intestinal epithelial cells.[59] Anti–*E coli* OmpC antibodies are found in high number in nearly half of CD patients.[59] The EnvX/OmpR pathway is also involved in biofilm formation. A more stable colonization of AIEC on intestinal epithelial cells would increase the chance of invasion, leading to more immune stimulation. Thus biofilm formation could be a major factor in AIEC's pathogenesis.[51]

Invasion

AIEC invade intestinal epithelial cells via a macropinocytosis-like entry.[53] The variant type 1 pili cause alterations in the host cell leading to bacterial internalization, a process dependent on host cytoskeletal rearrangements.[53] This entry is characterized by host cell membrane extensions that surround the invading bacteria. Once internalized, AIEC lyse the endocytic vacuole and replicate in the cytoplasm.[60]

The FimH subunit, as well as the naive fimbrial shaft, is necessary for epithelial cell invasion. Changes to the shaft prevent bacterial internalization, as does expressing LF82's variant type 1 pili on other bacteria.[56] This process suggests that other virulent factors are also involved in invasion. Flagella are also an essential virulence factor. Nonflagellated mutants cannot adhere or invade intestinal epithelial cells as efficiently as wild-type strains.[54] These mutants also were unable to induce inflammation as severely, or in some cases, at all.

Strains of AIEC are more likely to adhere and invade epithelial cells under conditions of increased osmolarity, characteristic of the intestinal tract.[59] It is proposed that increased osmolarity is sensed by the EnvZ/OmpR pathway, leading to overexpression of OmpC. This overexpression directly activates protease DegS, which acts to cleave RSA, freeing RpoE. RpoE increases its own expression and either directly or indirectly induces the expression of flagella, type 1 pili and, possibly, other virulence factors.[59]

AIEC and Macrophages

AIEC strains can survive and replicate in macrophage vacuoles.[61] AIEC are taken up by phagocytosis, and reside in phagosomes that mature into phagolysosomes where AIEC are exposed to low pH and cathepsin D. The acidic pH activates AIEC stress protein HtrA,[62] which is crucial for AIEC replication within the macrophage. HtrA not only protects AIEC from oxidative stress, but may also act as a chaperone for secreted proteins and the export of virulence factors.[62] Separate vacuoles within the same macrophage containing LF82 merge together to form one large vacuole.[60] The formation of the large vacuole could be a survival mechanism. Within a larger vacuole the toxic compounds are more dilute and the acidic pH is not as severe.[60]

Unlike the epithelial cell invasion, the uptake of LF82 by macrophages is not dependent on expression of the variant type 1 pili. Type 1 pili–negative mutants are taken up by macrophages, and were able to survive and replicate within the phagolysosome at similar rates as the wild-type strain.[60] It is hypothesized that continued replication of AIEC within macrophages causes secretion of a large amount of TNF-α.[60] TNF-α induces enterocytes to overexpress CEACAM6, which allows more AIEC to adhere to and invade enterocytes, enter the lamina propria, and be taken up by macrophages, producing more TNF-α.[63] Thus AIEC are capable of increasing their own colonization through this feedback loop.

E coli strains from both CD and UC induce the release of IL-8, a neutrophil chemoattractant.[50,54] Of note, LF82 was found to induce secretion of IL-8 from the apical surface of intestinal epithelial cells and another AIEC strain (O83:H1) induced the cells to secrete IL-8 from the basolateral surface.[54] The same study found that AIEC also induces the secretion of CCL20, a dendritic cell chemoattractant. The NF-kB pathway is responsible for IL-8 and CCL20 production along with other cytokines, which suggests that AIEC may recruit inflammatory cells in CD through this pathway.

Evolution

There are many hypotheses as to how AIEC evolved and what they evolved from. One study proposed that AIEC are extraintestinal pathogens that evolved to better suit their microenvironment, the intestinal tract.[55] Another study suggests that AIEC evolved from nonpathogenic *E coli* by developing adaptation mechanisms, and that high osmolarity or acidic macrophage environment act as signals to express virulence factors.[59,64]

There has been tremendous advancement in discovery of genes associated with the development of IBD, which has become a model for identifying polygenic disease susceptibilities.[65] Of importance, among these are host genes involved in bacterial sensing and degradation such as NOD2 (nucleotide oligomerization domain 2) and autophagy genes (IRGM and ATG16L1). Recently, autophagy-deficient epithelial cells were observed to have a significantly increased number of intracellular AIEC compared with cells with an active autophagic process.[66] The same study discovered a subpopulation of intracellular AIEC within epithelial cell autosomes, which suggests that active autophagy can limit AIEC replication. This possibility obviously adds credence to the theory of a microbial cause of IBD and genetically determined defects in the handling of invasive bacteria at the intestinal mucosa may be the link between IBD and AIEC. AIEC are harbored by healthy subjects, which suggests that AIEC are opportunistic pathogens that are capable of causing disease in susceptible hosts.[67]

SUMMARY

IBD is a prevalent and serious chronic disease in which gut microbes very likely have a major role in cause and development. Current therapies are focused on interrupting inflammatory signaling pathways, and greater specificity of this approach in recent years (eg, anti–TNF-α agents) has led to remarkable advancement in the treatment of these diseases. However, the essential microbial, environmental, and immunologic triggers remain elusive and therefore immunosuppressive treatments are generally required in these patients in the long term. Advanced molecular tools for characterizing complex microbial consortia in the gut have been applied over the past decade to identify microbial factors and host interplay that conspire to produce IBD. The overall goal remains to identify specific agents or dysbiotic states that are amenable to remediation by antibiotics or pharmabiotics (probiotics, prebiotics, and so forth) as primary or adjunctive therapies in IBD.

The long-known overabundance of *E coli* associated with IBD has led to identification of several aggressive strains of *E coli* in patients with IBD. AIEC has been a very productive and elegant line of investigation following rational paradigms for study of bacterial pathogenesis. Strong evidence of the disease causing potential of these strains has come from recent experiments in transgenic mice expressing human

CEACAMs in which infection with AIEC LF82 induced severe colitis.[68] These data will translate into mechanistically guided therapeutic trials of probiotics, bacterial adhesion antagonists or host receptor antagonists, or adhesin-based vaccines to treat or prevent CD. By comparison, the MAP story in CD has languished in recent years, and the recent anti-MAP antibiotics trials have not been a way forward. Going first to the bench to better understand basic mechanisms of MAP pathogenesis and improved means of clinical detection of MAP in the context of veterinary disease may yield new principles to revisit this putative agent of CD. A more focused search for MAP in highly selected, immunogenetically defined cases of CD, perhaps even looking outside the luminal gastrointestinal tract, may provide some clarity in this matter.[69,70]

As highlighted earlier, studying the microbiota in humans with IBD has many challenges. Host genetics determine to some degree the variability in intestinal microbiota observed among healthy individuals, and is compounded by day-to-day environmental influences of diet and exposure to other microbes. Factors involved in gut microbiota assembly and dynamics will best be defined in animal systems in which host genotype and diet can be constrained. In a similar vein, further study of identical twins that are concordant or discordant for IBD will control for genetic influences and enable dissection of microbial, environmental, and perhaps epigenetic factors that precede IBD. Further study of postoperative recurrence of IBD will likely yield important clues about early immunologic and microbial events in IBD pathogenesis in genetically defined and predisposed individuals. The Human Microbiome Project will substantially advance knowledge of the human gastrointestinal microbiota in health and IBD, and IBD metagenomics will continue to be informed by ever advancing sequencing capacity, phylogenetic resolution, and bioinformatics approaches. Systems biology will frontier new knowledge of the functional capabilities of gut microbial ecosystems by reconstructing and modeling host-bacterial networks from molecular data.

REFERENCES

1. Palmer C, Bik E, Digiulio D, et al. Development of the human infant intestinal microbiota. PLoS Biol 2007;5(7):e177.
2. Tamboli CP, Neut C, Desreumaux P, et al. Dysbiosis in inflammatory bowel disease. Gut 2004;53(1):1–4.
3. Zhang L, Man SM, Day AS, et al. Detection and isolation of *Campylobacter* species other than *C. jejuni* from children with Crohn's disease. J Clin Microbiol 2009;47(2):453–5.
4. Podolsky S. Cultural divergence: Elie Metchnikoff's *Bacillus bulgaricus* therapy and his underlying concept of health. Bull Hist Med 1998;72(1):1–27.
5. Van de Merwe JP, Schröder AM, Wensinck F, et al. The obligate anaerobic faecal flora of patients with Crohn's disease and their first-degree relatives. Scand J Gastroenterol 1988;23(9):1125–31.
6. Giaffer MH, Holdsworth CD, Duerden BI. The assessment of faecal flora in patients with inflammatory bowel disease by a simplified bacteriological technique. J Med Microbiol 1991;35(4):238–43.
7. van der Wiel-Korstanje JA, Winkler KC. The faecal flora in ulcerative colitis. J Med Microbiol 1975;8(4):491–501.
8. Sartor RB. Therapeutic correction of bacterial dysbiosis discovered by molecular techniques. Proc Natl Acad Sci U S A 2008;105(43):16413–4.

9. Seksik P, Rigottier-Gois L, Gramet G, et al. Alterations of the dominant faecal bacterial groups in patients with Crohn's disease of the colon. Gut 2003;52(2): 237–42.
10. Bullock NR, Booth JCL, Gibson GR. Comparative composition of bacteria in the human intestinal microflora during remission and active ulcerative colitis. Curr Issues Intest Microbiol 2004;5(2):59–64.
11. Mangin I, Bonnet R, Seksik P, et al. Molecular inventory of faecal microflora in patients with Crohn's disease. FEMS Microbiol Ecol 2004;50(1):25–36.
12. Prindiville T, Cantrell M, Wilson KH. Ribosomal DNA sequence analysis of mucosa-associated bacteria in Crohn's disease. Inflamm Bowel Dis 2004;10(6): 824–33.
13. Mylonaki M, Rayment NB, Rampton DS, et al. Molecular characterization of rectal mucosa-associated bacterial flora in inflammatory bowel disease. Inflamm Bowel Dis 2005;11(5):481–7.
14. Lepage P, Seksik P, Sutren M, et al. Biodiversity of the mucosa-associated microbiota is stable along the distal digestive tract in healthy individuals and patients with IBD. Inflamm Bowel Dis 2005;11(5):473–80.
15. Manichanh C, Rigottier-Gois L, Bonnaud E, et al. Reduced diversity of faecal microbiota in Crohn's disease revealed by a metagenomic approach. Gut 2006;55(2):205–11.
16. Bibiloni R, Mangold M, Madsen KL, et al. The bacteriology of biopsies differs between newly diagnosed, untreated, Crohn's disease and ulcerative colitis patients. J Med Microbiol 2006;55(Pt 8):1141–9.
17. Sokol H, Lepage P, Seksik P, et al. Temperature gradient gel electrophoresis of fecal 16S rRNA reveals active *Escherichia coli* in the microbiota of patients with ulcerative colitis. J Clin Microbiol 2006;44(9):3172–7.
18. Scanlan PD, Shanahan F, O'Mahony C, et al. Culture-independent analyses of temporal variation of the dominant fecal microbiota and targeted bacterial subgroups in Crohn's disease. J Clin Microbiol 2006;44(11):3980–8.
19. Gophna U, Sommerfeld K, Gophna S, et al. Differences between tissue-associated intestinal microfloras of patients with Crohn's disease and ulcerative colitis. J Clin Microbiol 2006;44(11):4136–41.
20. Martinez-Medina M, Aldeguer X, Gonzalez-Huix F, et al. Abnormal microbiota composition in the ileocolonic mucosa of Crohn's disease patients as revealed by polymerase chain reaction-denaturing gradient gel electrophoresis. Inflamm Bowel Dis 2006;12(12):1136–45.
21. Sokol H, Lepage P, Seksik P, et al. Molecular comparison of dominant microbiota associated with injured versus healthy mucosa in ulcerative colitis. Gut 2007; 56(1):152–4.
22. Vasquez N, Mangin I, Lepage P, et al. Patchy distribution of mucosal lesions in ileal Crohn's disease is not linked to differences in the dominant mucosa-associated bacteria: a study using fluorescence in situ hybridization and temporal temperature gradient gel electrophoresis. Inflamm Bowel Dis 2007;13(6): 684–92.
23. Frank DN, St Amand AL, Feldman RA, et al. Molecular-phylogenetic characterization of microbial community imbalances in human inflammatory bowel diseases. Proc Natl Acad Sci U S A 2007;104(34):13780–5.
24. Baumgart M, Dogan B, Rishniw M, et al. Culture independent analysis of ileal mucosa reveals a selective increase in invasive *Escherichia coli* of novel phylogeny relative to depletion of clostridiales in Crohn's disease involving the ileum. ISME J 2007;1(5):403–18.

25. Scanlan PD, Shanahan F, Marchesi JR. Human methanogen diversity and incidence in healthy and diseased colonic groups using McrA gene analysis. BMC Microbiol 2008;8:79.
26. Ott SJ, Kühbacher T, Musfeldt M, et al. Fungi and inflammatory bowel diseases: alterations of composition and diversity. Scand J Gastroenterol 2008;43(7): 831–41.
27. Swidsinski A, Loening-Baucke V, Vaneechoutte M, et al. Active Crohn's disease and ulcerative colitis can be specifically diagnosed and monitored based on the biostructure of the fecal flora. Inflamm Bowel Dis 2008;14(2):147–61.
28. Martinez C, Antolin M, Santos J, et al. Unstable composition of the fecal microbiota in ulcerative colitis during clinical remission. Am J Gastroenterol 2008; 103(3):643–8.
29. Dicksved J, Halfvarson J, Rosenquist M, et al. Molecular analysis of the gut microbiota of identical twins with Crohn's disease. ISME J 2008;2(7):716–27.
30. Nishikawa J, Kudo T, Sakata S, et al. Diversity of mucosa-associated microbiota in active and inactive ulcerative colitis. Scand J Gastroenterol 2009;44(2):180–6.
31. Schwiertz A, Jacobi M, Frick J-S, et al. Microbiota in pediatric inflammatory bowel disease. J Pediatr 2010;157: 240–4, e1.
32. Balamurugan R, Janardhan HP, George S, et al. Molecular studies of fecal anaerobic commensal bacteria in acute diarrhea in children. J Pediatr Gastroenterol Nutr 2008;46(5):514–9.
33. Manichanh C, Varela E, Martinez C, et al. The gut microbiota predispose to the pathophysiology of acute postradiotherapy diarrhea. Am J Gastroenterol 2008; 103(7):1754–61.
34. Swidsinski A, Loening-Baucke V, Verstraelen H, et al. Biostructure of fecal microbiota in healthy subjects and patients with chronic idiopathic diarrhea. Gastroenterology 2008;135(2):568–79.
35. Kassinen A, Krogius-Kurikka L, Mäkivuokko H, et al. The fecal microbiota of irritable bowel syndrome patients differs significantly from that of healthy subjects. Gastroenterology 2007;133(1):24–33.
36. Ley RE, Peterson DA, Gordon JI. Ecological and evolutionary forces shaping microbial diversity in the human intestine. Cell 2006;124(4):837–48.
37. Sokol H, Seksik P, Rigottier-Gois L, et al. Specificities of the fecal microbiota in inflammatory bowel disease. Inflamm Bowel Dis 2006;12(2):106–11.
38. Sokol H, Seksik P, Furet J, et al. Low counts of *Faecalibacterium prausnitzii* in colitis microbiota. Inflamm Bowel Dis 2009;15:1183–9.
39. Donachie SP, Foster JS, Brown MV. Culture clash: challenging the dogma of microbial diversity. ISME J 2007;1(2):97–9.
40. Neut C, Bulois P, Desreumaux P, et al. Changes in the bacterial flora of the neoterminal ileum after ileocolonic resection for Crohn's disease. Am J Gastroenterol 2002;97(4):939–46.
41. Feller M, Huwiler K, Stephan R, et al. *Mycobacterium avium* subspecies paratuberculosis and Crohn's disease: a systematic review and meta-analysis. Lancet Infect Dis 2007;7(9):607–13.
42. Cerf O, Griffiths M, Aziza F. Assessment of the prevalence of *Mycobacterium avium* subsp. *paratuberculosis* in commercially pasteurized milk. Foodborne Pathog Dis 2007;4(4):433–47.
43. Chamberlin W, Borody T, Naser S. Map-associated Crohn's disease map, Koch's postulates, causality and Crohn's disease. Dig Liver Dis 2007;39(8):792–4.
44. Borody TJ, Bilkey S, Wettstein AR, et al. Anti-mycobacterial therapy in Crohn's disease heals mucosa with longitudinal scars. Dig Liver Dis 2007;39(5):438–44.

45. Sartor RB. Does *Mycobacterium avium* subspecies *paratuberculosis* cause Crohn's disease? Gut 2005;54(7):896–8.
46. Shanahan F, O'mahony J. The mycobacteria story in Crohn's disease. Am J Gastroenterol 2005;100(7):1537–8.
47. Selby W, Pavli P, Crotty B, et al. Two-year combination antibiotic therapy with clarithromycin, rifabutin, and clofazimine for Crohn's disease. Gastroenterology 2007; 132(7):2313–9.
48. Kotlowski R, Bernstein CN, Sepehri S, et al. High prevalence of *Escherichia coli* belonging to the B2+D phylogenetic group in inflammatory bowel disease. Gut 2007;56(5):669–75.
49. Darfeuille-Michaud A, Neut C, Barnich N, et al. Presence of adherent *Escherichia coli* strains in ileal mucosa of patients with Crohn's disease. Gastroenterology 1998;115(6):1405–13.
50. Sasaki M, Sitaraman SV, Babbin BA, et al. Invasive *Escherichia coli* are a feature of Crohn's disease. Lab Invest 2007;87(10):1042–54.
51. Martinez-Medina M, Naves P, Blanco J, et al. Biofilm formation as a novel phenotypic feature of adherent-invasive *Escherichia coli* (AIEC). BMC Microbiol 2009; 9(1):202.
52. Barnich N, Carvalho FA, Glasser AL, et al. Ceacam6 acts as a receptor for adherent-invasive *E. coli*, supporting ileal mucosa colonization in Crohn disease. J Clin Invest 2007;117(6):1566–74.
53. Boudeau J, Glasser AL, Masseret E, et al. Invasive ability of an *Escherichia coli* strain isolated from the ileal mucosa of a patient with Crohn's disease. Infect Immun 1999;67(9):4499–509.
54. Eaves-Pyles T, Allen CA, Taormina J, et al. *Escherichia coli* isolated from a Crohn's disease patient adheres, invades, and induces inflammatory responses in polarized intestinal epithelial cells. Int J Med Microbiol 2008;298(5–6):397–409.
55. Sepehri S, Kotlowski R, Bernstein CN, et al. Phylogenetic analysis of inflammatory bowel disease associated *Escherichia coli* and the FimH virulence determinant. Inflamm Bowel Dis 2009;15:1737–45.
56. Boudeau J, Barnich N, Darfeuille-Michaud A. Type 1 pili-mediated adherence of *Escherichia coli* strain LF82 isolated from Crohn's disease is involved in bacterial invasion of intestinal epithelial cells. Mol Microbiol 2001;39(5):1272–84.
57. Martinez-Medina M, Aldeguer X, Lopez-Siles M, et al. Molecular diversity of *Escherichia coli* in the human gut: new ecological evidence supporting the role of adherent-invasive *E. coli* (AIEC) in Crohn's disease. Inflamm Bowel Dis 2009; 15(6):872–82.
58. Swidsinski A, Loening-Baucke V, Bengmark S, et al. Azathioprine and mesalazine-induced effects on the mucosal flora in patients with IBD colitis. Inflamm Bowel Dis 2007;13(1):51–6.
59. Rolhion N, Carvalho FA, Darfeuille-Michaud A. OMPC and the sigma(e) regulatory pathway are involved in adhesion and invasion of the Crohn's disease-associated *Escherichia coli* strain lf82. Mol Microbiol 2007;63(6):1684–700.
60. Glasser AL, Boudeau J, Barnich N, et al. Adherent invasive *Escherichia coli* strains from patients with Crohn's disease survive and replicate within macrophages without inducing host cell death. Infect Immun 2001;69(9): 5529–37.
61. Bringer MA, Rolhion N, Glasser AL, et al. The oxidoreductase DSBA plays a key role in the ability of the Crohn's disease-associated adherent-invasive *Escherichia coli* strain LF82 to resist macrophage killing. J Bacteriol 2007;189(13): 4860–71.

62. Bringer MA, Barnich N, Glasser AL, et al. Htra stress protein is involved in intra-macrophagic replication of adherent and invasive *Escherichia coli* strain LF82 isolated from a patient with Crohn's disease. Infect Immun 2005;73(2):712–21.
63. Glasser AL, Darfeuille-Michaud A. Abnormalities in the handling of intracellular bacteria in Crohn's disease: a link between infectious etiology and host genetic susceptibility. Arch Immunol Ther Exp (Warsz) 2008;56(4):237–44.
64. Bringer MA, Glasser AL, Tung CH, et al. The Crohn's disease-associated adherent-invasive *Escherichia coli* strain LF82 replicates in mature phagolysosomes within J774 macrophages. Cell Microbiol 2006;8(3):471–84.
65. Achkar JP, Duerr R. The expanding universe of inflammatory bowel disease genetics. Curr Opin Gastroenterol 2008;24(4):429–34.
66. Lapaquette P, Glasser AL, Huett A, et al. Crohn's disease-associated adherent-invasive *E. coli* are selectively favoured by impaired autophagy to replicate intracellularly. Cell Microbiol 2010;12(1):99–113.
67. Barnich N, Denizot J, Darfeuille-Michaud A. *E. coli*-mediated gut inflammation in genetically predisposed Crohn's disease patients. Pathol Biol (Paris) 2010. DOI: 10.1016/j.patbio.2010.01.004.
68. Carvalho FA, Barnich N, Sivignon A, et al. Crohn's disease adherent-invasive *Escherichia coli* colonize and induce strong gut inflammation in transgenic mice expressing human ceacam. J Exp Med 2009;206(10):2179–89.
69. Pierce E, Finlay B. Where are all the *Mycobacterium avium* subspecies *paratuberculosis* in patients with Crohn's disease? PLoS Pathog 2009;5(3):e1000234.
70. Behr MA. The path to Crohn's disease: is mucosal pathology a secondary event? Inflamm Bowel Dis 2010;16(5):896–902.

Infectious Causes of Appendicitis

Laura W. Lamps, MD

KEYWORDS

- Appendicitis • Infectious appendicitis
- Granulomatous appendicitis • Bacterial appendicitis
- Fungal appendicitis • Viral appendicitis • Parasitic appendicitis

The pathologic spectrum of the inflamed appendix encompasses a wide range of infectious entities, some with specific histologic findings, and others with nonspecific findings that may require an extensive diagnostic evaluation. The appendix is exclusively involved in some of these disorders, and in others may be involved through extension from other areas of the gastrointestinal (GI) tract. The numerous viral, bacterial, fungal, and parasitic organisms that may infect the appendix are summarized in **Table 1**.

VIRAL INFECTIONS OF THE APPENDIX

Adenovirus

Adenovirus is one of the more common viruses described in the appendix.[1–5] It is also associated with ileal and ileocecal intussusception, particularly in children.[1–4] The virus is believed to cause intussusception by producing lymphoid hyperplasia, altering intestinal motility, or a combination of both. Most patients do not have symptoms of appendicitis, and adenovirus is usually found after segmental resection for intussusception.[1–4] There is no specific antiviral therapy for treatment of enteric adenovirus, but most patients do well following surgery for intussusception.

Pathologic features

Morphologic changes are subtle, including lymphoid hyperplasia (**Fig. 1**) and overlying disorderly proliferation and degeneration of surface epithelium.[1–7] In the appendix, inclusions are reportedly found on routine stains in only one-third of patients with intussusception in which adenovirus is detected by other methods, such as immunohistochemistry, polymerase chain reaction (PCR), and in situ hybridization.[1–4] The most common adenovirus inclusions, known as smudge cells, have enlarged, basophilic nuclei without a clear nuclear membrane (**Fig. 2**).[2,4,6,7] Homogenous, eosinophilic inclusions surrounded by halos with distinct nuclear membranes (Cowdry A-type) are less common. Adenovirus inclusions are exclusively intranuclear, and fill

Department of Pathology, University of Arkansas for Medical Sciences, 4301 West Markham Street, Slot 517, Shorey Building, 4S/09, Little Rock, AR 72205, USA
E-mail address: lampslauraw@uams.edu

Infect Dis Clin N Am 24 (2010) 995–1018
doi:10.1016/j.idc.2010.07.012
id.theclinics.com
0891-5520/10/$ – see front matter

Table 1
Summary of Infections Involving the Appendix

Viruses	Bacteria	Fungi	Parasites
Measles	*Salmonella* sp (both typhoid and nontyphoid)	Mucormycosis	*Enterobius vermicularis* (pinworm)
Adenovirus	*Shigella* sp	Histoplasmosis	Schistosomes
CMV	*Yersinia* (both *Y enterocolitica* and *Y pseudotuberculosis*		*Entamoeba histolytica*
Epstein-Barr virus	*Actinomyces* sp		*Balantidium coli*
	Campylobacter sp		*Strongyloides stercoralis*
	Clostridium, including *Clostridium difficile*		*Toxoplasma*
	Mycobacteria (tuberculosis and atypical)		*Cryptosporidium*
	Rickettsia rickettsii		*Echinococcus*
			Trichuris sp (whipworms)
			Ascaris sp (roundworms)

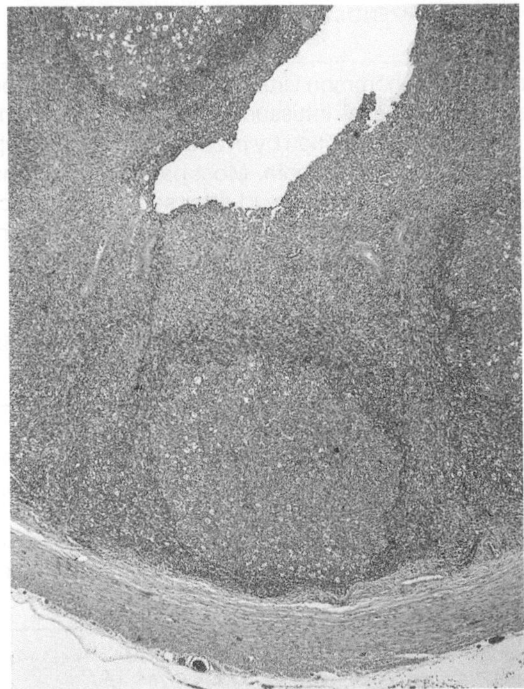

Fig. 1. Marked lymphoid hyperplasia with overlying ulceration and luminal narrowing in an appendix infected with adenovirus. Hematoxylin and eosin (H&E), original magnification ×40. To see full-color versions of all figures in this article, please go to http://www.id.theclinics.com/.

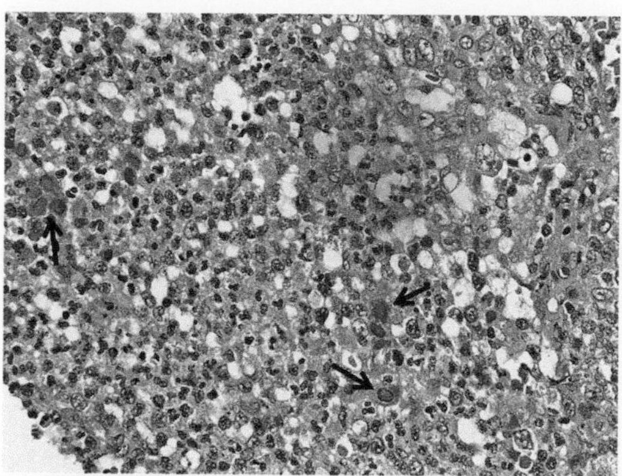

Fig. 2. Adenovirus inclusions, known as smudge cells, are seen within the nuclei of epithelial cells within the inflammatory debris. The smudge cells have homogenous basophilic nuclei with peripheral chromatin margination. H&E, original magnification ×100.

the entire nucleus; however, the cell itself is not enlarged. Inclusions are most often seen in areas with epithelial degenerative changes; inclusions may be widely scattered, with many apparently uninfected cells in between.

Useful aids in the diagnosis of adenovirus infection include immunohistochemistry (**Fig. 3**), stool and/or tissue examination by electron microscopy, and viral culture.[1–4] Positive serologies or fecal identification of the virus do not necessarily represent current infection, because viral shedding and increased serologic titers may persist for months.[5]

Differential diagnosis

The differential diagnosis of adenovirus infection is primarily with other viral infections, particularly cytomegalovirus (CMV). Adenovirus inclusions lack the owl's eye morphology of CMV, and are found primarily within epithelial rather than endothelial and stromal cells. In addition, the entire cell is enlarged in CMV infection, but not in adenovirus infection.

CMV

CMV is the most common GI pathogen in patients with AIDS. CMV is described in the appendix with increasing frequency in this population,[8–13] and it has been suggested

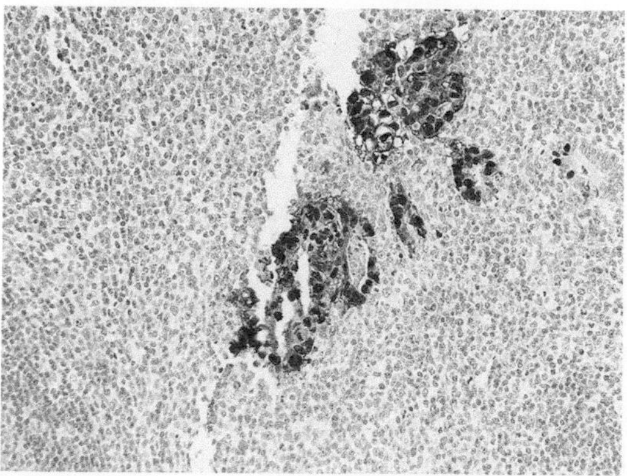

Fig. 3. Immunohistochemical stain for adenovirus highlights infected epithelial cells in the appendix. Adenovirus immunostain, original magnification ×200.

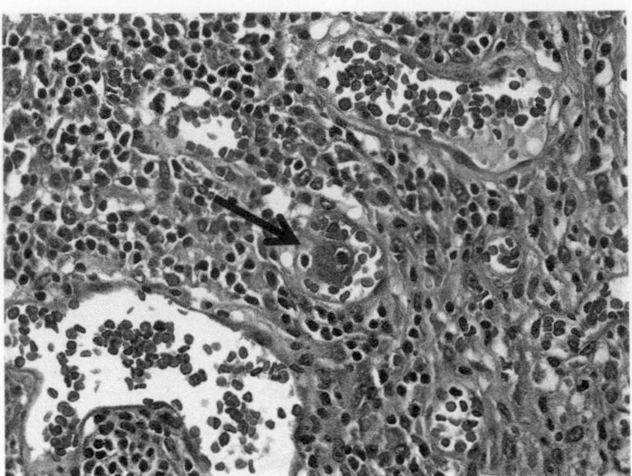

Fig. 4. The typical owl's eye inclusion of CMV, seen within a mucosal vessel. H&E, original magnification ×400.

that CMV appendicitis should be suspected in any human immunodeficiency virus (HIV)-positive patient who presents with localized right lower quadrant tenderness.[8] Patients typically present with a more prolonged prehospital course than that of immunocompetent patients with appendicitis, consisting of several weeks of fever, diarrhea, and abdominal pain and tenderness that ultimately localizes to the right lower quadrant.[8] Perforation is a common complication. In addition to surgical intervention for acute appendicitis, specific antiviral therapy (usually gancyclovir) is available, and GI CMV infection generally responds well.[14]

Pathologic features

Histologic findings include variably ulcerated appendiceal mucosa with a transmural mixed inflammatory infiltrate, including numerous histiocytes, plasma cells, and lymphocytes, in addition to neutrophils. The characteristic owl's eye inclusions (**Fig. 4**), as well as basophilic granular inclusions (**Fig. 5**), are typically seen in epithelial, endothelial, histiocytic, and stromal cells, either in intranuclear or intracytoplasmic locations.[8,9,14]

Useful diagnostic aids include immunohistochemistry, viral culture, PCR assays, in situ hybridization, and CMV serologic studies/antigen tests.[14] However, isolation of CMV in culture does not imply active infection, as virus may be excreted for months

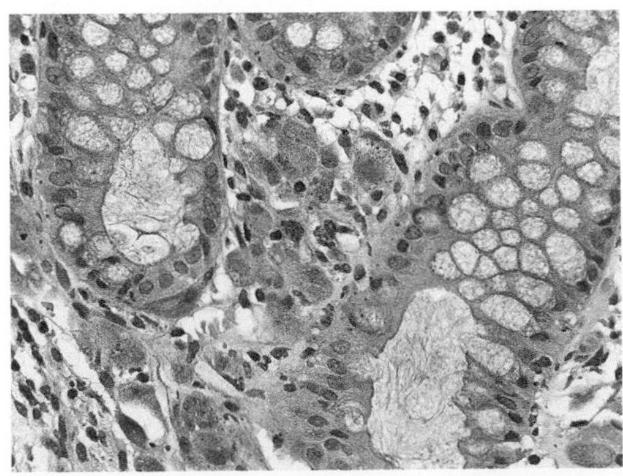

Fig. 5. Numerous basophilic CMV inclusions are seen within the lamina propria. H&E, original magnification ×200.

to years after a primary infection. The differential diagnosis is primarily that of other viral infections, particularly adenovirus (see earlier discussion).

Measles (Rubeola Virus)

Measles infection occasionally produces appendicitis and mesenteric lymphadenitis.[15–17] Histologic findings in measles-related appendicitis include lymphoid hyperplasia and multinucleate Warthin-Finkeldey giant cells (**Fig. 6**), predominantly within germinal centers; associated inflammation is variably present. Although the measles

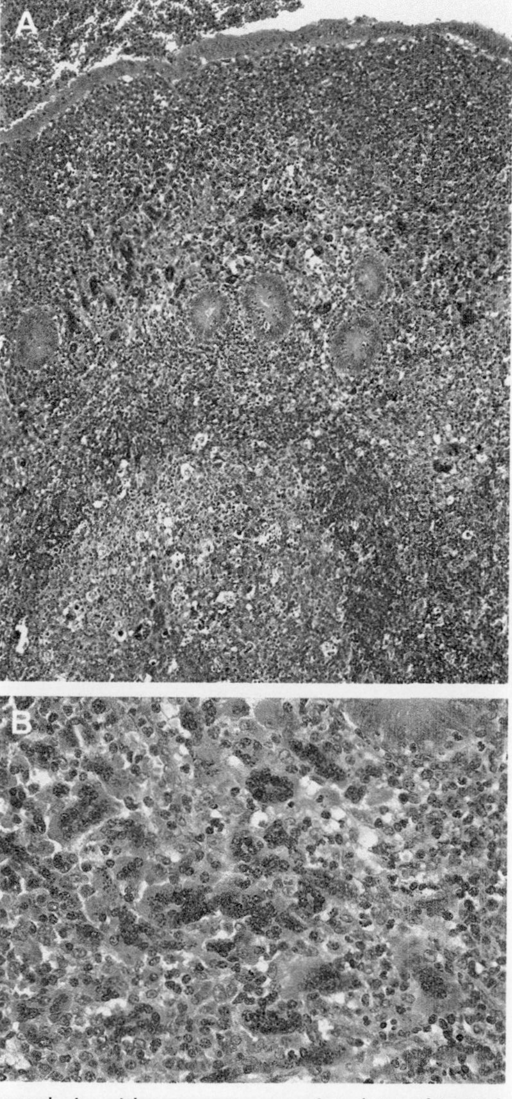

Fig. 6. Lymphoid hyperplasia with numerous associated Warthin-Finkeldey giant cells in a case of measles appendicitis. (*A*) H&E, original magnification ×40. Multinucleate Warthin-Finkeldey giant cells are seen within germinal centers. (*B*) H&E, original magnification ×400. (*Courtesy of* Dr David Owen.)

virus probably does not independently cause true appendicitis, the lymphoid hyperplasia may lead to obstruction, acute inflammation, and even gangrenous appendicitis. Patients often have a concomitant rash, although the GI morphologic findings may precede the viral xanthem, and serologic findings and immunohistochemistry can help confirm the diagnosis.

Acute appendicitis may also develop during the course of infectious mononucleosis as a result of Epstein-Barr virus infection, and changes in the appendiceal lymphoid tissue mimic those occurring in lymph nodes.[18]

SPECIFIC BACTERIAL INFECTIONS CAUSING APPENDICITIS

Numerous bacterial infections may cause appendicitis, with or without involvement of the surrounding bowel. In many of these cases, the infectious agent is determined only after removal of the appendix and careful examination for organisms, using special stains, microbiologic culture, and/or molecular methods.

Yersinia Species

Yersinia is one of the most common causes of bacterial enteritis in Western and Northern Europe. It has a worldwide distribution; the incidence of infection is rising within both Europe and the United States, although this may be due to better methods of detection and wider recognition of *Yersinia* as important enteric pathogens. *Yersinia* infection can be transmitted by both food and water, and is associated with meat, dairy products, chocolate, poultry, and produce. *Yersinia* has a preference for cold temperatures, thus there is a natural affinity for refrigerated food, and there is

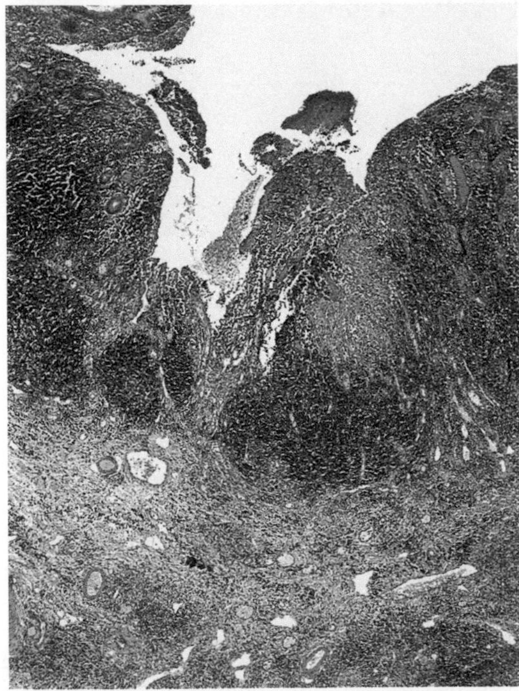

Fig. 7. Lymphoid hyperplasia, mucosal ulceration, and epithelioid granulomas in a case of *Y enterocolitica* appendicitis in a child. H&E, original magnification ×20.

speculation that infection is more common in cooler months.[19–23] *Y enterocolitica* and *Y pseudotuberculosis* are the species that cause human GI disease.[19,20,22,24]

These fastidious gram-negative coccobacilli have been implicated in numerous GI illnesses, including appendicitis (particularly granulomatous appendicitis) and mesenteric lymphadenitis.[19–22,24,25] Fever, pharyngitis, and leukocytosis may be present as well. Symptoms often have been present for weeks to months, leading to misdiagnosis as chronic idiopathic inflammatory bowel disease. Reactive polyarthritis and erythema nodosum are also associated with *Yersinia* infection. Infants, children, and young adults are most commonly infected. Patients with granulomatous appendicitis caused by *Yersinia* often present with signs and symptoms indistinguishable from acute nonspecific appendicitis. However, some patients with yersiniosis are initially believed to be suffering from appendicitis, but on exploration are found to have inflammation of the terminal ileum and mesenteric nodes that clinically mimics appendicitis (the pseudoappendicular syndrome).[19,22,24–28]

Pathologic features

The involved appendix has a thickened, edematous wall with nodular inflammatory masses centered on Peyer patches. Aphthoid and linear ulcers may be seen, and perforation is frequent. Involved lymph nodes may show grossly apparent foci of necrosis. Both suppurative and granulomatous patterns of inflammation are common, and are often mixed. *Y enterocolitica* typically features epithelioid granulomas, along with hyperplastic Peyer patches and overlying ulceration (**Fig. 7**).[20,29–32] GI infection with *Y pseudotuberculosis* has been described characteristically as a granulomatous process with central microabscesses (**Fig. 8**), almost always accompanied by mesenteric adenopathy.[20,26] However, there is significant overlap between the histologic features of *Y enterocolitica* and *Y pseudotuberculosis* infection, and either species may show epithelioid granulomas with prominent lymphoid cuffing (**Fig. 9**), lymphoid hyperplasia, transmural lymphoid aggregates (**Fig. 10**), mucosal ulceration, and lymph node involvement.[20] The transmural inflammation, fissuring and/or aphthoid ulcers, focal architectural distortion, skip lesions, and granulomas may closely mimic Crohn disease.

Special stains are usually not helpful in the diagnosis of *Yersinia*, because the organisms are small, usually present in low numbers, and are difficult to distinguish from normal nonpathogenic colonic flora. Because *Yersinia* is a fastidious organism that requires specific culture conditions, and serologic studies show significant cross-

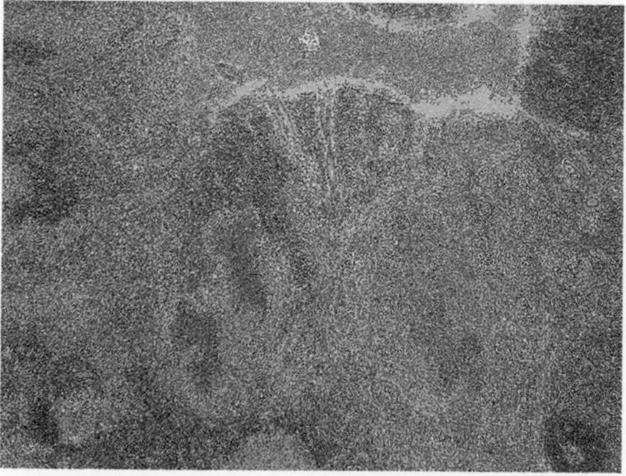

Fig. 8. *Y pseudotuberculosis* appendicitis, featuring granulomatous inflammation with prominent, irregular microabscesses and mucosal ulceration. H&E, original magnification ×40.

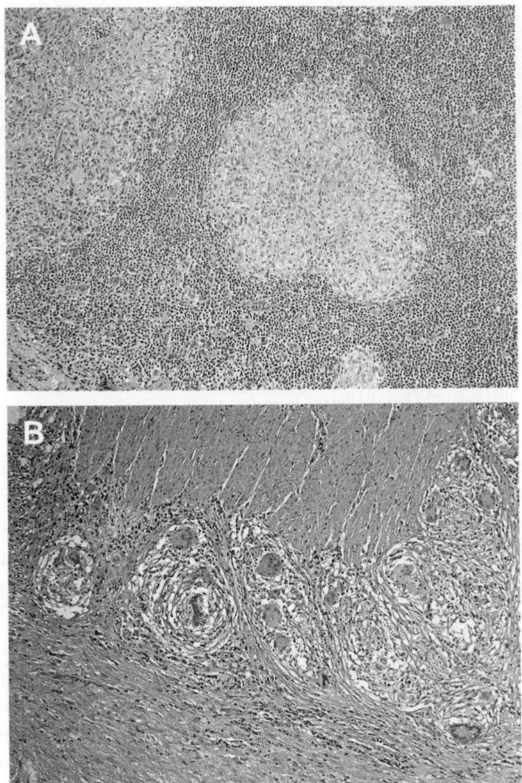

Fig. 9. Epithelioid granulomas typical of yersiniosis, with prominent surrounding lymphoid cuffs. (*A*) H&E, original magnification ×100. The granulomas are often present transmurally. (*B*) H&E, original magnification ×100.

reactivity with other gut pathogens, recognition of the histologic pattern of infection and molecular confirmation by PCR assay is the most reliable method of confirming the diagnosis.[19,20,22,29,33]

Uncomplicated cases of *Yersinia*-associated appendicitis and the pseudoappendicular syndrome usually resolve spontaneously without antibiotic therapy. Localized

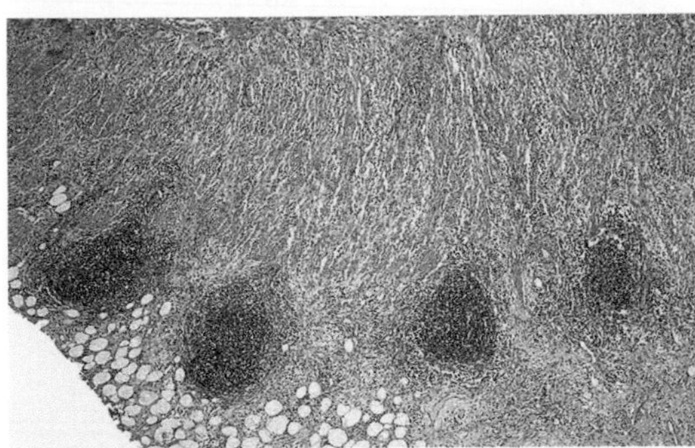

Fig. 10. Transmural lymphoid aggregates in *Yersinia*-associated appendicitis may mimic Crohn disease. H&E, original magnification ×100.

suppurative infections, bacteremic patients, and severe systemic infections may require antibiotics, especially in immunocompromised patients or patients at risk for severe yersiniosis (such as those on desferrioxamine therapy). However, optimal anti-Yersinial therapy has yet to be determined. *Y enterocolitica* is susceptible to many broad-spectrum antibiotics, although there is resistance to ampicillin and first-generation cephalosporins. Fluoroquinolones are the treatment of choice for *Y pseudotuberculosis*.[34–37]

Differential diagnosis

The major differential diagnosis includes other infectious processes, particularly *Mycobacteria*. Acid-fast stains and culture results help distinguish mycobacterial infection from yersiniosis. Sarcoidosis, foreign body reaction to fecal material, and granulomatous inflammation secondary to delayed (interval) appendectomy with antibiotic therapy are also in the differential diagnosis of *Yersinia*-associated granulomatous appendicitis.[38–41]

Crohn disease and yersiniosis may be difficult to distinguish from one another. Features favoring Crohn disease include fistula formation, cobblestoning of mucosa, presence of creeping fat, and histologic changes of chronicity including crypt distortion, thickening of the muscularis mucosa, and prominent neural hyperplasia. However, some cases are simply indistinguishable on histologic grounds alone.

Although Crohn disease and yersiniosis may be indistinguishable on histologic grounds alone, patients with isolated granulomatous appendicitis develop generalized inflammatory bowel disease less than 10% of the time.[29,42,43] In addition, many cases of granulomatous appendicitis previously considered to be either a limited form of Crohn disease or idiopathic are probably caused by infection. Features that suggest an underlying infectious cause include a large number of granulomas, confluent granulomas, and necrosis or central abscess formation.[42,43] Ultimately, because either species of *Yersinia* may mimic Crohn disease histologically and clinically, it is important to carefully consider other potential causes of granulomatous appendicitis before rendering a diagnosis of Crohn disease.[29,42,43]

Actinomycosis (Actinomyces Israelii)

This filamentous anaerobic gram-positive bacterium is a normal inhabitant of the oral cavity and upper GI tract that occasionally produces chronic, usually granulomatous appendicitis. Patients frequently present with fever, weight loss, abdominal pain, and, occasionally, a palpable mass that may mimic malignancy.[44–47] The correct diagnosis is usually not established preoperatively, but is discovered only once the appendix has been resected for a suspected neoplasm.[45]

Pathologic features

The appendix is the most common intra-abdominal organ involved by actinomycosis, followed by the right colon.[44–46] Grossly, appendices are often markedly enlarged, indurated, and adherent to adjacent structures, mimicking malignancy. Mucosal ulceration is variably present. The inflammatory reaction is predominantly neutrophilic.[44–46] Palisading histiocytes and giant cells, as well as frank granulomas, often surround the neutrophilic inflammation. Transmural inflammation, lymphoid hyperplasia, and marked fibrosis (**Fig. 11**) are common histologic features,[44–47] along with mucosal ulceration and architectural distortion. Small sinuses may track from the lumen into the wall of the appendix, and there is often marked fibrosis with variable abscess formation.

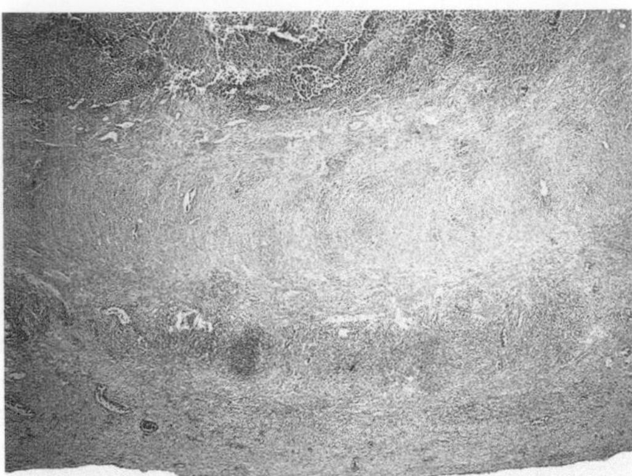

Fig. 11. Appendiceal actinomycosis, featuring marked mural fibrosis with overlying lymphoid hyperplasia and transmural lymphoid aggregates. H&E, original magnification ×40. (*Courtesy of* Dr Dianne Johnson.)

The organism typically produces actinomycotic (sulfur) granules, consisting of irregular round clusters of bacteria rimmed by eosinophilic, clublike projections of proteinaceous material (Splendore-Hoeppli material) (**Fig. 12**). Gram stain reveals the filamentous, gram-positive organisms (**Fig. 13**). Actinomyces may stain with Grocott methenamine silver (GMS) stain and Warthin-Starry stain.

Commensal actinomyces may be present at the lumenal surface of the appendix, and these do not necessarily imply invasive infection, particularly if there is no inflammatory response. A definite diagnosis of invasive actinomycosis (rather than the presence of commensal organisms) is important, given the therapeutic implications discussed later, and requires evidence of the organisms within the wall of the bowel with an associated inflammatory response. This process may require multiple levels of lesional tissue sections.[44,48]

Combined surgical and medical therapy produces good results in most cases of invasive actinomycosis. After resection and/or drainage of abscesses, long-term antibiotic therapy is necessary, because of both the difficulty of achieving good antibiotic penetration in fibrous tissue, and the propensity of the infection to recur. Actinomyces are sensitive to penicillins, but tetracycline and clindamycin are also effective. Intravenous antibiotics are usually given initially, followed by oral administration.[44,45,47]

Differential diagnosis

Macroscopically, the infiltrative, fibrotic masses produced by actinomycosis can mimic malignancy. The histologic differential primarily includes other infectious processes, particularly *Nocardia*. *Nocardia* are partially acid-fast and do not form the typical sulfur granules of actinomycosis; however, cultures may be required to distinguish these 2 filamentous organisms. Even although actinomyces are GMS positive, they have a more slender morphology than fungi, and do not bud or produce hyphae. Care should be taken not to confuse actinomycosis with other bacteria that form clusters and chains but are not truly filamentous, such as *Pseudomonas* and *Escherichia coli.* Occasionally, the transmural inflammation, fibrosis, and granulomatous inflammation produced by actinomycotic infection may mimic Crohn disease.

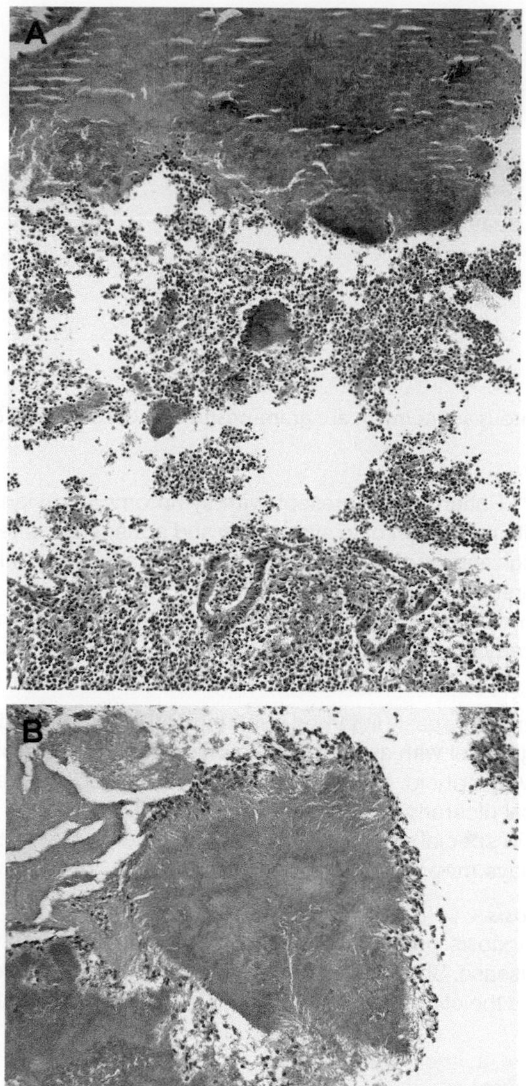

Fig. 12. Appendiceal actinomycosis, showing mucosal ulceration with overlying acute inflammation and admixed actinomycotic granules. (*A*) H&E, original magnification ×100. Actinomycotic granules are often associated with proteinaceous debris at the periphery (Splendore-Hoeppli material) and acute inflammation. (*B*) H&E, original magnification ×200.

Tuberculous Appendicitis

Despite the proximity of the appendix to the ileocecum, tuberculosis of the appendix is rare, and usually secondary to infection elsewhere in the abdomen.[49–51] Although the ileocecum is involved in more than 40% of cases of abdominal tuberculosis, the appendix is involved in only about 1%.[30] In nonendemic countries, many patients with intestinal and appendiceal tuberculosis are immunocompromised.[49] Mechanisms of involvement include extension from ileocecal or genital tuberculosis, hematogenous spread from a distant focus of infection, and contact with intestinal contents

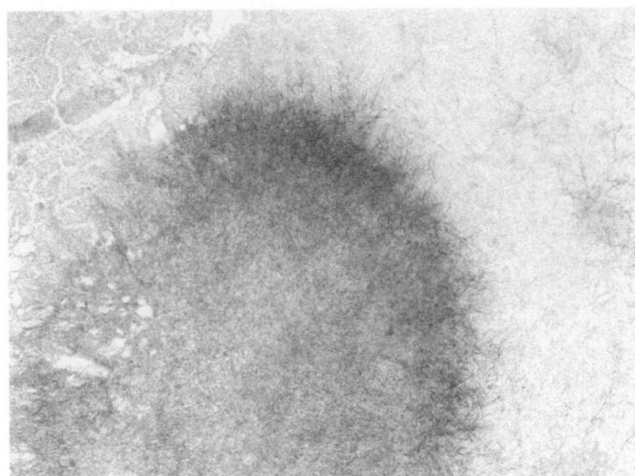

Fig. 13. The filamentous actinomyces are gram-positive on Gram stain. H&E, original magnification ×200.

containing bacilli.[50] Patients may present with symptoms and signs typical of acute appendicitis, or with milder, chronic symptoms and nonspecific intermittent right iliac fossa pain.[50] A high index of suspicion is required, and appendiceal tuberculosis should be considered in immigrants presenting with the symptoms mentioned earlier who are from regions where tuberculosis is endemic. Patients need several months of antitubercular therapy after appendectomy.[52,53]

Pathologic features

The appendix is usually grossly inflamed, with mural thickening, and is often adherent to the surrounding bowel with associated lymphadenitis.[49–51] Histologically, involved appendices show lymphoid hyperplasia with associated caseating granulomas (**Fig. 14**).[51] Mucosal ulceration may be present as well. Organisms may be rare, and even multiple sets of special stains may fail to reveal acid-fast bacilli; therefore, culture and molecular assays may be invaluable to diagnosis.

Differential diagnosis

The differential diagnosis primarily includes other granulomatous infectious process, and rarely Crohn disease. Showing organisms by histochemical, microbial, or molecular methods, as well as the clinical context, helps to resolve the differential in most cases.

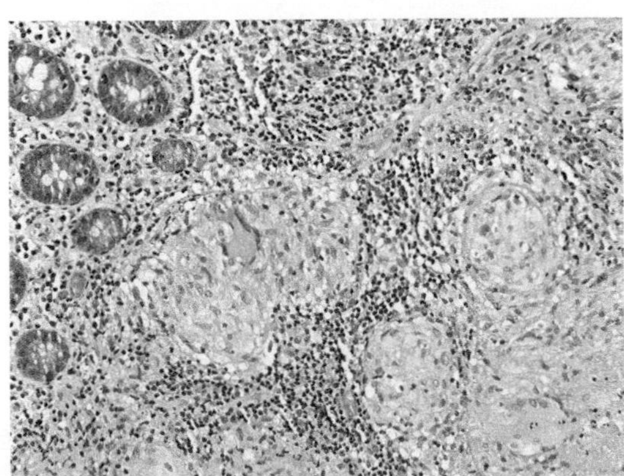

Fig. 14. Confluent, epithelioid granulomas with giant cells and a surrounding lymphoid infiltrate are seen in tuberculosis. H&E, original magnification ×200.

Atypical mycobacteria (particularly *Mycobacterium avium-intracellulare* [*MAI*]) only rarely cause appendicitis, and this scenario occurs almost exclusively in immunocompromised patients.[54,55] The diffuse histiocytic infiltrate typical of GI *MAI* infection may be seen, and discrete granulomas are variably present. Numerous acid-fast bacilli are usually detectable with appropriate acid-fast stains. Mycobacterial spindle cell pseudotumors have also been reported rarely in patients with AIDS.[56]

Campylobacter Species

Campylobacter species, particularly *Campylobacter jejuni*, have been isolated from resected appendices using molecular, microbiological, immunohistochemical, and electron microscopic methods.[57–59] Grossly, appendices are often normal. Histologic findings are similar to those of early nonspecific acute suppurative appendicitis, although inflammatory changes may be limited to the mucosa (without transmural inflammation or periappendicitis) in some cases. Most patients do not require postappendectomy antibiotic therapy.

Clostridium Difficile

Appendiceal involvement by *Clostridium difficile* is usually associated with more widespread colonic involvement by pseudomembranous colitis.[60,61] The *Clostridium difficile* toxin assay is helpful in confirming the diagnosis, and patients require antimicrobial therapy, usually oral vancomycin or flagyl.

Pathologic features

Grossly, appendices may contain pseudomembranes similar to those seen in the colon,[60] or may have nonspecific suppurative inflammation.[61] Histologic changes are also similar to those seen in the colon, and include volcano or mushroom mucosal lesions (**Fig. 15**) with intercrypt necrosis and ballooned crypts, giving rise to the laminated pseudomembrane composed of fibrin, mucin, and neutrophils. The ballooned glands are filled with neutrophils and mucin, and the superficial epithelial cells are often lost.

Other bacterial infections that may cause appendicitis are listed in **Table 1**. *Salmonella* species (both typhoid and nontyphoid) are rarely isolated from acutely inflamed appendices; clinical presentation and histologic findings are identical to acute

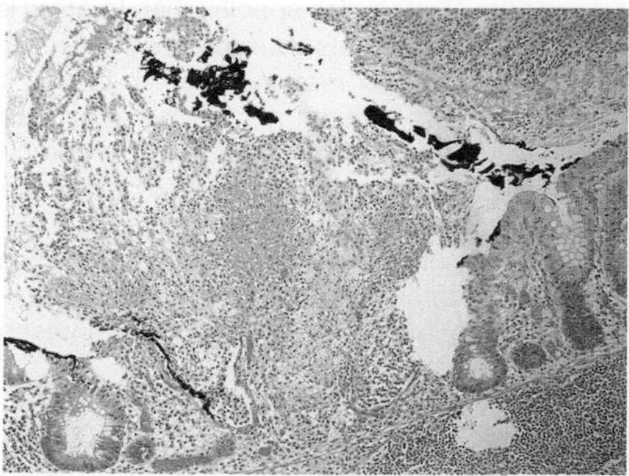

Fig. 15. *Clostridium difficile* infection of the appendix. Note the attenuated, exploding crypts giving rise to an inflammatory pseudomembrane composed of mucin, neutrophils, and fibrinous debris. H&E, original magnification ×100.

nonspecific appendicitis.[62,63] Patients often remain febrile postoperatively, and *Salmonella* infection requires antibiotic treatment following appendectomy. Appendicitis has been reported rarely associated with dysentery caused by *Shigella*.[64]

Bacterial Infection and Acute Nonspecific Appendicitis

Although the appendix is the most commonly resected and examined intra-abdominal organ in surgical pathology practice, the pathogenesis of acute nonspecific appendicitis (the most common diagnosis made in this organ) and its association with specific bacterial causes remain enigmatic. Historically, obstruction of the appendiceal lumen, with subsequent secondary infection, has been the most popular theory regarding the pathogenesis of acute nonspecific appendicitis.[48,65] Proponents of this theory argue that obstruction, either by fecalith, lymphoid hyperplasia, or adhesions, leads to an increase in intraluminal pressure, which in turn causes vascular compromise, mucosal ischemia, mucosal ulceration, and ultimately infection by luminal microorganisms. However, evidence of obstruction can be shown in only a minority of resected appendices,[48,65] and some investigators have argued that obstruction is the result, rather than the cause, of appendiceal inflammation.[66] Other purported risk factors that may lead to bacterial superinfection include mucosal ulceration from viral infection, and low-fiber diets with slowing of intestinal transit time and retention of stool in the appendix.[48,65,67,68] No single theory can explain all cases of acute nonspecific appendicitis, and it is likely that multiple causes, varying with the individual patient, may lead to invasion of the appendiceal wall by intraluminal bacteria and associated mucosal ulceration.[65,69]

The possible role of gut bacteria in both the development and the sequelae of acute appendicitis has also been a subject of discussion. Bacteriologic studies, usually historically performed using microbiologic culture techniques, reveal a wide variety of anaerobic and aerobic bacteria.[70,71] When correlated with histologic findings, it seems that aerobic infection predominates in early appendicitis, with a shift toward a mixture of aerobes and anaerobes later in the course of disease.[48] *Bacteroides* species are the most common isolate, particularly *Bacteroides fragilis*, and their role in the pathogenesis of acute appendicitis has been hotly debated.[70,72] Some studies have found a higher incidence of *Bacteroides fragilis* in inflamed appendices when compared with normal, whereas others have found no difference.[70,71] Studies examining the immunologic response to commonly isolated bacteria have shown a greater serologic antibody response to *Bacteroides* species than to other isolated organisms in gangrenous and perforated appendices, but this may reflect a greater extent of organ destruction and tissue immune response rather than a true pathogenetic role.[70,73] In addition, other workers showed similar serologic results when patients with noninflamed appendices were studied.[73] The possible contributions that any of these organisms might make to the pathogenesis of acute appendicitis remain unclear, but it is important to be aware of the mixture of anaerobic and aerobic bacteria that can exist within an inflamed appendix. If antibiotic therapy is necessary for either wound infections or peritonitis secondary to perforation, the antimicrobials selected should cover the variety of organisms that may be present.[48,70]

FUNGAL INFECTIONS CAUSING APPENDICITIS

Fungal infection of the appendix is rare. Mucormycosis has been reported to cause inflammatory masses of the right lower quadrant involving the appendix, ileum, and cecum in patients undergoing chemotherapy.[74] Histoplasmosis may involve the appendix as part of generalized infection of the GI tract, usually in immunocompromised patients (**Fig. 16**).[75] Patients usually require antifungal therapy following resection.

PARASITIC INFECTIONS CAUSING APPENDICITIS

Many parasites can be found in the lumen of the appendix, including pinworms (most commonly), *Ascaris* (roundworms), *Giardia*, and *Entamoeba histolytica*. Clinicians should be alerted when parasites are found in the appendix that could affect other parts of the GI tract.

Enterobius Vermicularis (Pinworms)

Pinworms are one of the most common human parasites. These nematodes have a worldwide distribution, but are more common in cold or temperate climates and in developed countries. Prevalence is highest among children ages 5 to 10 years, and it has been reported that pinworm infections of the GI tract affect 4% to 28% of children around the globe.[76–78] These infections are common in the United States and Northwestern Europe. The infective egg resides in dust and soil, and transmission is believed to be via the fecal-oral route. Pinworms are known as *Oxyuris vermicularis* in the older literature.

The worms live and reproduce in the ileum, cecum, proximal colon, and appendix, and the female migrates to the anus to deposit eggs and die. The perianal eggs and worms produce the characteristic symptoms of pruritis ani, which often leads to perianal scratching and insomnia. Many infections are asymptomatic.

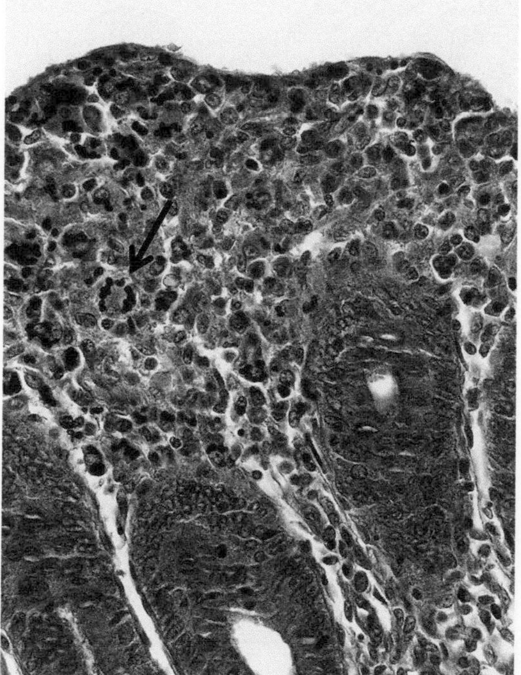

Fig. 16. Numerous silver-stained *Histoplasma* are seen within macrophages in this appendix. H&E/methenamine silver, original magnification ×400.

The causal role of *Enterobius* in appendicitis remains controversial. Although pinworms are detected in approximately 0.6% to 13% of resected appendices, they are usually not invasive, and their ability to cause mucosal damage has been a subject of intense debate.[76–79] The relationship between pinworm infection and the symptoms of acute appendicitis also remains unclear. Some authorities believe that the lack of inflammation surrounding invasive pinworms indicates that the organism invades only after the appendix has been removed to escape the decrease in oxygen tension.[76] However, invasion has been documented occasionally, with associated mucosal ulceration and inflammation, and it has been suggested that if additional sections were submitted from appendices containing lumenal pinworms, more cases of invasive enterobiasis would be found. In addition, both worms and ova may obstruct the appendiceal lumen and cause inflammation similar to that caused by fecaliths.[48,76–79]

Pathologic findings

In the appendix, the mucosa usually seems normal, and pinworms are most often found in the appendiceal lumen (**Fig. 17**). Even invasive pinworms incite little, or no, inflammatory reaction, but rarely an inflammatory infiltrate composed of neutrophils and eosinophils may occur,[76–79] along with hemorrhage and ulceration. Granulomas, sometimes with necrosis, may develop rarely as a reaction to degenerating worms or eggs.

The worms are 2 to 5 mm long, white or ivory, and pointed at both ends; the posterior end is curved. They may be seen with the naked eye. Morphologically, pinworms have prominent lateral alae with easily visible internal organs (**Fig. 18**); eggs are ovoid with one flat side, and a bilayered refractile shell.

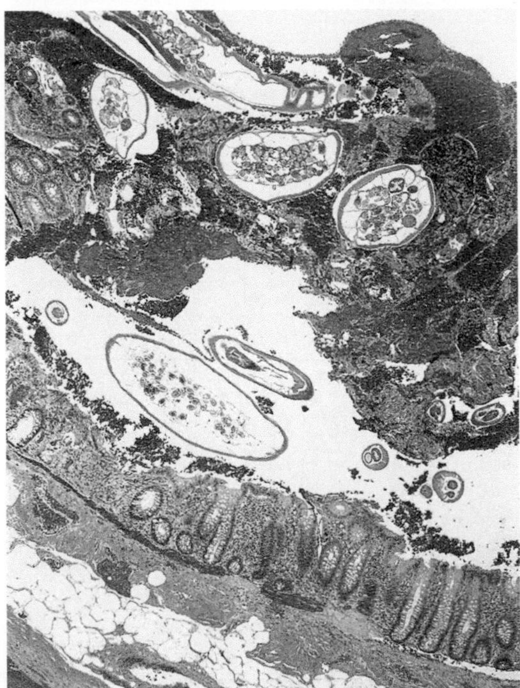

Fig. 17. Multiple pinworms are present in the lumen of a resected appendix. H&E, original magnification ×100.

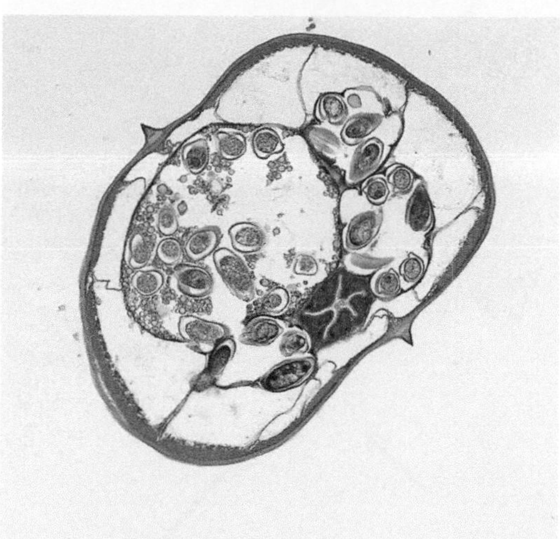

Fig. 18. *Enterobius vermicularis* has lateral alae with easily visible organs. H&E, original magnification ×200.

Differential diagnosis

The morphologic features of the worm, described earlier, are characteristic of enterobiasis. As discussed earlier, it may be difficult to distinguish between primary *Enterobius* infection and the presence of worms complicating or existing within the context of preexisting acute appendicitis.

Strongyloides stercoralis is a nematode with a worldwide distribution. It is endemic in tropical climates; in the United States, it is endemic in the southeast, urban areas with large immigrant populations, and mental institutions.[80–84] *Strongyloides stercoralis* is contracted from soil containing the organism, and infection occurs primarily in adults, many of whom are hospitalized, suffer from chronic illnesses, or are immunocompromised. Corticosteroids and human T-lymphotropic virus 1 viral infection are also associated with strongyloidiasis. Patients with AIDS do not seem to be unusually susceptible. *Strongyloides stercoralis* is a rare cause of appendicitis, and the diagnosis of strongyloidiasis is almost always made postsurgically.[84]

Patients may have symptoms that are clinically indistinguishable from acute nonspecific appendicitis.[80–82] Some patients have a more protracted course of nonspecific chronic abdominal pain.[84] GI manifestations may be accompanied by mesenteric adenopathy, rash, urticaria, pruritis, mild anemia, peripheral eosinophilia and leukocytosis, and concomitant pulmonary symptoms.[83]

Pathologic features

Affected appendices typically show a marked transmural eosinophilic and neutrophilic infiltrate. Granulomas are occasionally present as well. Larvae may be found within granulomas.[80,82,83] Both adult worms and larvae may be found in the crypts (**Figs. 19** and **20**), but they may be difficult to detect. Worms typically have sharply pointed tails that may be curved. In severe infections, larvae may be seen transmurally, and in lymphatics and small vessels. Examination of stool may be an invaluable aid to diagnosis.

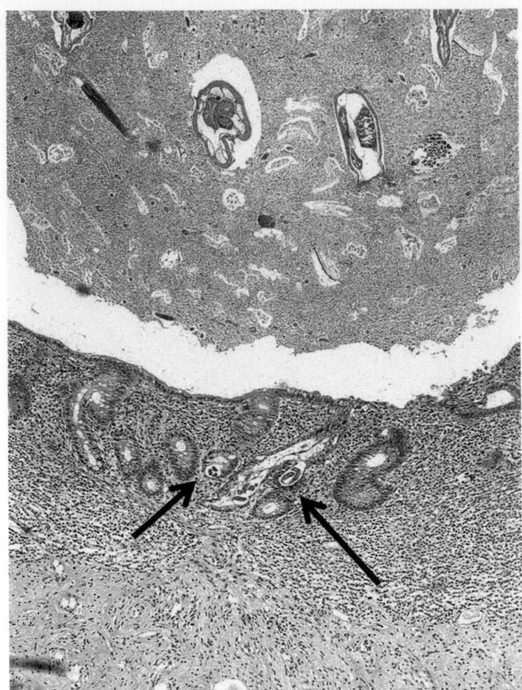

Fig. 19. *Strongyloides* are seen in the crypts of an appendix; note also that there are pinworms in the overlying debris. H&E, original magnification ×100. (*Courtesy of* Dr Dennis Baroni-Cruz.)

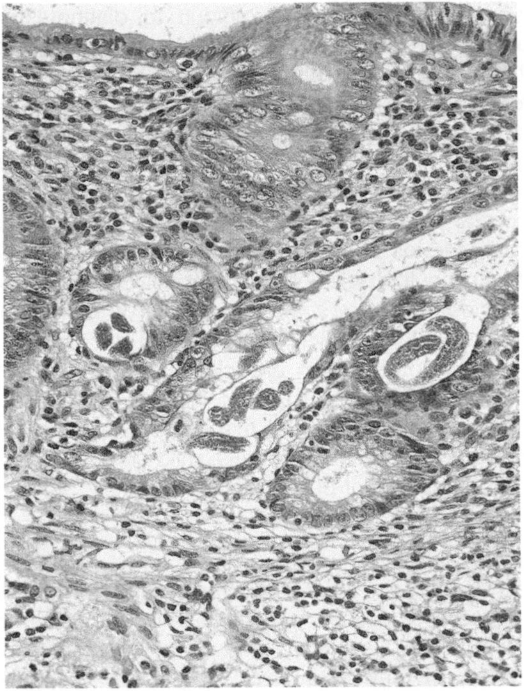

Fig. 20. High-power view of *Strongyloides* in the appendiceal crypts. The surrounding inflammatory infiltrate contains numerous eosinophils. H&E, original magnification ×400. (*Courtesy of* Dr Dennis Baroni-Cruz.)

Differential diagnosis

The presence of larvae with sharply pointed, sometimes curved tails within the glands of the GI mucosa is essentially diagnostic of strongyloidiasis. Ancillary diagnostic tests include stool examination for larvae, worms, or eggs, and serologic tests.

Schistosomiasis

Schistosomes, most commonly *Schistosoma haematobium*, only rarely cause appendicitis even in nations where schistosomiasis is endemic.[85–88] Patients usually present with signs and symptoms typical of acute appendicitis, although some present with inflammatory masses. Patients may require antischistosomal therapy in addition to appendectomy.[88]

Pathologic features

Histologically, appendices may show transmural inflammation rich in eosinophils, with a granulomatous reaction to ova. Older granulomas may be fibrotic and hyalinized,[85–87] with numerous calcified eggs (**Fig. 21**). Similar to earlier discussion, arguments regarding the pathogenicity of *Enterobius* in the appendix have also occurred pertaining to schistosomes. However, it has been shown at least in some cases that schistosomes do cause acute appendicitis, either by inducing granulomatous inflammation, or by producing such marked fibrosis that lumenal obstruction leads to signs and symptoms of acute appendicitis.[86,87]

Entamoeba Histolytica

Entamoeba histolytica are occasionally found in the appendix, usually in the lumen without accompanying inflammation, and rarely with associated acute appendicitis.

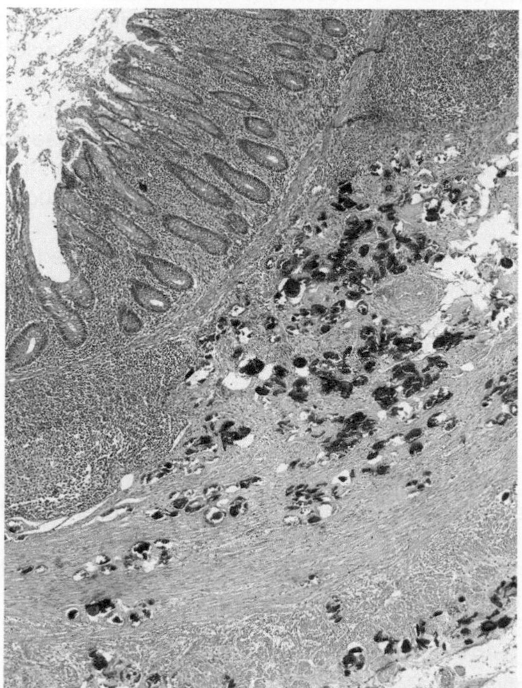

Fig. 21. Schistosome eggs in the wall of the appendix, with surrounding marked fibrosis and calcification of eggs. H&E, original magnification ×40. (*Courtesy of* Dr Joseph Misdraji.)

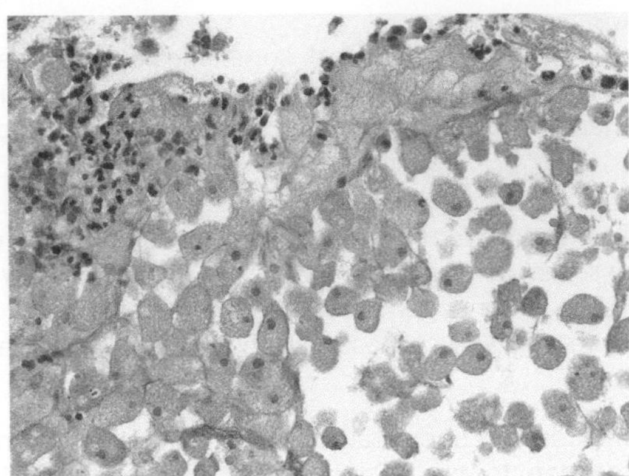

Fig. 22. *Entamoeba histolytica* feature foamy cytoplasm, a round, eccentric nucleus with homogeneous chromatin, and ingested red blood cells. H&E, original magnification ×400.

These cases are usually associated with heavy infection of the right colon,[48,81,89–91] and patients may require antiparasitic therapy in addition to surgery.

When amoebae are found in the appendix, pathogenic *Entamoeba histolytica* must be distinguished from nonpathogenic amoeba such as *Entamoeba coli*,[48] and from macrophages. Amebic trophozoites have distinct cell membranes with foamy cytoplasm, round and eccentrically located nuclei with peripheral margination of chromatin, and a central karyosome. The presence of ingested red blood cells is essentially pathognomonic of *Entamoeba histolytica,* and helps to distinguish it from other amoebae (see later discussion) (**Fig. 22**). Distinction of trophozoites from macrophages within inflammatory exudates may be difficult, particularly in poorly fixed tissue sections. Amoebae are trichrome and periodic acid-Schiff positive; in addition, their nuclei are usually more rounded, smaller, paler, and have a more open nuclear chromatin pattern than those of macrophages. Macrophages stain with CD68, α_1-antitrypsin, and chymotrypsin, whereas amoebae do not. Useful diagnostic tests for *Entamoeba histolytica* include stool examination for cysts and trophozoites, stool culture, serologic tests, and PCR assays, although the latter are not widely available.

Other parasites that may affect the appendix (summarized in **Table 1**) include *Trichuris* species (whipworms)[92,93] and *Ascaris lumbricoides* (roundworms).[48,94] Rarely, coccidians such as *Cryptosporidium* have been found in the appendix, primarily in immunocompromised patients.[95]

REFERENCES

1. Guarner J, de Leon-Bojorge B, Lopez-Corella E, et al. Intestinal intussusception associated with adenovirus infection in Mexican children. Am J Clin Pathol 2003; 120:845–50.
2. Yunis EJ, Atchison RW, Michaels RH, et al. Adenovirus and ileocecal intussusception. Lab Invest 1975;33:347–51.
3. Montgomery EA, Popek EJ. Intussusception, adenovirus, and children: a brief reaffirmation. Hum Pathol 1994;25:169–74.
4. Porter HJ, Padfield CJ, Peres LC, et al. Adenovirus and intranuclear inclusions in appendices in intussusception. J Clin Pathol 1993;46:154–8.
5. Reif RM. Viral appendicitis. Hum Pathol 1981;12:193–6.

6. Lamps LW. Appendicitis and infection of the appendix. Semin Diagn Pathol 2004; 21:86–97.
7. Lamps LW. Beyond acute inflammation: a review of appendicitis and infections of the appendix. Diagn Histopathol 2008;14:68–77.
8. Neumayer LA, Makar R, Ampel N, et al. Cytomegalovirus appendicitis in a patient with human immunodeficiency virus infection: case report and review of the literature. Arch Surg 1993;128:467–8.
9. Valerdiz-Casasola S, Pardo-Mindan FJ. Cytomegalovirus infection of the appendix in a patient with the acquired immunodeficiency syndrome. Gastroenterology 1991;101:247–9.
10. Tucker RM, Swanson S, Wenzel RP. Cytomegalovirus and appendiceal perforation in a patient with acquired immunodeficiency syndrome. South Med J 1989;82:1056–7.
11. Lin J, Bleiweiss IJ, Mendelson MH, et al. Cytomegalovirus-associated appendicitis in a patient with the acquired immunodeficiency syndrome. Am J Med 1990;89:377–9.
12. Dieterich DT, Kim MH, McMeeding A, et al. Cytomegalovirus appendicitis in a patient with acquired immune deficiency syndrome. Am J Gastroenterol 1991;86:904–6.
13. Davidson T, Allen-Mersh TG, Miles AJG, et al. Emergency laparotomy in patients with AIDS. Br J Surg 1991;78:924–6.
14. Chetty R, Roskell DE. Cytomegalovirus infection in the gastrointestinal tract. J Clin Pathol 1994;47:968–72.
15. Paik SY, Oh JT, Choi YJ, et al. Measles-related appendicitis. Arch Pathol Lab Med 2002;126:82–4.
16. Pancharoen C, Ruttanamongkol P, Suwangool P, et al. Measles-associated appendicitis: two case reports and literature review. Scand J Infect Dis 2001; 33:632–3.
17. Whalen TV, Klos JR, Kovalcik PJ, et al. Measles and appendicitis. Am Surg 1980; 46:412–3.
18. Lopez-Navidad A, Domingo P, Cadafalch J, et al. Acute appendicitis complicating infectious mononucleosis: case report and review. Rev Infect Dis 1990; 12:297–302.
19. Natkin J, Beavis KG. *Yersinia enterocolitica* and *Yersinia pseudotuberculosis*. Clin Lab Med 1999;19:523–36.
20. Lamps LW, Madhusudhan KT, Greenson JK, et al. The role of *Y. enterocolitica* and *Y. pseudotuberculosis* in granulomatous appendicitis: a histologic and molecular study. Am J Surg Pathol 2001;25:508–15.
21. Saebo A, Lassen J. Acute and chronic gastrointestinal manifestations associated with *Yersinia enterocolitica* infection: a Norwegian 10-year follow-up study on 458 hospitalized patients. Ann Surg 1992;215:250–5.
22. Baert F, Peetermans W, Knockaert D. Yersiniosis: the clinical spectrum. Acta Clin Belg 1994;49:76–84.
23. Bennion RS, Thompson JE, Gil J, et al. The role of *Yersinia enterocolitica* in appendicitis in the southwestern United States. Am Surg 1991;57:766–8.
24. Attwood SEA, Cafferkey MT, West AB, et al. *Yersinia* infection and acute abdominal pain. Lancet 1987;1(8532):529–33.
25. Van Noyen R, Selderslaghs R, Bekaert J, et al. Causative role of *Yersinia* and other enteric pathogens in the appendicular syndrome. Eur J Clin Microbiol Infect Dis 1991;10:735–41.
26. El-Maraghi NR, Mair N. The histopathology of enteric infection with *Yersinia pseudotuberculosis*. Am J Clin Pathol 1979;71:631–9.

27. Simmonds SD, Noble MA, Freeman HJ. Gastrointestinal features of culture-positive *Yersinia enterocolitica* infection. Gastroenterology 1987;92:112–7.
28. Schapers RF, Renate R, Lennert K, et al. Mesenteric lymphadenopathy due to *Yersinia enterocolitica*. Virchows Arch A Pathol Anat Histol 1981;390:127–38.
29. Lamps LW, Madhusudhan KT, Havens JM, et al. Pathogenic *Yersinia enterocolitica* and *Yersinia pseudotuberculosis* DNA is detected in bowel and mesenteric nodes from Crohn's disease patients. Am J Surg Pathol 2003;27(2):220–7.
30. Gleason TH, Patterson SD. The pathology of *Yersinia enterocolitica* ileocolitis. Am J Surg Pathol 1982;6:347–55.
31. Bradford ND, Noce PS, Gutman LT. Pathologic features of enteric infection with *Yersinia enterocolitica*. Arch Pathol 1974;98:17–22.
32. Vantrappen G, Agg HO, Ponette E, et al. *Yersinia* enteritis and enterocolitis: gastroenterological aspects. Gastroenterology 1977;72:220–7.
33. Paff JR, Triplett DA, Saari TN. Clinical and laboratory aspects of *Yersinia pseudotuberculosis* infections, with a report of two cases. Am J Clin Pathol 1976;66:101–10.
34. Gayraud M, Scavizzi MR, Mollaret HH, et al. Antibiotic treatment of *Yersinia enterocolitica* septicemia: a retrospective review of 43 cases. Clin Infect Dis 1993;17:405–10.
35. Pham JN, Bell SM, Lanzarone JY. Biotype and antibiotic sensitivity of 100 clinical isolates of *Yersinia enterocolitica*. J Antimicrob Chemother 1991;28:13–8.
36. Pham JN, Bell SM, Lanzarone JY. A study of the b-lactamases of 100 clinical isolates of *Yersinia enterocolitica*. J Antimicrob Chemother 1991;28:19–24.
37. Lemaitre BC, Mazigh DA, Scavizzi MR. Failure of b-lactam antibiotics and marked efficacy of fluoroquinolones in treatment of murine *Yersinia pseudotuberculosis* infection. Antimicrobial Agents Chemother 1987;35:1785–90.
38. Bronner MP. Granulomatous appendicitis and the appendix in idiopathic inflammatory bowel disease. Semin Diagn Pathol 2004;21:98–107.
39. Guo G, Greenson JK. Histopathology of interval (delayed) appendectomy specimens: strong association with granulomatous and xanthogranulomatous appendicitis. Am J Surg Pathol 2003;27:1147–51.
40. Clarke H, Pollett W, Chittal S, et al. Sarcoidosis with involvement of the appendix. Arch Intern Med 1983;143:1603–4.
41. Veress B, Alafuzoff I, Juliusson G. Granulomatous peritonitis and appendicitis of food starch origin. Gut 1991;32:718–20.
42. Dudley TH, Dean PJ. Idiopathic granulomatous appendicitis, or Crohn's disease of the appendix revisited. Hum Pathol 1993;24:595–601.
43. Huang JC, Appelman HD. Another look at chronic appendicitis resembling Crohn's disease. Mod Pathol 1996;9(10):975–81.
44. Ferrari TC, Couto CA, Murta-Oliveira C, et al. Actinomycosis of the colon: a rare form of presentation. Scand J Gastroenterol 2000;35:108–9.
45. Mueller MC, Ihrler S, Degenhart C, et al. Abdominal actinomycosis. Infection 2008;36:191.
46. Schmidt P, Koltai JL, Weltzien A. Actinomycosis of the appendix in childhood. Pediatr Surg Int 1999;15:63–5.
47. Waadegaard P, Pziegiel M. Actinomycosis mimicking abdominal neoplasm. Acta Chir Scand 1988;154:315–6.
48. Williams RA. Inflammatory disorders of the appendix. In: Williams RA, Myers P, editors. Pathology of the appendix and its surgical treatment. London: Chapman and Hall Medical Press; 1994. p. 63.
49. Horvath KD, Whelan RL. Intestinal tuberculosis: return of an old disease. Am J Gastroenterol 1998;93:692–6.

50. Singh MK, Arunabh, Kapoor VK. Tuberculosis of the appendix–a report of 17 cases and a suggested aetiopathological classification. Postgrad Med J 1987;63:855–7.
51. Mittal VK, Khanna SK, Gupta M, et al. Isolated tuberculosis of the appendix. Am Surg 1975;41:172–4.
52. Agarwal P, Sharma D, Agarwal A, et al. Tuberculous appendicitis in India. Trop Doct 2004;34:36–8.
53. Walia HS, Khafagy AR, al-Sayer HM, et al. Unusual presentations of abdominal tuberculosis. Can J Surg 1994;37:300–6.
54. Domingo P, Ris J, Lopez-Contreras J, et al. Appendicitis due to *Mycobacterium avium* complex in a patient with AIDS. Arch Intern Med 1996;156:1114.
55. Livingston RA, Siberry GK, Paidas CN, et al. Appendicitis due to *Mycobacterium avium* complex in an adolescent infected with the human immunodeficiency virus. Clin Infect Dis 1995;20:1579–80.
56. Basilio-de-Oliveira C, Eyer-Silva WA, Valle HA, et al. Mycobacterial spindle cell pseudotumor of the appendix vermiformis in a patient with AIDS. Braz J Infect Dis 2001;5:98–100.
57. van Spreeuwel JP, Lindeman J, Bax R, et al. *Campylobacter*-associated appendicitis: prevalence and clinicopathologic features. Pathol Annu 1987;22(Pt 1): 55–65.
58. Chan FT, Stringel G, MacKenzie AM. Isolation of *C. jejuni* from an appendix. J Clin Microbiol 1983;18:422–4.
59. Campbell LK, Havens JM, Scott MA, et al. Molecular detection of *Campylobacter jejuni* in archival cases of acute appendicitis. Mod Pathol 2006;19:1042–6.
60. Coyne JK, Dervan PA, Haboubi NY. Involvement of the appendix in pseudomembranous colitis. J Clin Pathol 1997;50:70–1.
61. Brown TA, Rajappannair L, Dalton AB, et al. Acute appendicitis in the setting of *Clostridium difficile* colitis: case report and review of the literature. Clin Gastroenterol Hepatol 2007;5:969–71.
62. Kazlow PG, Freed J, Rosh JR, et al. *Salmonella typhimurium* appendicitis. J Pediatr Gastroenterol Nutr 1991;13:101–3.
63. Golakai VK, Makunike R. Perforation of terminal ileum and appendix in typhoid enteritis: report of two cases. East Afr Med J 1997;74:796–9.
64. Lending RE, Buchsbaum HW, Hyland RN. Shigellosis complicated by acute appendicitis. South Med J 1986;l79:1046–7.
65. Carr NJ. The pathology of acute appendicitis. Ann Diagn Pathol 2000;4:46–58.
66. Wangensteen OH, Bowers WF. Significance of the obstructive factor in the genesis of acute appendicitis. Arch Surg 1937;34:496.
67. Arnbjornsson E, Bengmark S. Role of obstruction in the pathogenesis of acute appendicitis. Am J Surg 1984;147:390–2.
68. Arnbjornsson E. Acute appendicitis and dietary fiber. Arch Surg 1983;118: 868–70.
69. Sisson RG, Ahlvin RC, Harlow MC. Superficial mucosal ulceration and the pathogenesis of acute appendicitis. Am J Surg 1971;122:378–80.
70. Jindal N, Kaur GD, Rajiv SA. Bacteriology of acute appendicitis with special reference to anaerobes. Indian J Pathol Microbiol 1994;37:299–305.
71. Roberts JP. Quantitative bacterial flora of acute appendicitis. Arch Dis Child 1988;63:536–40.
72. Pieper R, Kager L, Weintraub A, et al. The role of *Bacteroides fragilis* in the pathogenesis of acute appendicitis. Acta Chir Scand 1982;148:39–44.
73. Elhag EM, Alwan MH, Al-Adnan MS, et al. *Bacteroides fragilis* is a silent pathogen in acute appendicitis. J Med Microbiol 1986;21:245–9.

74. ter Borg F, Kuijper EJ, van der Lelie H. Fatal mucormycosis presenting as an appendiceal mass with metastatic spread to the liver during chemotherapy-induced granulocytopenia. Scand J Infect Dis 1990;22:499–501.
75. Lamps LW, Molina CP, Haggitt RC, et al. The pathologic spectrum of gastrointestinal and hepatic histoplasmosis. Am J Clin Pathol 2000;113:64–72.
76. Sinniah B, Leopairut J, Neafie RC, et al. Enterobiasis: a histopathological study of 259 patients. Ann Trop Med Parasitol 1991;85:625–35.
77. Wiebe BM. Appendicitis and *Enterobius vermicularis*. Scand J Gastroenterol 1991;26:336–8.
78. Arca MJ, Gates RL, Groner JI, et al. Clinical manifestations of appendiceal pinworms in children: an institutional experience and a review of the literature. Pediatr Surg Int 2004;20:372–5.
79. Moggensen K, Pahle E, Kowalski K. *Enterobius vermicularis* and acute appendicitis. Acta Chir Scand 1985;151:705–7.
80. Shakir AA, Youngberg G, Alvarez S. *Strongyloides* infestation as a cause of acute appendicitis. J Tenn Med Assoc 1986;79:543–4.
81. Nadler S, Cappell MS, Bhatt B, et al. Appendiceal infection by *Entamoeba histolytica* and *Strongyloides stercoralis* presenting like acute appendicitis. Dig Dis Sci 1990;35:603–8.
82. Noodleman JS. Eosinophilic appendicitis: demonstration of *Strongyloides stercoralis* as a causative agent. Arch Pathol Lab Med 1981;105:148–9.
83. Genta RM, Haque AK. Strongyloidiasis. In: Connor DH, Chandler FW, Schwartz DA, et al, editors. Pathology of infectious diseases. Stamford (CT): Appleton and Lange; 1997. p. 1567–76.
84. Komenaka IK, Wu GC, Lazar EL, et al. *Strongyloides* appendicitis: unusual etiology in two siblings with chronic abdominal pain. J Pediatr Surg 2003;38: E8–10.
85. Adebamowo CA, Akang EE, Ladipo JK, et al. Schistosomiasis of the appendix. Br J Surg 1991;78:1219–21.
86. Satti MB, Tamimi DM, Al Sohaibani M, et al. Appendicular schistosomiasis: a cause of clinical acute appendicitis? J Clin Pathol 1987;40:424–8.
87. Badmos KB, Komolafe AO, Rotimi O. Schistosomiasis presenting as acute appendicitis. East Afr Med J 2006;83:528–32.
88. Doudier B, Parola B, Dales JP, et al. Schistosomiasis as an unusual cause of appendicitis. Clin Microbiol Infect 2004;10:89–91.
89. Ramdial PK, Madiba TE, Kharwa S, et al. Isolated amoebic appendicitis. Virchows Arch 2002;441:63–8.
90. Gotohda N, Itano S, Okada Y, et al. Acute appendicitis caused by amoebiasis. J Gastroenterol 2000;135:861–3.
91. Yildirim S, Nursal T, Tarim A, et al. A rare cause of acute appendicitis: parasitic infection. Scand J Infect Dis 2005;37:757–9.
92. Cook GC. The clinical significance of gastrointestinal helminths – a review. Trans R Soc Trop Med Hyg 1986;80:675–85.
93. Kenney M, Yermakov V. Infection of man with *Trichuris vulpis*, the whipworm of dogs. Am J Trop Med Hyg 1980;29:1205–8.
94. Sinha SN, Sinha BN. Appendicular perforation due to *Ascaris lumbricoides*. J Indian Med Assoc 1974;63:396–7.
95. Oberhuber G, Lauer E, Stolte M, et al. Cryptosporidiosis of the appendix vermiformis: a case report. Z Gastroenterol 1991;29:606–8.

Infectious Causes of Colorectal Cancer

Nazia Hasan, MD, MPH[a], Ari Pollack, BA[b], Ilseung Cho, MD, MS[c,*]

KEYWORDS

• Gut microbes • Microbiome • Colorectal cancer

Colorectal cancer is a major cause of cancer-related morbidity and mortality in the United States and many other regions of the world. Approximately 150,000 new cases of colorectal cancer are diagnosed annually in the United States and more than 50,000 Americans die each year of colorectal cancer.[1] Although the incidence of colorectal cancer declined in the United States by 3% between 1998 and 2005 as a result of increased screening and surveillance efforts,[1] colorectal cancer remains the second leading cause of cancer death in the United States.[1] This situation is despite the $6.4 billion spent on treatment annually and the roughly $90 billion spent on primary screening per decade.[2]

Our understanding of the pathogenesis of colorectal cancer, from the precursor adenomatous polyp to adenocarcinoma, has evolved rapidly. Colorectal carcinogenesis is a sequential process characterized by the accumulation of multiple genetic and molecular alterations in colonic epithelial cells (**Fig. 1**). These specific alterations result in the inactivation of tumor suppressor genes such as APC, DCC, DPC4, and p53 along with the activation of oncogenes such as those in the Ras family.[3] These genetic mutations lead to the transformation of normal epithelium into dysplastic epithelium with increased proliferation, resulting in the development of the adenomatous polyp, which has malignant potential.[3] However, the development of colorectal cancer involves more then just a genetic predisposition. Familial adenomatous polyposis (FAP) and hereditary nonpolyposis colorectal cancer are the most common of the familial colon cancer syndromes, but combined account for fewer than 5% of all colorectal cancers.[4] Even with the characterization of specific genetic alterations, other potential contributory factors behind the development of sporadic colorectal cancer remain ambiguous. External or environmental factors presumably play a significant role, and inflammatory bowel diseases, obesity, alcohol consumption, and a diet

[a] Department of Medicine, NYU School of Medicine, 462 First Avenue, New Bellevue 16N27, New York, NY 10016, USA
[b] Department of Medicine, Columbia University School of Medicine, New York City, NY, USA
[c] Division of Gastroenterology, Department of Medicine, NYU School of Medicine, 423 East 23rd Street, GI Suite, 11 North, New York, NY 10010, USA
* Corresponding author.
E-mail address: ilseung.cho@nyumc.org

Infect Dis Clin N Am 24 (2010) 1019–1039
doi:10.1016/j.idc.2010.07.009
0891-5520/10/$ – see front matter. Published by Elsevier Inc.

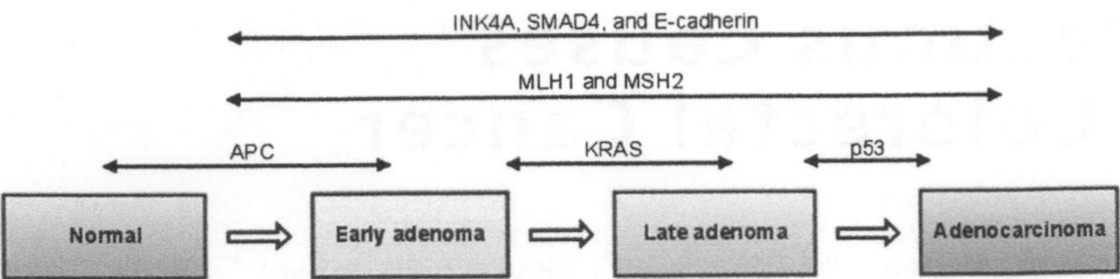

Fig. 1. Sequence of mutational events that characterize the transition from normal colonic mucosa to colonic adenocarcinoma first described by Vogelstein. The APC and KRAS gene mutations are the most common found in sporadic colorectal cancers.

high in fat and low in fiber have all been implicated as risk factors for the development of either colonic adenomas or carcinomas.[5]

We are becoming increasingly aware of microbes as causes of malignancies. The best-known examples are *Helicobacter pylori* with gastric cancer and human papillomavirus (HPV) with cervical cancer. This article reviews the various microbes that have been associated with the development of colorectal carcinomas.

INFLAMMATION, MICROBES, AND THE DEVELOPMENT OF COLON CANCER IN MURINE MODELS

Chronic inflammation in the human colon leads to increased risk of colorectal cancer, best shown in individuals with ulcerative colitis. Inflammation has been proposed as a possible mechanism for tumorigenesis, by inhibiting apoptosis, damaging DNA, and chronically stimulating mucosal proliferation.[6] Cyclooxygenase 2 (COX-2) was found to be highly expressed in tumor specimens of patients with colorectal cancer[7] and the inhibition of COX-2 activity is believed to account for the chemopreventive activity of nonsteroidal antiinflammatory drugs against colorectal neoplasia in patients with FAP.[8] COX-2 mRNA is overexpressed in 80% to 90% of human colorectal carcinomas and in 40% to 50% of premalignant adenomas.[9] Specific cytokines, such as interleukin 1β (IL-1β) and IL-6, which are associated with COX-2 induction, have also been found at high levels within colorectal neoplasia cells[10] and serum concentrations of IL-6 and tumor necrosis factor α have been associated with an increased prevalence of colorectal adenomas,[11] suggesting that inflammation plays a significant role in the early development of colonic neoplasia. Inflammation stimulates the release of proinflammatory cytokines from lymphocytes, which subsequently can lead to the production of reactive oxygen species and other genotoxic compounds in the epithelial milieu.

In the normal colon, the microbiota keeps the mucosa in a continuous state of physiologic, low-grade inflammation and stimulates release of proinflammatory cytokines.[12] The best example of the role of colonic microbiota in the development of colon neoplasia is in the T-cell receptor β (TCRβ)/p53 double knock-out (KO) mouse. This model mimics the development of adenocarcinoma in a background of ulcerative colitis. In conventional TCRβ/p53-KO mice, adenocarcinoma of the colon develops in 70% of animals by 4 months. In contrast, TCRβ/p53-KO mice that are raised under germ-free conditions do not develop adenocarcinoma.[13] Similar results have also been noted in IL-10 KO[14] and Gpx1/Gpx2 double KO mice.[15] In addition, treatment of IL-10-KO with the probiotic *Lactobacillus salivarius* ssp *Salivarius* UCC118 reduces the intensity of mucosal inflammation, decreases the incidence of colon cancer from 50% to 10%, and reduces the census of enterococci, fecal coliforms, and *Clostridium perfringens*.[16] A similar phenomenon has also been noted in the ApcMin model, in which mice raised in a germ-free environment develop 50% fewer adenomas than conventionally raised mice,[17] suggesting that gut microbes play an important role in modulating tumorigenesis. More recent research has suggested that tumorigenesis in some of the ApcMin models may be mediated via selective activation of colonic signal transducer and activator of transcription-3 and TH-17 T-cell responses.[18] Alterations in the colonic microbiota have significant effects on the development of colonic neoplasia, potentially through the production of compounds such as N-nitroso compounds, heterocyclic aromatic amines,[19] and superoxides.[20] Investigators have shown that some microbes can substantially increase the damage related to these compounds whereas others can metabolize and mitigate the damaging effects.[16,21] It seems plausible that changes in the microbial population, either in particular species or in the overall composition of the gut microbiome, may lead to increased chronic inflammation that increases the risk of adenoma and carcinoma development (**Fig. 2**).

Specific bacteria have been shown to induce carcinogenesis in genetically susceptible mice. *Helicobacter hepaticus* is a noncarcinogenic bacterium in most mouse models but has been shown to have significant effects on the transforming growth factor β1 (TGFβ1)/Rag-2 deficient mouse model. These mice do not develop inflammation or cancers in germ-free or specific pathogen-free environments but when colonized with *H hepaticus* they develop both colonic adenomas and carcinomas.[22,23] Recent research suggests that type VI secretion systems may be one mechanism by which *H hepaticus* interacts with intestinal epithelial cells.[24] *Enterococcus faecalis* is an opportunistic microbe that is found in both animals and humans, often as a clinical infection. However, in addition to its role in infectious pathogen, it has been shown to cause dysplasia in the IL-10 KO mouse model, in which 25% of mice colonized with *Enterococcus faecalis* develop rectal dysplasia or carcinoma, whereas germ-free or *Lactococcus lactis* colonized control mice did not.[14] Not all interactions with bacteria are pathogenic, and ongoing research has shown that some microbes have antitumorigenic properties.[25–29]

STREPTOCOCCUS BOVIS

Streptococcus bovis is a gram-positive, nonenterococcal, group D *Streptococcus*, the most well known of which is type I, also known as *Streptococcus gallolyticus*.[30] Approximately 5% to 16% of adults carry *S bovis* as a part of their normal gastrointestinal tract flora.[31] In humans, the clinical manifestations occur when the organism invades the blood stream and causes bacteremia and infective endocarditis. Eleven percent to 12% of infective endocarditis is attributable to *S bovis*,[32,33] making it the second most common streptococcal cause of endocarditis after *Streptococcus viridans*.[34]

The association between colorectal carcinoma and *S bovis* endocarditis was first published in a case report in 1951.[35] Since then, there have been numerous other case reports illustrating the same association.[36–49] A retrospective review in 2004 reported that 6% to 71% of patients with *S bovis* bacteremia had an associated colonic malignancy, as well as an increased number of extracolonic malignancies.[48] This review was confirmed by a more recent systematic review that showed significant variation in reported colorectal cases, ranging from 6% to 67%.[50] Furthermore, 12 studies also included significant associations with either extracolonic malignancies or liver disease. Most studies included in these meta-analyses were limited in size. The largest study was a retrospective analysis by Zarkin[44] that included 92 patients with *S bovis* endocarditis or bacteremia who were evaluated using various modalities, including endoscopy, barium enema, and pathologic specimens. In this study, 58% of

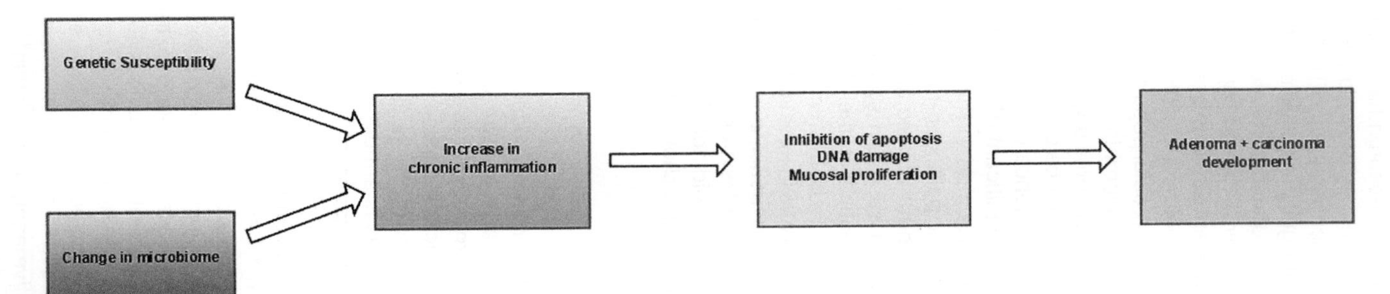

Fig. 2. Possible mechanism by which microbes may induce tumorigenesis. The gut microbiome maintains the colonic epithelium in a state of low-grade physiologic inflammation. Changes in the microbiome, either at a species level or in overall composition, may lead to increased inflammation. Chronic inflammation has been proposed as a mechanism for tumorigenesis.

patients with endocarditis and 46% of patients with bacteremia had colonic disease (defined as polyp, carcinoma, or acute inflammatory conditions such as diverticulitis, colon ischemia, and colitis) and 52% of patients with endocarditis and 57% of patients with bacteremia had liver disease (defined as abnormal liver function tests, chronic passive congestion, cirrhosis, metastatic infiltration, central lobular necrosis, abscess, or nonspecific changes on liver biopsy).[44]

Several studies have compared the rates of colorectal neoplasia between individuals with *S bovis* endocarditis and other forms of infective endocarditis. Leport and colleagues[43] compared the prevalence of colonic polyps and neoplasia in 34 patients with *S bovis* endocarditis against 43 patients with endocarditis from other bacteria and found that there was a significant difference between the 2 groups with respect to both polyps (35% vs 7%) and cancer (26% vs 2%). Two other studies confirmed these findings,[45,46] suggesting that *S bovis* endocarditis is unlike the other forms of infective endocarditis with respect to its association with colorectal neoplasia.

Serologic and stool studies of *S bovis* have shown sometimes conflicting results. Two studies evaluated serum IgG antibody titers to *S bovis* between patients with colorectal cancer and age-matched controls and have shown that antibody titers are significantly higher in individuals with colorectal malignancies than controls, although both of these studies were limited by a small sample size.[51,52] Stool studies have not shown convincing evidence of any association, with studies showing either a positive association[36,53] or no association at all.[51,52,54]

S bovis is hypothesized to induce oncogenesis through an immune-mediated response in the host. Studies have shown that antigens extracted from the cell wall of *S bovis* are able to induce release of CXC chemokines, such as IL-8 (humans) or CINC/GRO (mice), in cell culture as well as overexpression of COX-2.[55–57] These same antigens have also been shown to significantly increase the development of preneoplastic lesions in azoxymethane-treated rats.[55]

Although some studies have failed to show a significant association between *S bovis* infections and colorectal cancers, most published data suggest that *S bovis* is at least an associative risk factor for colorectal neoplasia, with some data suggesting that the organism may have direct oncogenic effects. Based on the available evidence, it is currently recommended that a screening colonoscopy be performed on all individuals with clinically proven *S bovis* endocarditis or bacteremia. Furthermore, with evidence that *S bovis* exposure may be associated with extracolonic malignancies, further care should be taken to monitor for such clinical findings in the appropriate context.

H PYLORI

H pylori is a gram-negative bacterium that is a well-known pathogen in the human stomach.[58] Chronic infection and subsequent inflammation from *H pylori* in the stomach is a known cause of peptic ulcer disease, and its association with gastric cancer has led to it being classified as a class 1 carcinogen by the World Health Organization.[59–61] *H pylori* is believed to be transmitted mostly via a fecal-oral route,[62] with high worldwide infection rates. The EUROGAST study group has reported infection rates as high as 49% through 17 populations throughout the world.[63] Although the relationship between *H pylori* and gastric pathologies has been extensively studied, the association between this bacterium and colorectal cancer is not so well understood.

The association between the presence of *H pylori* antibodies in the serum and colorectal neoplasia has been examined by 16 studies. In 6 of these studies, a statistically significant association was found with an odds ratio (OR) ranging from 1.4 to 4.0,[64–69] although one study showed an inverse association (OR 0.7).[70] The remaining 9 studies revealed no significant associations between *H pylori* seropositivity and colorectal cancer.[71–79] The use of serum antibodies to study the association with colorectal cancer is problematic because of the high prevalence of *H pylori* in the general population, particularly in endemic regions, and because seropositivity does not necessarily indicate active colonization by this microbe.

Because *H pylori* is a difficult microbe to culture, polymerase chain reaction (PCR) studies have also been used to evaluate the presence of *H pylori* in colorectal malignancies. Like the serologic studies, studies using PCR methods have been similarly equivocal. Two studies found that detection of *H pylori* via PCR to be significantly higher in colorectal adenocarcinoma tissue when compared with normal colorectal tissue[80,81] but a third study found that only 1.2% of malignant colorectal tissue samples were positive for *H pylori* compared with 6% of normal tissues.[82]

The C-urea breath test, which has a 97% sensitivity and specificity in *H pylori* detection, has also been used in study[83] but like the PCR-based studies, the evidence is not convincing. One study showed significantly increasing rates of *H pylori* positivity from controls (72.3%) to adenomas (80.7%) to carcinomas (82.5%) in controls versus 80.7% in adenomas (P = .037) versus 82.5% in adenocarcinomas (P = .029) that resulted in OR of 1.6 (95% confidence interval [CI], 1.18–2.02) for adenomas and 1.8 (95% CI, 1.28–2.32) for adenocarcinomas.[84] However, other studies have also shown that there is no significant association between *H pylori* positivity by C-urea breath tests and colorectal adenomas.[85]

The proposed mechanism of carcinogenesis is believed to be caused by inflammation and disruption of the cell cycle. *H pylori* contains a pathogenicity island, cytotoxin-associated gene A (CagA) that binds and activates human phosphatase (SHP2), which acts as an oncoprotein, promoting cell growth.[59] Studies in gastric cancer have shown that the presence of CagA leads to a higher risk of gastric cancer[86,87] and a single study by Shmuely and colleagues[74] did show that the presence of CagA had a significantly increased risk of colorectal cancer with an OR 10.6 (95% CI, 2.7–41.3), although the results of this study have not been replicated. Hypergastrinemia, which is associated with *H pylori* colonization, has also been hypothesized as a possible mechanism for tumorigenesis because of its trophic effect on the intestinal mucosa.[66,88,89] Several studies have evaluated this hypothesis and have found that gastrin levels are increased in patients colonized with *H pylori* who are diagnosed with colorectal cancer.[66,72,77] The results of these studies are difficult to interpret, as it is unclear if the hypergastrinemia is a result of *H pylori* colonization and independent of the colorectal neoplasia.

CLOSTRIDIUM SEPTICUM

Clostridium septicum is a gram-positive, anaerobic spore-forming rod that is a rare but dangerous cause of infection in humans with high rates of mortality.[90] Clinically, in addition to fever, chills, and abdominal pain, it can present with the abrupt onset of nontraumatic myonecrosis, also referred to as gas gangrene, in healthy tissues along with abscess formation, cellulites, and fasciitis.[91] It has been linked with hematologic malignancies, specifically leukemia. However, several case reports have illustrated the association between the development of spontaneous *C septicum* infection and occult colorectal cancer, particularly in patients with diabetes.[91] A systematic review by Panwalker[92] showed an associated colorectal carcinoma is found in roughly 25% of patients with *C septicum* bacteremia, with 75% of all patients diagnosed with some form of malignancy. It is thought that the compromised mucosa overlying a gastrointestinal malignancy serves as an entry point for the organism into the bloodstream.[90] There are no data to suggest that *C septicum* itself has any tumorigenic properties but the development of *C septicum* infection in a patient mandates an investigation for underlying colorectal carcinoma.[90]

ESCHERICHIA COLI

Escherichia coli are rod-shaped, gram-negative bacteria that are normal inhabitants of the human gastrointestinal tract and are among the bacterial species most commonly isolated from stool cultures. Although typically nonpathogenic, *E coli* can become pathogenic through the acquisition of genetic material and is one of the most frequent bacterial causes of diarrhea.[93] *E coli* residing in the lumen of the gastrointestinal tract is considered to be a normal constituent of the gut microbiome but mucosally adherent species may not be.[94] Studies have shown that mucosa-associated and intraepithelial *E coli* are routinely found in the colonic mucosa of patients with colorectal adenocarcinoma, but not in healthy controls.[94,95] Swidsinski and colleagues[94] reported that, in a series of 125 patients, only 3% of colonic mucosal biopsies from asymptomatic controls tested positive for mucosa-adherent bacteria compared with more than 90% of patients with colonic adenomas or carcinomas, with *E coli* and coliform bacteria being the principal organisms in 80% of these patients. In addition, the gentamicin protection assay indicated that *E coli* was partially intracellular in 87% of patients with adenoma and carcinoma and in none of the controls.[94]

A recent mechanistic study by Maddocks and colleagues[96] explored the role of the bacterial adhesion protein intimin produced by enteropathogenic *E coli* and discovered that it could facilitate carcinogenesis by downregulating DNA mismatch repair proteins in colorectal cell lines in vitro, thereby increasing the susceptibility of colonic epithelial cells to developing tumor-promoting mutations. This finding could provide some insight into the mechanisms by which *E coli* may be related to colonic neoplasia.

OTHER STREPTOCOCCAL SPECIES

As discussed earlier, the association between *S bovis* bacteremia, specifically type I, and underlying colonic malignancy is widely recognized. However, some studies have examined the relationship between other streptococcal species and their association with colorectal malignancy, including *Streptococcus salivarius* and *Streptococcus sanguis*. Corredoira and colleagues[97] reported on the clinical significance of *S salivarius* and *S bovis* biotypes I and II recovered from blood cultures and found that bacteremia caused by *S salivarius*, a component of the oral flora in humans,[98] occurred predominantly in patients who developed significant disruption of their mucous membranes and/or serious underlying diseases, specifically cancer. The study failed to show any significantly increased rates of colorectal cancer in patients with *S salivarius* bacteremia when compared with *S bovis* type I or II, indicating that there does not seem to a significant association between this microbe and colorectal malignancies.[97]

Other examples of streptococcal bacteremia in association with underlying colorectal malignancy aside from *S bovis* have been limited apart from a few case reports. Kampe and colleagues[99] reported the first case of *S sanguis* bacteremia in a patient with a liver abscess and a well-differentiated adenocarcinoma of the cecum. *S sanguis* is a normally a commensal organism of the upper aerodigestive tract and rarely the source of positive blood cultures aside from patients with underlying respiratory or oropharyngeal conditions.[100] Since then, there have been several case reports with *S sanguis* bacteremia in association with colorectal malignancy.[99,101–103] In all of these reports, it was presumed that the portal of entry for *S sanguis* into the blood stream was the gastrointestinal tract as a result of breaches in the mucosa from tumor ulceration. No controlled studies have been performed to evaluate the association of *S sanguis* with colorectal malignancies.

ENTEROCOCCUS FAECALIS

Intestinal commensals have long been viewed as a potential contributor to the development of sporadic colorectal cancer in human beings through a variety of mechanisms. *Enterococcus faecalis* is part of the human intestinal microbiota that produces oxygen free radicals including extracellular superoxide that can damage colonic epithelial cell DNA, both in vitro and in vivo.[104] *Enterococcus faecalis* is known to cause increased inflammation as well as colorectal cancer in IL-10 KO mice,[14,105] and this species of bacteria is capable of promoting genomic rearrangements in the form of chromosomal instability in mammalian cells[106] as well as aneuploidy and tetraploidy in colonic epithelial cells.[107] Despite these profound mechanisms by which *Enterococcus faecalis* has been shown to create an environment ripe for malignancy, no studies have shown an association between intestinal colonization with this enterococci and the development of colorectal cancer. A prospective cohort study by Winters and colleagues[108] found that 40% of human stool samples from adults undergoing colonoscopy contained enterococci that produced extracellular superoxide but no association could be established between colonization with extracellular superoxide-producing enterococci and an increased risk for colorectal adenomas or cancer. In addition, follow-up stool studies of these patients 1 year later showed remarkable changes in the enterococcal flora, suggesting that pathologic changes and risk associated with this bacterium are difficult to measure at any single point in time.[108] Despite the impressive mechanisms by which *Enterococcus faecalis* has been shown to induce pathologic changes in colonic epithelium in the laboratory setting, the clinical evidence has not been convincing

HPV

HPV is a double-stranded DNA virus with more than 100 subtypes, some of which infect genital epithelial cells through microscopic abrasions.[109,110] It is the most common sexually transmitted disease among the 15- to 49-year-old age group in the United States.[111] Although most HPV infections are asymptomatic and self-limited, certain types of persistent HPV infections in women have been shown to lead to cancer.[112] The following types have been linked to carcinogenesis: 16, 18, 31, 33, 35, 39, 45, 51, 52, 56, 58, 59, 68, 73, and 82.[110] HPV-16 and HPV-18 have been shown to be the most high risk, with a review by Munoz and colleagues[113] revealing that 70% of cervical cancer cases were positive for type 16, 18, or both. Although HPV is a necessary substrate for cervical cancer, various other types have also been linked to oropharyngeal and urogenital malignancies.[113–115]

Early case reports of an association between HPV infection and colorectal cancers were not supported by the first case studies, which were unable to detect HPV DNA in colorectal cancer tissue.[116–119] However, improvements in detection methods for HPV, specifically with PCR or immunohistochemistry, led to several studies that re-examined the association. These studies compared HPV detection rates between control tissue specimens and colorectal carcinomas. Although the control specimen varied from normal mucosa and simple adenomatous polyps in disease-free patients to normal mucosa from patients with colorectal cancer,[120–127] the results of the studies all showed a positive association between HPV infection and colorectal cancer. The presence of HPV confirmed either by PCR or immunohistochemistry conferred an OR ranging from 2.7 (95% CI, 1.1–6.2) to 9.1 (95% CI, 3.7–22.3).[122,123]

Three large cohort studies have examined the longitudinal risk of colorectal cancer in women with cervical cancer versus the general population.[128–130] The number of patients in these studies ranged from 21,222 to 104,760. Chaturvedi and colleagues[130] reported that cervical cancer survivors who received radiation therapy had an increased risk of anal and rectal cancers. However, the study failed to show an increased risk of cancer in individuals who did not receive radiation therapy, and therefore it is unclear if the increased risk of anorectal cancer was due to HPV or radiation exposure. This finding was supported by 2 other studies that also found no association between cervical cancer and development of colorectal cancer.[128,129]

The tumor suppressor protein p53 plays a significant role in numerous malignancies and has been shown to be mutated in approximately 50% of all colorectal cancers.[131] However, a study by Buyru and colleagues[132] found that in a cohort of 56 HPV-positive colorectal cancers, only 3.6% had mutations in p53, suggesting that HPV may have direct oncogenic effects independent of any mutations in p53. Although HPV-associated tumors often do not have p53 mutations,[133] it was hypothesized by the investigators that HPV may promote carcinogenesis by functionally inactivating p53.[132] Further studies have also suggested that HPV interferes with the tumor suppressor protein, pRb, to promote uncontrolled cell growth via expression of viral proteins E6 and E7.[114] Both these mechanism have been proposed as mechanisms of colorectal carcinogenesis by HPV.

Although several case-control studies have suggested that there is an association between HPV and colorectal carcinoma, most of the data regarding this association are inconclusive. The suggestion that HPV may be directly associated with carcinogenesis, even in the absence of p53 mutations, is an interesting observation that warrants further study.

JC VIRUS

JC virus (JCV) is a polyomavirus that is common in the general population, infecting 70% to 90% of all humans.[134] Most individuals acquire JCV in childhood or adolescence. Although the route of transmission is not known, high levels of JCV in sewage systems suggests fecal-oral transmission as a possible mechanism. The virus remains latent in the gastrointestinal tract and the tubular epithelial cells of the kidney.[135] In immunocompromised patients, the reactivation of the virus can lead to progressive multifocal leukoencephalopathy, a progressive and typically fatal disease.[136]

Most data on the association of JCV and cancer arise from the detection of JCV in central nervous system tumors.[137–139] However, recent studies have examined the potential association between JCV and colorectal cancer.[140–143] In 1999, a study published by Laghi and colleagues[140] compared JCV loads in neoplastic and normal colonic tissue and showed that neoplastic tissue had 1 log higher copies of JCV compared with controls by a semiquantitative PCR method. Two subsequent studies had similar findings with regard to adenomatous tissue.[142,143] Theodoropoulos and colleagues[142] detected JCV in 61% of cancer tissue and 60% of adenomatous tissue versus 30% in normal control tissue. The JCV viral load was also significantly higher in cancer and adenomatous tissue, with a range of 9×10^3 to 20×10^3 copies/μg DNA (mean $\pm$ standard deviation, $14{,}235.16 \pm 3920.59$) compared with normal tissue with a range of 50 to 450 copies/μg DNA (mean value, 242 ± 127.23). Some studies have not been able to confirm these findings.[144,145]

Two studies used JCV serologic testing. Lundstig and colleagues[146] studied JCV seropositivity and colorectal cancer in a nested case-control study. Blood samples were examined from male cases of colorectal cancer and compared with matched controls. There were 386 patients in each arm, and the samples from the cases were collected at least 3 months before the cancer diagnosis. There was no association between JCV seropositivity and the presence of colorectal cancer, with OR of 0.9 (95% CI, 0.7–1.3). This conclusion was supported by another recent nested case-control study[147] in which IgG antibody to JC virus was measured in 611 colorectal cancer cases, 123 adenomatous polyp cases, and matched controls. There was no association between antibodies to JCV and colorectal cancer, with OR 0.91 (95% CI, 0.71–1.17). There was a statistically significant positive association between JCV seropositivity and adenoma diagnosis in men with OR 2.31 (95% CI, 1.20–4.46) and an inverse association in women with OR 0.31 (95% CI, 0.14–0.67) after adjustments for baseline smoking and body mass index (calculated as weight in kilograms divided by the square of height in meters).

There has been some evidence that specific strains of JCV may be more pathogenic. Specifically, a particular variant of the Mad-1 strain of JCV has been shown to have tropism for colorectal tissue.[148] There are several studies that have suggested that one of the viral protein products, the large T-antigen, may be pivotal in JCV oncogenesis.[149,150] An in vitro study showed that the JCV large T-antigen causes chromosomal mutations specifically in colonic epithelial cell lines[151] and that the chromosomal instability is believed to be the result of inhibition of tumor suppression via the binding of large T-antigen with p53 and pRb proteins[152–154]

There seem to be emerging data that JCV may be associated with colorectal malignancies. Many of the studies are more recent, reflecting newer and more reliable methods for detection of the virus. However, until further studies are reported, no specific clinical recommendations regarding the association between JCV and colorectal cancers can be made.

EPSTEIN-BARR VIRUS

Epstein-Barr virus (EBV), also known as human herpesvirus 4 (HHV-4), is a DNA virus known to cause infectious mononucleosis via entry into the orophayngeal epithelium.[155,156] It has strong associations with various Hodgkin and non-Hodgkin lymphomas[157] as well as lymphoepitheliomalike carcinomas of the pharynx, colon, and other sites.[158–160] In addition, studies have linked EBV with conventional epithelial cancers of breast,[161–163] lung,[164–166] and gastric carcinomas.[167,168] The role of EBV in other malignancies has prompted studies of potential associations with colorectal adenocarcinomas.

Three early studies used PCR, immunohistochemistry, and/or fluorescence in situ hybridization (FISH) to detect EBV in primary colorectal carcinoma tissue. Although all 3 studies detected high rates of EBV infection in the colorectal carcinoma tissue,[169–171] only one compared the rates with adjacent normal tissue and found a significant difference in EBV detection.[169] Follow-up studies were unable to show any evidence that EBV was detected at a significantly higher rate in colorectal carcinoma,[172,173] even in higher-risk populations such as patients with inflammatory bowel disease.[174]

There is no convincing evidence that EBV is associated with the development of colorectal carcinoma.

CYTOMEGALOVIRUS

Cytomegalovirus (CMV), also known as human herpes virus 5 (HHV-5), can cause life-threatening infections in immunocompromised patients.[175] The role of CMV in adenocarcinoma of the colon was first suggested by 2 early studies. In 1978, Huang and Roche[176] analyzed 7 adenocarcinoma cases from the colon with cRNA-DNA hybridization and found that 4 of the 7 samples contained more than 2 genome equivalents per cell, whereas controls from normal colons and cases of Crohn disease were negative. A study published soon after detected CMV in 3 of 16 cell cultures derived from colorectal malignancies.[177] A study evaluating serologic patterns in 37 patients with adenocarcinoma of the colon found only that there was a significantly increased IgG antibody titer to CMV in patients treated with chemotherapy,[178] which likely represented infections secondary to the immunosuppression by the chemotherapy rather than an association with the colorectal malignancy. Further studies then showed that CMV was not detected at a significantly higher rate in carcinoma tissue than normal tissue by multiple detection methods, such as FISH, immunohistochemistry, or DNA hybridization.[179,180]

FUTURE DIRECTIONS

The inability to fully characterize the gut microbes has been a significant shortcoming of most of the studies relating to microbial causes of colorectal cancer. Until recently, most studies were limited to studying organisms that are identified by culture-based methods. Advances in sequence-based microbial identification have led to the development of culture-independent characterizations of the gut microbes but given the complexity of the gut microbiome, these methods have been time-consuming and inefficient. Studies using certain techniques, such as 16S rRNA gene denaturing gradient gel electrophoresis, have shown promising results, indicating that alterations of the gut microbiome may be associated with the presence of colorectal cancers.[181]

Investigation of ssrRNA gene sequences has revolutionized the study of microbial ecology, leading to fundamental new insights into the diversity present in the prokaryotic world. Furthermore, it has underscored the major differences between the numbers and type of microbes cultured in the laboratory versus those present in the environment; thus, it has become a well-accepted method for interrogating diversity in environmental samples.[182,183] Diversity measurements using ssrRNA analyses also can be complemented with whole community or metagenomic sequencing. New approaches are constantly being developed to address diversity questions with respect to microbial communities by focusing on the regions of the ribosomal operons that have the highest information content.[184–186] In this setting, molecular analysis of the human microbiome has great potential.[187,188] In particular, 454 sequencing technology has revolutionized our ability to sequence large population samples. This approach allows for parallel sequencing of hundreds of thousands of templates immobilized on microbeads. This technology allows for the generation of more than 100 MB of raw sequence data in a single run, and with forthcoming technical improvements, will approach 0.5GB of data. From the sequence data, phylogenetic relationships can be developed and microbial patterns can be established for bacterial populations of interest. Using this technology, studies have already examined fecal samples from the human gastrointestinal tract,[189,190] highlighting the diversity of microbes associated with the human body and new investigations are under way to evaluate the relationship between the gut microbiome and human disease.[191,192] We anticipate that these techniques will be used to study the relationship between the gut microbes and colorectal cancer in the near future.

SUMMARY

Many infectious agents have been hypothesized to play a role in the development of sporadic colorectal carcinomas, primary by an immune-mediated inflammatory response in the host. *S bovis* is the most well known of the microbes believed to be associated with colorectal cancer, and sufficient evidence exists that patients with *S bovis* infections should be evaluated for colorectal cancer. The data regarding other microbes are limited. Emerging technologies that allow us to comprehensively characterize the gut microbiome may lead to a greater understanding of which organisms or patterns of organisms may be associated with the development of colorectal cancer.

REFERENCES

1. Jemal A, Siegel R, Ward E, et al. Cancer statistics, 2008. CA Cancer J Clin 2008; 58(2):71–96.
2. Jemal A, Thun MJ, Ries LA, et al. Annual report to the nation on the status of cancer, 1975-2005, featuring trends in lung cancer, tobacco use, and tobacco control. J Natl Cancer Inst 2008;100(23):1672–94.
3. Fearon ER, Vogelstein B. A genetic model for colorectal tumorigenesis. Cell 1990;61(5):759–67.
4. Ponz de Leon M, Sassatelli R, Benatti P, et al. Identification of hereditary nonpolyposis colorectal cancer in the general population. The 6-year experience of a population-based registry. Cancer 1993;71(11):3493–501.
5. Potter JD. Colorectal cancer: molecules and populations. J Natl Cancer Inst 1999;91(11):916–32.
6. Balkwill F, Mantovani A. Inflammation and cancer: back to Virchow? Lancet 2001;357(9255):539–45.
7. Eberhart CE, Coffey RJ, Radhika A, et al. Up-regulation of cyclooxygenase 2 gene expression in human colorectal adenomas and adenocarcinomas. Gastroenterology 1994;107(4):1183–8.
8. Sheng H, Shao J, Kirkland SC, et al. Inhibition of human colon cancer cell growth by selective inhibition of cyclooxygenase-2. J Clin Invest 1997;99(9):2254–9.
9. Sano H, Kawahito Y, Wilder RL, et al. Expression of cyclooxygenase-1 and -2 in human colorectal cancer. Cancer Res 1995;55(17):3785–9.
10. Maihofner C, Charalambous MP, Bhambra U, et al. Expression of cyclooxygenase-2 parallels expression of interleukin-1beta, interleukin-6 and NF-kappaB in human colorectal cancer. Carcinogenesis 2003;24(4):665–71.
11. Kim S, Keku TO, Martin C, et al. Circulating levels of inflammatory cytokines and risk of colorectal adenomas. Cancer Res 2008;68(1):323–8.
12. Rhodes JM, Campbell BJ. Inflammation and colorectal cancer: IBD-associated and sporadic cancer compared. Trends Mol Med 2002;8(1):10–6.
13. Kado S, Uchida K, Funabashi H, et al. Intestinal microflora are necessary for development of spontaneous adenocarcinoma of the large intestine in T-cell receptor beta chain and p53 double-knockout mice. Cancer Res 2001;61(6): 2395–8.
14. Balish E, Warner T. Enterococcus faecalis induces inflammatory bowel disease in interleukin-10 knockout mice. Am J Pathol 2002;160(6):2253–7.
15. Chu FF, Esworthy RS, Chu PG, et al. Bacteria-induced intestinal cancer in mice with disrupted Gpx1 and Gpx2 genes. Cancer Res 2004;64(3):962–8.
16. O'Mahony L, Feeney M, O'Halloran S, et al. Probiotic impact on microbial flora, inflammation and tumour development in IL-10 knockout mice. Aliment Pharmacol Ther 2001;15(8):1219–25.
17. Dove WF, Clipson L, Gould KA, et al. Intestinal neoplasia in the ApcMin mouse: independence from the microbial and natural killer (beige locus) status. Cancer Res 1997;57(5):812–4.

18. Wu S, Rhee KJ, Albesiano E, et al. A human colonic commensal promotes colon tumorigenesis via activation of T helper type 17 T cell responses. Nat Med 2009; 15(9):1016–22.
19. Hughes R, Cross AJ, Pollock JR, et al. Dose-dependent effect of dietary meat on endogenous colonic N-nitrosation. Carcinogenesis 2001;22(1):199–202.
20. Huycke MM, Gaskins HR. Commensal bacteria, redox stress, and colorectal cancer: mechanisms and models. Exp Biol Med (Maywood) 2004;229(7):586–97.
21. Horie H, Kanazawa K, Okada M, et al. Effects of intestinal bacteria on the development of colonic neoplasm: an experimental study. Eur J Cancer Prev 1999; 8(3):237–45.
22. Engle SJ, Ormsby I, Pawlowski S, et al. Elimination of colon cancer in germ-free transforming growth factor beta 1-deficient mice. Cancer Res 2002;62(22): 6362–6.
23. Erdman SE, Poutahidis T, Tomczak M, et al. CD4+ CD25+ regulatory T lymphocytes inhibit microbially induced colon cancer in Rag2-deficient mice. Am J Pathol 2003;162(2):691–702.
24. Chow J, Mazmanian SK. A pathobiont of the microbiota balances host colonization and intestinal inflammation. Cell Host Microbe 2010;7(4):265–76.
25. Kim Y, Oh S, Yun HS, et al. Cell-bound exopolysaccharide from probiotic bacteria induces autophagic cell death of tumour cells. Lett Appl Microbiol 2010;51:123–30.
26. Altonsy MO, Andrews SC, Tuohy KM. Differential induction of apoptosis in human colonic carcinoma cells (Caco-2) by Atopobium, and commensal, probiotic and enteropathogenic bacteria: mediation by the mitochondrial pathway. Int J Food Microbiol 2010;137(2-3):190–203.
27. Paolillo R, Romano Carratelli C, Sorrentino S, et al. Immunomodulatory effects of *Lactobacillus plantarum* on human colon cancer cells. Int Immunopharmacol 2009;9(11):1265–71.
28. Jiang SN, Phan TX, Nam TK, et al. Inhibition of tumor growth and metastasis by a combination of *Escherichia coli*-mediated cytolytic therapy and radiotherapy. Mol Ther 2010;18(3):635–42.
29. Ma EL, Choi YJ, Choi J, et al. The anticancer effect of probiotic *Bacillus polyfermenticus* on human colon cancer cells is mediated through ErbB2 and ErbB3 inhibition. Int J Cancer 2010;127(4):780–90.
30. Facklam R. What happened to the streptococci: overview of taxonomic and nomenclature changes. Clin Microbiol Rev 2002;15(4):613–30.
31. Noble CJ. Carriage of group D streptococci in the human bowel. J Clin Pathol 1978;31(12):1182–6.
32. Ballet M, Gevigney G, Gare JP, et al. Infective endocarditis due to *Streptococcus bovis*. A report of 53 cases. Eur Heart J 1995;16(12):1975–80.
33. Kupferwasser I, Darius H, Muller AM, et al. Clinical and morphological characteristics in *Streptococcus bovis* endocarditis: a comparison with other causative microorganisms in 177 cases. Heart 1998;80(3):276–80.
34. Dunham WR, Simpson JH, Feest TG, et al. *Streptococcus bovis* endocarditis and colorectal disease. Lancet 1980;1(8165):421–2.
35. Wc M, Mason JM 3rd. Enterococcal endocarditis associated with carcinoma of the sigmoid; report of a case. J Med Assoc State Ala 1951;21(6):162–6.
36. Klein RS, Recco RA, Catalano MT, et al. Association of *Streptococcus bovis* with carcinoma of the colon. N Engl J Med 1977;297(15):800–2.
37. Klein RS, Catalano MT, Edberg SC, et al. Streptococcus bovis septicemia and carcinoma of the colon. Ann Intern Med 1979;91(4):560–2.

38. Murray HW, Roberts RB. *Streptococcus bovis* bacteremia and underlying gastrointestinal disease. Arch Intern Med 1978;138(7):1097–9.
39. Marshall JB, Gerhardt DC. Polyposis coli presenting with *Streptococcus bovis* endocarditis. Am J Gastroenterol 1981;75(4):314–6.
40. Friedrich IA, Wormser GP, Gottfried EB. The association of recent *Streptococcus bovis* bacteremia with colonic neoplasia. Mil Med 1982;147(7):584–5.
41. Reynolds JG, Silva E, McCormack WM. Association of *Streptococcus bovis* bacteremia with bowel disease. J Clin Microbiol 1983;17(4):696–7.
42. Beeching NJ, Christmas TI, Ellis-Pegler RB, et al. *Streptococcus bovis* bacteraemia requires rigorous exclusion of colonic neoplasia and endocarditis. Q J Med 1985;56(220):439–50.
43. Leport C, Bure A, Leport J, et al. Incidence of colonic lesions in *Streptococcus bovis* and enterococcal endocarditis. Lancet 1987;1(8535):748.
44. Zarkin BA, Lillemoe KD, Cameron JL, et al. The triad of *Streptococcus bovis* bacteremia, colonic pathology, and liver disease. Ann Surg 1990;211(6): 786–91 [discussion: 91–2].
45. Hoen B, Briancon S, Delahaye F, et al. Tumors of the colon increase the risk of developing *Streptococcus bovis* endocarditis: case-control study. Clin Infect Dis 1994;19(2):361–2.
46. Pergola V, Di Salvo G, Habib G, et al. Comparison of clinical and echocardiographic characteristics of *Streptococcus bovis* endocarditis with that caused by other pathogens. Am J Cardiol 2001;88(8):871–5.
47. Waisberg J, Matheus Cde O, Pimenta J. Infectious endocarditis from *Streptococcus bovis* associated with colonic carcinoma: case report and literature review. Arq Gastroenterol 2002;39(3):177–80.
48. Gold JS, Bayar S, Salem RR. Association of *Streptococcus bovis* bacteremia with colonic neoplasia and extracolonic malignancy. Arch Surg 2004;139(7): 760–5.
49. Alazmi W, Bustamante M, O'Loughlin C, et al. The association of *Streptococcus bovis* bacteremia and gastrointestinal diseases: a retrospective analysis. Dig Dis Sci 2006;51(4):732–6.
50. Gupta A, Madani R, Mukhtar H. *Streptococcus bovis* endocarditis; a silent sign for colonic tumour. Colorectal Dis 2010;12:164–71.
51. Darjee R, Gibb AP. Serological investigation into the association between *Streptococcus bovis* and colonic cancer. J Clin Pathol 1993;46(12):1116–9.
52. Tjalsma H, Scholler-Guinard M, Lasonder E, et al. Profiling the humoral immune response in colon cancer patients: diagnostic antigens from *Streptococcus bovis*. Int J Cancer 2006;119(9):2127–35.
53. Burns CA, McCaughey R, Lauter CB. The association of *Streptococcus bovis* fecal carriage and colon neoplasia: possible relationship with polyps and their premalignant potential. Am J Gastroenterol 1985;80(1):42–6.
54. Potter MA, Cunliffe NA, Smith M, et al. A prospective controlled study of the association of *Streptococcus bovis* with colorectal carcinoma. J Clin Pathol 1998;51(6):473–4.
55. Biarc J, Nguyen IS, Pini A, et al. Carcinogenic properties of proteins with proinflammatory activity from *Streptococcus infantarius* (formerly *S. bovis*). Carcinogenesis 2004;25(8):1477–84.
56. Ellmerich S, Scholler M, Duranton B, et al. Promotion of intestinal carcinogenesis by *Streptococcus bovis*. Carcinogenesis 2000;21(4):753–6.
57. Harris RE. Cyclooxygenase-2 (COX-2) and the inflammogenesis of cancer. Subcell Biochem 2007;42:93–126.

58. De Luca A, Iaquinto G. *Helicobacter pylori* and gastric diseases: a dangerous association. Cancer Lett 2004;213(1):1–10.
59. Lochhead P, El-Omar EM. *Helicobacter pylori* infection and gastric cancer. Best Pract Res Clin Gastroenterol 2007;21(2):281–97.
60. Logan RP. *Helicobacter pylori* and gastric cancer. Lancet 1994;344(8929): 1078–9.
61. Parsonnet J, Friedman GD, Vandersteen DP, et al. *Helicobacter pylori* infection and the risk of gastric carcinoma. N Engl J Med 1991;325(16):1127–31.
62. Malaty HM. Epidemiology of *Helicobacter pylori* infection. Best Pract Res Clin Gastroenterol 2007;21(2):205–14.
63. EuroGAST. An international association between *Helicobacter pylori* infection and gastric cancer. The EUROGAST Study Group. Lancet 1993;341(8857): 1359–62.
64. Aydin A, Karasu Z, Zeytinoglu A, et al. Colorectal adenomateous polyps and *Helicobacter pylori* infection. Am J Gastroenterol 1999;94(4):1121–2.
65. Breuer-Katschinski B, Nemes K, Marr A, et al. *Helicobacter pylori* and the risk of colonic adenomas. Colorectal Adenoma Study Group. Digestion 1999;60(3): 210–5.
66. Hartwich A, Konturek SJ, Pierzchalski P, et al. *Helicobacter pylori* infection, gastrin, cyclooxygenase-2, and apoptosis in colorectal cancer. Int J Colorectal Dis 2001;16(4):202–10.
67. Meucci G, Tatarella M, Vecchi M, et al. High prevalence of *Helicobacter pylori* infection in patients with colonic adenomas and carcinomas. J Clin Gastroenterol 1997;25(4):605–7.
68. Mizuno S, Morita Y, Inui T, et al. *Helicobacter pylori* infection is associated with colon adenomatous polyps detected by high-resolution colonoscopy. Int J Cancer 2005;117(6):1058–9.
69. Zumkeller N, Brenner H, Chang-Claude J, et al. *Helicobacter pylori* infection, interleukin-1 gene polymorphisms and the risk of colorectal cancer: evidence from a case-control study in Germany. Eur J Cancer 2007;43(8):1283–9.
70. Moss SF, Neugut AI, Garbowski GC, et al. *Helicobacter pylori* seroprevalence and colorectal neoplasia: evidence against an association. J Natl Cancer Inst 1995;87(10):762–3.
71. Penman ID, el-Omar E, Ardill JE, et al. Plasma gastrin concentrations are normal in patients with colorectal neoplasia and unaltered following tumor resection. Gastroenterology 1994;106(5):1263–70.
72. Thorburn CM, Friedman GD, Dickinson CJ, et al. Gastrin and colorectal cancer: a prospective study. Gastroenterology 1998;115(2):275–80.
73. Fireman Z, Trost L, Kopelman Y, et al. *Helicobacter pylori*: seroprevalence and colorectal cancer. Isr Med Assoc J 2000;2(1):6–9.
74. Shmuely H, Passaro D, Figer A, et al. Relationship between *Helicobacter pylori* CagA status and colorectal cancer. Am J Gastroenterol 2001;96(12): 3406–10.
75. Siddheshwar RK, Muhammad KB, Gray JC, et al. Seroprevalence of *Helicobacter pylori* in patients with colorectal polyps and colorectal carcinoma. Am J Gastroenterol 2001;96(1):84–8.
76. Limburg PJ, Stolzenberg-Solomon RZ, Colbert LH, et al. *Helicobacter pylori* seropositivity and colorectal cancer risk: a prospective study of male smokers. Cancer Epidemiol Biomarkers Prev 2002;11(10 Pt 1):1095–9.
77. Georgopoulos SD, Polymeros D, Triantafyllou K, et al. Hypergastrinemia is associated with increased risk of distal colon adenomas. Digestion 2006;74(1):42–6.

78. Machida-Montani A, Sasazuki S, Inoue M, et al. Atrophic gastritis, *Helicobacter pylori*, and colorectal cancer risk: a case-control study. Helicobacter 2007;12(4): 328–32.
79. D'Onghia V, Leoncini R, Carli R, et al. Circulating gastrin and ghrelin levels in patients with colorectal cancer: correlation with tumour stage, *Helicobacter pylori* infection and BMI. Biomed Pharmacother 2007;61(2–3):137–41.
80. Jones M, Helliwell P, Pritchard C, et al. *Helicobacter pylori* in colorectal neoplasms: is there an aetiological relationship? World J Surg Oncol 2007;5:51.
81. Grahn N, Hmani-Aifa M, Fransen K, et al. Molecular identification of *Helicobacter* DNA present in human colorectal adenocarcinomas by 16s rDNA PCR amplification and pyrosequencing analysis. J Med Microbiol 2005;54(Pt 11): 1031–5.
82. Bulajic M, Stimec B, Jesenofsky R, et al. *Helicobacter pylori* in colorectal carcinoma tissue. Cancer Epidemiol Biomarkers Prev 2007;16(3):631–3.
83. Chen TS, Chang FY, Chen PC, et al. Simplified ^{13}C-urea breath test with a new infrared spectrometer for diagnosis of *Helicobacter pylori* infection. J Gastroenterol Hepatol 2003;18(11):1237–43.
84. Fujimori S, Kishida T, Kobayashi T, et al. *Helicobacter pylori* infection increases the risk of colorectal adenoma and adenocarcinoma, especially in women. J Gastroenterol 2005;40(9):887–93.
85. Liou JM, Lin JW, Huang SP, et al. *Helicobacter pylori* infection is not associated with increased risk of colorectal polyps in Taiwanese. Int J Cancer 2006;119(8): 1999–2000.
86. Beales IL, Crabtree JE, Scunes D, et al. Antibodies to CagA protein are associated with gastric atrophy in *Helicobacter pylori* infection. Eur J Gastroenterol Hepatol 1996;8(7):645–9.
87. Maeda S, Mentis AF. Pathogenesis of *Helicobacter pylori* infection. Helicobacter 2007;12(Suppl 1):10–4.
88. Mulholland G, Ardill JE, Fillmore D, et al. *Helicobacter pylori* related hypergastrinaemia is the result of a selective increase in gastrin 17. Gut 1993;34(6): 757–61.
89. Sobhani I, Lehy T, Laurent-Puig P, et al. Chronic endogenous hypergastrinemia in humans: evidence for a mitogenic effect on the colonic mucosa. Gastroenterology 1993;105(1):22–30.
90. Wentling GK, Metzger PP, Dozois EJ, et al. Unusual bacterial infections and colorectal carcinoma–*Streptococcus bovis* and *Clostridium septicum*: report of three cases. Dis Colon Rectum 2006;49(8):1223–7.
91. Lorimer JW, Eidus LB. Invasive *Clostridium septicum* infection in association with colorectal carcinoma. Can J Surg 1994;37(3):245–9.
92. Panwalker AP. Unusual infections associated with colorectal cancer. Rev Infect Dis 1988;10(2):347–64.
93. Nataro JP, Kaper JB. Diarrheagenic *Escherichia coli*. Clin Microbiol Rev 1998; 11(1):142–201.
94. Swidsinski A, Khilkin M, Kerjaschki D, et al. Association between intraepithelial *Escherichia coli* and colorectal cancer. Gastroenterology 1998;115(2):281–6.
95. Martin HM, Campbell BJ, Hart CA, et al. Enhanced *Escherichia coli* adherence and invasion in Crohn's disease and colon cancer. Gastroenterology 2004; 127(1):80–93.
96. Maddocks OD, Short AJ, Donnenberg MS, et al. Attaching and effacing *Escherichia coli* downregulate DNA mismatch repair protein in vitro and are associated with colorectal adenocarcinomas in humans. PLoS One 2009;4(5):e5517.

97. Corredoira JC, Alonso MP, Garcia JF, et al. Clinical characteristics and significance of *Streptococcus salivarius* bacteremia and *Streptococcus bovis* bacteremia: a prospective 16-year study. Eur J Clin Microbiol Infect Dis 2005;24(4):250–5.
98. Whiley RA, Beighton D. Current classification of the oral streptococci. Oral Microbiol Immunol 1998;13(4):195–216.
99. Kampe CE, Vovan T, Alim A, et al. *Streptococcus sanguis* bacteremia and colorectal cancer: a case report. Med Pediatr Oncol 1995;24(1):67–8.
100. Klein RS, Warman SW, Knackmuhs GG, et al. Lack of association of *Streptococcus bovis* with noncolonic gastrointestinal carcinoma. Am J Gastroenterol 1987;82(6):540–3.
101. Fass R, Alim A, Kaunitz JD. Adenocarcinoma of the colon presenting as *Streptococcus sanguis* bacteremia. Am J Gastroenterol 1995;90(8):1343–5.
102. Macaluso A, Simmang C, Anthony T. *Streptococcus sanguis* bacteremia and colorectal cancer. South Med J 1998;91(2):206–7.
103. Siegert CE, Overbosch D. Carcinoma of the colon presenting as *Streptococcus sanguis* bacteremia. Am J Gastroenterol 1995;90(9):1528–9.
104. Huycke MM, Abrams V, Moore DR. *Enterococcus faecalis* produces extracellular superoxide and hydrogen peroxide that damages colonic epithelial cell DNA. Carcinogenesis 2002;23(3):529–36.
105. Kim SC, Tonkonogy SL, Albright CA, et al. Variable phenotypes of enterocolitis in interleukin 10-deficient mice monoassociated with two different commensal bacteria. Gastroenterology 2005;128(4):891–906.
106. Wang X, Huycke MM. Extracellular superoxide production by *Enterococcus faecalis* promotes chromosomal instability in mammalian cells. Gastroenterology 2007;132(2):551–61.
107. Wang X, Allen TD, May RJ, et al. *Enterococcus faecalis* induces aneuploidy and tetraploidy in colonic epithelial cells through a bystander effect. Cancer Res 2008;68(23):9909–17.
108. Winters MD, Schlinke TL, Joyce WA, et al. Prospective case-cohort study of intestinal colonization with enterococci that produce extracellular superoxide and the risk for colorectal adenomas or cancer. Am J Gastroenterol 1998; 93(12):2491–500.
109. Schiffman M, Kjaer SK. Chapter 2: natural history of anogenital human papillomavirus infection and neoplasia. J Natl Cancer Inst Monogr 2003;31:14–9.
110. Wiley D, Masongsong E. Human papillomavirus: the burden of infection. Obstet Gynecol Surv 2006;61(6 Suppl 1):S3–14.
111. Koutsky L. Epidemiology of genital human papillomavirus infection. Am J Med 1997;102(5A):3–8.
112. Giuliano AR, Harris R, Sedjo RL, et al. Incidence, prevalence, and clearance of type-specific human papillomavirus infections: the Young Women's Health Study. J Infect Dis 2002;186(4):462–9.
113. Munoz N, Bosch FX, de Sanjose S, et al. Epidemiologic classification of human papillomavirus types associated with cervical cancer. N Engl J Med 2003; 348(6):518–27.
114. Steenbergen RD, de Wilde J, Wilting SM, et al. HPV-mediated transformation of the anogenital tract. J Clin Virol 2005;32(Suppl 1):S25–33.
115. D'Souza G, Kreimer AR, Viscidi R, et al. Case-control study of human papillomavirus and oropharyngeal cancer. N Engl J Med 2007;356(19):1944–56.
116. Boguszakova L, Hirsch I, Brichacek B, et al. Absence of cytomegalovirus, Epstein-Barr virus, and papillomavirus DNA from adenoma and adenocarcinoma of the colon. Acta Virol 1988;32(4):303–8.

117. Koulos J, Symmans F, Chumas J, et al. Human papillomavirus detection in adenocarcinoma of the anus. Mod Pathol 1991;4(1):58–61.
118. Shah KV, Daniel RW, Simons JW, et al. Investigation of colon cancers for human papillomavirus genomic sequences by polymerase chain reaction. J Surg Oncol 1992;51(1):5–7.
119. Shroyer KR, Kim JG, Manos MM, et al. Papillomavirus found in anorectal squamous carcinoma, not in colon adenocarcinoma. Arch Surg 1992;127(6):741–4.
120. Bodaghi S, Yamanegi K, Xiao SY, et al. Colorectal papillomavirus infection in patients with colorectal cancer. Clin Cancer Res 2005;11(8):2862–7.
121. Buyru N, Tezol A, Dalay N. Coexistence of K-ras mutations and HPV infection in colon cancer. BMC Cancer 2006;6:115.
122. Cheng JY, Sheu LF, Lin JC, et al. Detection of human papillomavirus DNA in colorectal adenomas. Arch Surg 1995;130(1):73–6.
123. Kirgan D, Manalo P, Hall M, et al. Association of human papillomavirus and colon neoplasms. Arch Surg 1990;125(7):862–5.
124. Lee YM, Leu SY, Chiang H, et al. Human papillomavirus type 18 in colorectal cancer. J Microbiol Immunol Infect 2001;34(2):87–91.
125. McGregor B, Byrne P, Kirgan D, et al. Confirmation of the association of human papillomavirus with human colon cancer. Am J Surg 1993;166(6):738–40 [discussion: 41–2].
126. Perez LO, Abba MC, Laguens RM, et al. Analysis of adenocarcinoma of the colon and rectum: detection of human papillomavirus (HPV) DNA by polymerase chain reaction. Colorectal Dis 2005;7(5):492–5.
127. Zhu Q, Cao J, Li S. [Detection of human papillomavirus gene in biopsies from colon carcinoma by PCR]. Zhonghua Shi Yan He Lin Chuang Bing Du Xue Za Zhi 1999;13(4):352–4 [in Chinese].
128. Weinberg DS, Newschaffer CJ, Topham A. Risk for colorectal cancer after gynecologic cancer. Ann Intern Med 1999;131(3):189–93.
129. Rex D. Should we colonoscope women with gynecologic cancer? Am J Gastroenterol 2000;95(3):812–3.
130. Chaturvedi AK, Engels EA, Gilbert ES, et al. Second cancers among 104,760 survivors of cervical cancer: evaluation of long-term risk. J Natl Cancer Inst 2007;99(21):1634–43.
131. Slattery ML, Curtin K, Schaffer D, et al. Associations between family history of colorectal cancer and genetic alterations in tumors. Int J Cancer 2002;97(6):823–7.
132. Buyru N, Budak M, Yazici H, et al. P53 gene mutations are rare in human papillomavirus-associated colon cancer. Oncol Rep 2003;10(6):2089–92.
133. Tommasino M, Accardi R, Caldeira S, et al. The role of TP53 in cervical carcinogenesis. Hum Mutat 2003;21(3):307–12.
134. Walker DL, Padgett BL. The epidemiology of human polyomaviruses. Prog Clin Biol Res 1983;105:99–106.
135. Khalili K, Del Valle L, Otte J, et al. Human neurotropic polyomavirus, JCV, and its role in carcinogenesis. Oncogene 2003;22(33):5181–91.
136. Hou J, Major EO. Progressive multifocal leukoencephalopathy: JC virus induced demyelination in the immune compromised host. J Neurovirol 2000;6(Suppl 2): S98–100.
137. Krynska B, Del Valle L, Croul S, et al. Detection of human neurotropic JC virus DNA sequence and expression of the viral oncogenic protein in pediatric medulloblastomas. Proc Natl Acad Sci U S A 1999;96(20):11519–24.
138. Caldarelli-Stefano R, Boldorini R, Monga G, et al. JC virus in human glial-derived tumors. Hum Pathol 2000;31(3):394–5.

139. Del Valle L, Gordon J, Assimakopoulou M, et al. Detection of JC virus DNA sequences and expression of the viral regulatory protein T-antigen in tumors of the central nervous system. Cancer Res 2001;61(10):4287–93.
140. Laghi L, Randolph AE, Chauhan DP, et al. JC virus DNA is present in the mucosa of the human colon and in colorectal cancers. Proc Natl Acad Sci U S A 1999; 96(13):7484–9.
141. Ricciardiello L, Laghi L, Ramamirtham P, et al. JC virus DNA sequences are frequently present in the human upper and lower gastrointestinal tract. Gastroenterology 2000;119(5):1228–35.
142. Theodoropoulos G, Panoussopoulos D, Papaconstantinou I, et al. Assessment of JC polyoma virus in colon neoplasms. Dis Colon Rectum 2005;48(1):86–91.
143. Hori R, Murai Y, Tsuneyama K, et al. Detection of JC virus DNA sequences in colorectal cancers in Japan. Virchows Arch 2005;447(4):723–30.
144. Hernandez Losa J, Fernandez-Soria V, Parada C, et al. JC virus and human colon carcinoma: an intriguing and inconclusive association. Gastroenterology 2003;124(1):268–9 [author reply: 69–70].
145. Newcomb PA, Bush AC, Stoner GL, et al. No evidence of an association of JC virus and colon neoplasia. Cancer Epidemiol Biomarkers Prev 2004;13(4):662–6.
146. Lundstig A, Stattin P, Persson K, et al. No excess risk for colorectal cancer among subjects seropositive for the JC polyomavirus. Int J Cancer 2007; 121(5):1098–102.
147. Rollison DE, Helzlsouer KJ, Lee JH, et al. Prospective study of JC virus seroreactivity and the development of colorectal cancers and adenomas. Cancer Epidemiol Biomarkers Prev 2009;18(5):1515–23.
148. Ricciardiello L, Chang DK, Laghi L, et al. Mad-1 is the exclusive JC virus strain present in the human colon, and its transcriptional control region has a deleted 98-base-pair sequence in colon cancer tissues. J Virol 2001;75(4):1996–2001.
149. Haggerty S, Walker DL, Frisque RJ. JC virus-simian virus 40 genomes containing heterologous regulatory signals and chimeric early regions: identification of regions restricting transformation by JC virus. J Virol 1989;63(5):2180–90.
150. Bollag B, Chuke WF, Frisque RJ. Hybrid genomes of the polyomaviruses JC virus, BK virus, and simian virus 40: identification of sequences important for efficient transformation. J Virol 1989;63(2):863–72.
151. Ricciardiello L, Baglioni M, Giovannini C, et al. Induction of chromosomal instability in colonic cells by the human polyomavirus JC virus. Cancer Res 2003; 63(21):7256–62.
152. Niv Y, Goel A, Boland CR. JC virus and colorectal cancer: a possible trigger in the chromosomal instability pathways. Curr Opin Gastroenterol 2005;21(1): 85–9.
153. Staib C, Pesch J, Gerwig R, et al. P53 inhibits JC virus DNA replication in vivo and interacts with JC virus large T-antigen. Virology 1996;219(1):237–46.
154. Khalili K, Del Valle L, Wang JY, et al. T-antigen of human polyomavirus JC cooperates with IGF-IR signaling system in cerebellar tumors of the childhood-medulloblastomas. Anticancer Res 2003;23(3A):2035–41.
155. Epstein MA, Achong BG, Barr YM. Virus particles in cultured lymphoblasts from Burkitt's lymphoma. Lancet 1964;1(7335):702–3.
156. Niederman JC, McCollum RW, Henle G, et al. Infectious mononucleosis. Clinical manifestations in relation to EB virus antibodies. JAMA 1968;203(3):205–9.
157. Preciado MV, De Matteo E, Diez B, et al. Presence of Epstein-Barr virus and strain type assignment in Argentine childhood Hodgkin's disease. Blood 1995; 86(10):3922–9.

158. Kieff E. Epstein-Barr virus–increasing evidence of a link to carcinoma. N Engl J Med 1995;333(11):724–6.
159. Samaha S, Tawfik O, Horvat R, et al. Lymphoepithelioma-like carcinoma of the colon: report of a case with histologic, immunohistochemical, and molecular studies for Epstein-Barr virus. Dis Colon Rectum 1998;41(7):925–8.
160. Zubizarreta PA, D'Antonio G, Raslawski E, et al. Nasopharyngeal carcinoma in childhood and adolescence: a single-institution experience with combined therapy. Cancer 2000;89(3):690–5.
161. Labrecque LG, Barnes DM, Fentiman IS, et al. Epstein-Barr virus in epithelial cell tumors: a breast cancer study. Cancer Res 1995;55(1):39–45.
162. Bonnet M, Guinebretiere JM, Kremmer E, et al. Detection of Epstein-Barr virus in invasive breast cancers. J Natl Cancer Inst 1999;91(16):1376–81.
163. Fina F, Romain S, Ouafik L, et al. Frequency and genome load of Epstein-Barr virus in 509 breast cancers from different geographical areas. Br J Cancer 2001;84(6):783–90.
164. Castro CY, Ostrowski ML, Barrios R, et al. Relationship between Epstein-Barr virus and lymphoepithelioma-like carcinoma of the lung: a clinicopathologic study of 6 cases and review of the literature. Hum Pathol 2001;32(8):863–72.
165. Han AJ, Xiong M, Gu YY, et al. Lymphoepithelioma-like carcinoma of the lung with a better prognosis. A clinicopathologic study of 32 cases. Am J Clin Pathol 2001;115(6):841–50.
166. Wong MP, Chung LP, Yuen ST, et al. In situ detection of Epstein-Barr virus in non-small cell lung carcinomas. J Pathol 1995;177(3):233–40.
167. Koriyama C, Akiba S, Iriya K, et al. Epstein-Barr virus-associated gastric carcinoma in Japanese Brazilians and non-Japanese Brazilians in Sao Paulo. Jpn J Cancer Res 2001;92(9):911–7.
168. Takada K. Epstein-Barr virus and gastric carcinoma. Mol Pathol 2000;53(5):255–61.
169. Song LB, Zhang X, Zhang CQ, et al. Infection of Epstein-Barr virus in colorectal cancer in Chinese. Ai Zheng 2006;25(11):1356–60.
170. Liu HX, Ding YQ, Li X, et al. Investigation of Epstein-Barr virus in Chinese colorectal tumors. World J Gastroenterol 2003;9(11):2464–8.
171. Liu HX, Ding YQ, Sun YO, et al. Detection of Epstein-Barr virus in human colorectal cancer by in situ hybridization. Di Yi Jun Yi Da Xue Xue Bao 2002;22(10):915–7.
172. Grinstein S, Preciado MV, Gattuso P, et al. Demonstration of Epstein-Barr virus in carcinomas of various sites. Cancer Res 2002;62(17):4876–8.
173. Yuen ST, Chung LP, Leung SY, et al. In situ detection of Epstein-Barr virus in gastric and colorectal adenocarcinomas. Am J Surg Pathol 1994;18(11):1158–63.
174. Wong NA, Herbst H, Herrmann K, et al. Epstein-Barr virus infection in colorectal neoplasms associated with inflammatory bowel disease: detection of the virus in lymphomas but not in adenocarcinomas. J Pathol 2003;201(2):312–8.
175. Griffiths PD, Walter S. Cytomegalovirus. Curr Opin Infect Dis 2005;18(3):241–5.
176. Huang ES, Roche JK. Cytomegalovirus D.N.A. and adenocarcinoma of the colon: evidence for latent viral infection. Lancet 1978;1(8071):957–60.
177. Hashiro GM, Horikami S, Loh PC. Cytomegalovirus isolations from cell cultures of human adenocarcinomas of the colon. Intervirology 1979;12(2):84–8.
178. Avni A, Haikin H, Feuchtwanger MM, et al. Antibody pattern to human cytomegalovirus in patients with adenocarcinoma of the colon. Intervirology 1981;16(4):244–9.

179. Hart H, Neill WA, Norval M. Lack of association of cytomegalovirus with adenocarcinoma of the colon. Gut 1982;23(1):21–30.
180. Ruger R, Fleckenstein B. Cytomegalovirus DNA in colorectal carcinoma tissues. Klin Wochenschr 1985;63(9):405–8.
181. Scanlan PD, Shanahan F, Clune Y, et al. Culture-independent analysis of the gut microbiota in colorectal cancer and polyposis. Environ Microbiol 2008;10(3):789–98.
182. DeLong EF, Preston CM, Mincer T, et al. Community genomics among stratified microbial assemblages in the ocean's interior. Science 2006;311(5760):496–503.
183. Schloss PD, Handelsman J. Metagenomics for studying unculturable microorganisms: cutting the Gordian knot. Genome Biol 2005;6(8):229.
184. Chakravorty S, Helb D, Burday M, et al. A detailed analysis of 16s ribosomal RNA gene segments for the diagnosis of pathogenic bacteria. J Microbiol Methods 2007;69(2):330–9.
185. Kysela DT, Palacios C, Sogin ML. Serial analysis of V6 ribosomal sequence tags (SARST-V6): a method for efficient, high-throughput analysis of microbial community composition. Environ Microbiol 2005;7(3):356–64.
186. Sogin ML, Morrison HG, Huber JA, et al. Microbial diversity in the deep sea and the underexplored "rare biosphere". Proc Natl Acad Sci U S A 2006;103(32):12115–20.
187. Weng L, Rubin EM, Bristow J. Application of sequence-based methods in human microbial ecology. Genome Res 2006;16(3):316–22.
188. Turnbaugh PJ, Ley RE, Hamady M, et al. The human microbiome project. Nature 2007;449(7164):804–10.
189. Eckburg PB, Bik EM, Bernstein CN, et al. Diversity of the human intestinal microbial flora. Science 2005;308(5728):1635–8.
190. Gill SR, Pop M, Deboy RT, et al. Metagenomic analysis of the human distal gut microbiome. Science 2006;312(5778):1355–9.
191. Ley RE, Backhed F, Turnbaugh P, et al. Obesity alters gut microbial ecology. Proc Natl Acad Sci U S A 2005;102(31):11070–5.
192. Ley RE, Turnbaugh PJ, Klein S, et al. Microbial ecology: human gut microbes associated with obesity. Nature 2006;444(7122):1022–3.

Future Perspectives on Infections Associated with Gastrointestinal Tract Diseases

Guy D. Eslick, PhD, MMedSc(Clin Epi), MMedStat

KEYWORDS

• Gastrointestinal • Infection • Molecular techniques • Future
• Technology

CHANGING BURDEN OF GASTROINTESTINAL DISEASE

In 2004, in the United States, there were 72 million presentations with a primary diagnosis of a digestive disease and 104 million presentations with combined gastrointestinal (GI) tract diseases and other diseases (**Table 1**).[1] It was also found that those who are older tend to have more GI problems, there was no difference in the rates of digestive disease between the African Americans and the whites, and women were 20% more likely to present than men with digestive diseases. Thus, more than one-third (35%) of all presentations are for digestive diseases. In 2009, in the United States, the cancer statistics revealed 275,720 new cases of GI cancer, with colorectal and pancreatic cancer in the top 10 for both men and women.[2] There were 135,830 deaths due to GI cancer, with colorectal, pancreatic, hepatic, and esophageal cancers in the top 10 for both men and women, except for esophageal cancer, which was only listed for men (**Fig. 1**).[2] Furthermore, 2 of these 3 cancers that have an increasing mortality were GI tract cancers for both genders, with esophageal and hepatic cancers among men and pancreatic and hepatic cancers among women. Worldwide the rates of digestive diseases are staggering.

From 1979 to 1989, in the United States, a decrease was observed in the ambulatory care visits and hospital discharges for digestive diseases. These rates remained constant between 1990 and 1999, until 2000 when the rates climbed dramatically and was still increasing in 2004 (**Fig. 2**).[1] During this period, substantial increases in the

Conflict of Interest: None.
The Whiteley-Martin Research Centre, Discipline of Surgery, Nepean Hospital, The University of Sydney, Level 5, South Block, PO Box 63, Penrith, New South Wales 2751, Australia
E-mail address: eslickg@med.usyd.edu.au

Infect Dis Clin N Am 24 (2010) 1041–1058
doi:10.1016/j.idc.2010.08.002 **id.theclinics.com**
0891-5520/10/$ – see front matter

Table 1
Burden of selected digestive diseases in the United States, 2004

Digestive Disease	Deaths, Underlying Cause[a]	Years of Potential Life Lost to Age 75 Years[a]	Ambulatory Care Visits, All-Listed Diagnoses[b]	Hospital Discharges, All-Listed Diagnoses[c]
All Digestive Diseases	236,164	2,007,500	104,790,000	13,533,000
All Digestive Cancers	135,107	945,200	4,198,000	726,000
Colorectal Cancer	53,226	333,000	2,589,000	255,000
Pancreatic Cancer	31,800	206,800	415,000	68,000
Esophageal Cancer	13,667	113,800	372,000	44,000
Gastric Cancer	11,253	84,200	141,000	31,000
Primary Liver Cancer	6323	72,400	63,000	33,000
Bile Duct Cancer	4954	32,900	—	17,000
Gall Bladder Cancer	1939	10,900	—	6000
Cancer of the Small Intestine	1115	9300	—	9000
Liver Disease	36,090	559,100	2,398,000	759,000
All Viral Hepatitis	5393	101,800	3,510,000	475,000
Hepatitis C	4595	87,500	2,747,000	419,000
Hepatitis B	645	11,800	729,000	69,000
Hepatitis A	58	800	—	10,000
GI Infections	4396	12,800	2,365,000	450,000
Peptic Ulcer Disease	3692	19,700	1,473,000	489,000
Pancreatitis	3480	42,800	881,000	454,000

Diverticular Disease	3372	8600	3,269,000	815,000
Abdominal Wall Hernia	1172	6900	4,787,000	372,000
Gastroesophageal Reflux Disease	1150	6000	18,342,000	3,189,000
Gallstones	1092	4400	1,836,000	622,000
All Inflammatory Bowel Disease	933	9100	1,892,000	221,000
Crohn Disease	622	7000	1,176,000	141,000
Ulcerative Colitis	311	2000	716,000	82,000
Appendicitis	453	5000	782,000	325,000
All Functional Intestinal Disorders	423	2500	11,648,000	1,241,000
Chronic Constipation	137	900	6,306,000	700,000
Irritable Bowel Syndrome	20	0	3,054,000	212,000
Hemorrhoids	14	200	3,275,000	306,000

[a] Vital statistics of the United States.
[b] The National Ambulatory Medical Care Survey and the National Hospital Ambulatory Medical Care Survey.
[c] The Healthcare Cost and Use Project Nationwide Inpatient Sample.

Data from Everhart JE, editor. The burden of digestive diseases in the United States. US Department of Health and Human Services, Public Health Service, National Institutes of Health, National Institute of Diabetes and Digestive and Kidney Diseases. Washington, DC: US Government Printing Office, 2008; NIH Publication No. 09–6443; p. 6–7.

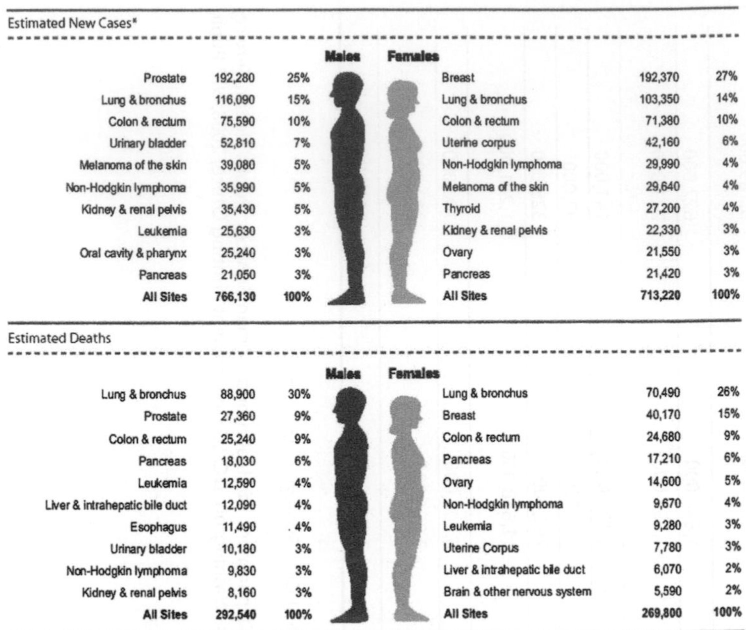

Estimated New Cases*

Males			Females		
Prostate	192,280	25%	Breast	192,370	27%
Lung & bronchus	116,090	15%	Lung & bronchus	103,350	14%
Colon & rectum	75,590	10%	Colon & rectum	71,380	10%
Urinary bladder	52,810	7%	Uterine corpus	42,160	6%
Melanoma of the skin	39,080	5%	Non-Hodgkin lymphoma	29,990	4%
Non-Hodgkin lymphoma	35,990	5%	Melanoma of the skin	29,640	4%
Kidney & renal pelvis	35,430	5%	Thyroid	27,200	4%
Leukemia	25,630	3%	Kidney & renal pelvis	22,330	3%
Oral cavity & pharynx	25,240	3%	Ovary	21,550	3%
Pancreas	21,050	3%	Pancreas	21,420	3%
All Sites	**766,130**	**100%**	**All Sites**	**713,220**	**100%**

Estimated Deaths

Males			Females		
Lung & bronchus	88,900	30%	Lung & bronchus	70,490	26%
Prostate	27,360	9%	Breast	40,170	15%
Colon & rectum	25,240	9%	Colon & rectum	24,680	9%
Pancreas	18,030	6%	Pancreas	17,210	6%
Leukemia	12,590	4%	Ovary	14,600	5%
Liver & intrahepatic bile duct	12,090	4%	Non-Hodgkin lymphoma	9,670	4%
Esophagus	11,490	4%	Leukemia	9,280	3%
Urinary bladder	10,180	3%	Uterine Corpus	7,780	3%
Non-Hodgkin lymphoma	9,830	3%	Liver & intrahepatic bile duct	6,070	2%
Kidney & renal pelvis	8,160	3%	Brain & other nervous system	5,590	2%
All Sites	**292,540**	**100%**	**All Sites**	**269,800**	**100%**

Fig. 1. The 10 leading cancer types among the estimated new cancer cases and deaths, by sex, in the United States in 2009. (*From* Jemal A, Siegel R, Ward E, et al. Cancer statistics, 2009. CA Cancer J Clin 2009;59:225–49; with permission.)

prevalence were observed for certain GI tract diseases, including gastroesophageal reflux disease (GERD) with an increase of 376 per 100,000 population, hepatitis C with 79 per 100,000 population, chronic constipation with 62 per 100,000 population, intestinal infections with 41 per 100,000 population, and pancreatitis with 23 per 100,000 population.[1]

The prevalence of digestive diseases around the world is enormous and varies from country to country (**Table 2**). Worldwide there has been a dynamic shift in the epidemiology of GI tract diseases, with some diseases such as peptic ulcer decreasing dramatically since the discovery of *Helicobacter pylori* infection and a larger number of conditions increasing, such as GERD, nonalcoholic fatty liver disease, diverticular disease, Barrett esophagus, cholelithiasis, alcoholic liver disease, hepatitis C, chronic pancreatitis, esophageal cancer and colorectal cancer.[3–8] In conjunction with this increasing incidence of digestive diseases are the re-emergence of certain infectious agents (**Box 1**) (eg, cholera) and the identification of new agents (eg, *H pylori*, *Laribacter*, *Campylobacter concisus*), which are associated with GI tract diseases.[9] Since the discovery of *H pylori* there has been an enormous interest in the relationship between microorganisms and GI tract diseases, including cancers.

CAUSE-AND-EFFECT ISSUES

One of the main issues associated with infections and disease is determining the relationship of the cause and effect. The landmark article by Sir Austin Bradford Hill in 1965 titled The environment and disease: association or causation? became widely known as the Bradford Hill's criteria.[10] There were 8 criteria that were required to

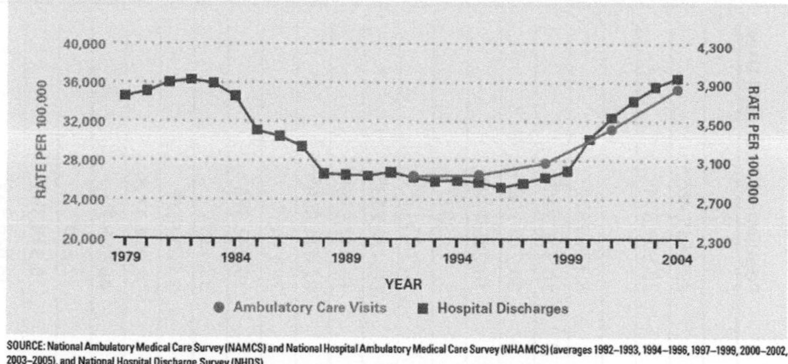

Fig. 2. For all digestive diseases, age-adjusted rates of ambulatory care visits and hospital discharges with all-listed diagnoses in the United States from 1979 to 2004. (*From* Everhart JE, editor. The burden of digestive diseases in the United States. US Department of Health and Human Services, Public Health Service, National Institutes of Health, National Institute of Diabetes and Digestive and Kidney Diseases. Washington, DC: US Government Printing Office, 2008; NIH Publication No. 09–6443 p. 6–7.

be met to determine a cause-and-effect relationship (**Box 2**). It is usually difficult to meet all these criteria, particularly when trying to find the cause-and-effect relationships between organisms in the small intestine or colon because of the large number of organisms living in these environments. Even for *H pylori* infection and the relationship with gastric cancer, although it is currently the only bacterium classified as a class I carcinogen, the evidence supporting this relationship is not complete in terms of Bradford Hill's criteria.

ORGANISMS ASSOCIATED WITH GI TRACT DISEASES

There are a large number of organisms believed to be responsible for diseases of the digestive system. Some of these organisms are true pathogens, whereas others are merely commensal in nature and are unlikely to ever produce any pathologic condition. **Table 3** shows the various types of microbes that are associated with diseases of the GI tract covered in this issue; it is by no means all-inclusive but provides the current magnitude of an ever-increasing field of research. At present, some of these diseases are only associated with a single group of organisms (eg, irritable bowel syndrome), whereas other diseases are affected by all groups of organisms (eg, appendicitis).

FUTURE CHALLENGES

There are a variety of methodological and technical issues related to infectious agents and their role in digestive diseases. For diseases of the colon, the major limitation remains the inability to completely identify these organisms. Identification of bacteria was mainly conducted using culture-based methods. Now, the focus in identification of bacteria is increasingly based on using molecular techniques. Many of these techniques allow the detection and identification of viable but nonculturable cells that are metabolically active but not reproducing. Gene sequencing using single-stranded RNA has been a key method in being able to elucidate multitudes of organisms that remain unknown. At present, there are approximately 9000 bacterial species, and this number is estimated as just the tip of the iceberg. The development of molecular

Table 2
Estimates of digestive disease burden around the world

Country/Region	Extrapolated Prevalence	Population Estimated Used
Digestive Diseases in North America (Extrapolated Statistics)		
United States of America	64,776,924	293,655,405[a]
Canada	7,170,854	32,507,874[b]
Digestive Diseases in Europe (Extrapolated Statistics)		
Austria	1,803,256	8,174,7622
Belgium	2,282,707	10,348,276[b]
Britain (United Kingdom)	13,295,008	60,270,708 for UK[b]
Czech Republic	274,892	10,246,178[b]
Denmark	1,194,130	5,413,392[b]
Finland	1,150,259	5,214,512[b]
France	13,328,869	60,424,213[b]
Greece	2,348,719	10,647,529[b]
Germany	18,181,898	82,424,609[b]
Iceland	64,845	293,966[b]
Hungary	2,213,023	10,032,375[b]
Liechtenstein	7375	33,436[b]
Ireland	875,637	3,969,558[b]
Italy	12,806,795	58,057,477[b]
Luxembourg	102,063	462,690[b]
Monaco	7118	32,270[b]
Netherlands (Holland)	3,599,602	16,318,199[b]
Poland	8,520,517	38,626,349[b]
Portugal	2,321,502	10,524,145[b]
Spain	8,885,465	40,280,780[b]

Sweden	1,982,294	8,986,400[b]
Switzerland	1,643,573	7,450,867[b]
United Kingdom	13,295,008	60,270,708[b]
Wales	643,676	2,918,000[b]
Digestive Diseases in the Balkans (Extrapolated Statistics)		
Albania	781,942	3,544,808[b]
Bosnia and Herzegovina	89,913	407,608[b]
Croatia	991,956	4,496,869[b]
Macedonia	450,018	2,040,085[b]
Serbia and Montenegro	2,388,066	10,825,900[b]
Digestive Diseases in Asia (Extrapolated Statistics)		
Bangladesh	31,178,044	141,340,476[b]
Bhutan	482,110	2,185,569[b]
China	286,510,493	1,298,847,624[b]
East Timor	224,834	1,019,252[b]
Hong Kong SAR	1,512,159	6,855,125[b]
India	234,942,036	1,065,070,607[b]
Indonesia	52,599,913	238,452,952[b]
Japan	28,088,161	127,333,002[b]
Laos	1,338,555	6,068,117[b]
Macau SAR	98,224	445,286[b]
Malaysia	5,188,782	23,522,482[b]
Mongolia	606,907	2,751,314[b]
Philippines	19,023,902	86,241,697[b]
Papua New Guinea	1,195,649	5,420,280[b]
Vietnam	18,234,440	82,662,800[b]
Singapore	960,417	4,353,893[b]

(continued on next page)

Table 2
(*continued*)

Country/Region	Extrapolated Prevalence	Population Estimated Used
Pakistan	35,116,837	159,196,336[b]
North Korea	5,006,812	22,697,553[b]
South Korea	10,639,799	48,233,760[b]
Sri Lanka	4,390,845	19,905,165[b]
Taiwan	5,018,346	22,749,838[b]
Thailand	14,308,570	64,865,523[b]
Digestive Diseases in Eastern Europe (Extrapolated Statistics)		
Azerbaijan	1,735,673	7,868,385[b]
Belarus	2,274,379	10,310,520[b]
Bulgaria	1,658,376	7,517,973[b]
Estonia	295,955	1,341,664[b]
Georgia	1,035,417	4,693,892[b]
Kazakhstan	3,340,522	15,143,704[b]
Latvia	508,743	2,306,306[b]
Lithuania	795,860	3,607,899[b]
Romania	4,931,371	22,355,551[b]
Russia	31,758,982	143,974,059[b]
Slovakia	1,196,375	5,423,567[b]
Slovenia	443,707	2,011,473[b]
Tajikistan	1,546,666	7,011,556[b]
Ukraine	10,529,134	47,732,079[b]
Uzbekistan	5,825,826	26,410,416[b]
Digestive Diseases in Australasia and Southern Pacific (Extrapolated Statistics)		
Australia	4,392,605	19,913,144[b]
New Zealand	880,989	3,993,817[b]

Digestive Diseases in the Middle East (Extrapolated Statistics)		
Afghanistan	6,289,781	28,513,677[b]
Egypt	16,790,606	76,117,421[b]
Gaza Strip	292,277	1,324,991[b]
Iran	14,890,412	67,503,205[b]
Iraq	5,597,358	25,374,691[b]
Israel	1,367,428	6,199,008[b]
Jordan	1,237,765	5,611,202[b]
Kuwait	497,988	2,257,549[b]
Lebanon	833,209	3,777,218[b]
Libya	1,242,261	5,631,585[b]
Saudi Arabia	5,690,280	25,795,938[b]
Syria	3,974,310	18,016,874[b]
Turkey	15,197,187	68,893,918[b]
United Arab Emirates	556,745	2,523,915[b]
West Bank	509,824	2,311,204[b]
Yemen	4,417,249	20,024,867[b]
Digestive Diseases in South America (Extrapolated Statistics)		
Belize	60,208	272,945[b]
Brazil	40,610,537	184,101,109[b]
Chile	3,490,578	15,823,957[b]
Colombia	9,333,258	42,310,775[b]
Guatemala	3,150,131	14,280,596[b]
Mexico	23,152,850	104,959,594[b]
Nicaragua	1,182,299	5,359,759[b]
Paraguay	1,365,742	6,191,368[b]
Peru	6,075,949	27,544,305[b]
Puerto Rico	859,844	3,897,960[b]
Venezuela	5,518,541	25,017,387[b]

(continued on next page)

Table 2
(continued)

Country/Region	Extrapolated Prevalence	Population Estimated Used
Digestive Diseases in Africa (Extrapolated Statistics)		
Angola	2,421,739	10,978,552[b]
Botswana	361,595	1,639,231[b]
Central African Republic	825,547	3,742,482[b]
Chad	2,104,090	9,538,544[b]
Congo Brazzaville	661,332	2,998,040[b]
Congo Kinshasa	12,864,050	58,317,030[b]
Ethiopia	15,736,007	71,336,571[b]
Ghana	4,578,756	20,757,032[b]
Kenya	7,275,464	32,982,109[b]
Liberia	747,934	3,390,635[b]
Niger	2,506,000	11,360,538[b]
Nigeria	3,915,519	125,750,356[b]
Rwanda	1,817,354	8,238,673[b]
Senegal	2,393,855	10,852,147[b]
Sierra Leone	1,297,916	5,883,889[b]
Somalia	1,831,897	8,304,601[b]
Sudan	8,635,623	39,148,162[b]
South Africa	9,804,809	44,448,470[b]
Swaziland	257,920	1,169,241[b]
Tanzania	7,956,793	36,070,799[b]
Uganda	5,821,380	26,390,258[b]
Zambia	2,432,137	11,025,690[b]
Zimbabwe	809,969	12,671,860[b]

Abbreviation: SAR, special administrative region.
[a] US Census Bureau, population estimates, 2004.
[b] US Census Bureau, international database, 2004.

Box 1
List of the National Institute of Allergy and Infectious Diseases on emerging and re-emerging diseases

Group I: pathogens newly recognized in the past 2 decades

Acanthamebiasis

Australian bat Lyssavirus

Babesia, atypical

Bartonella henselae

Ehrlichiosis

Encephalitozoon cuniculi

Encephalitozoon hellem

Enterocytozoon bieneusi

H pylori

Hendra or equine *morbillivirus*

Hepatitis C

Hepatitis E

Human herpesvirus 8

Human herpesvirus 6

Lyme borreliosis

Parvovirus B19

Group II: re-emerging pathogens

Enterovirus 71

Clostridium difficile

Mumps virus

Streptococcus, group A

Staphylococcus aureus

Group III: Agents with bioterrorism potential

National Institute of Allergy and Infectious Diseases (NIAID): category A

- *Bacillus anthracis* (anthrax)
- *Clostridium botulinum* toxin (botulism)
- *Yersinia pestis* (plague)
- Variola major (smallpox) and other related poxviruses
- *Francisella tularensis* (tularemia)
- Viral hemorrhagic fevers
- Arenaviruses: lymphocytic choriomeningitis virus, Junin virus, Machupo virus, Guanarito virus, Lassa fever
- Bunyaviruses: Hantaviruses, Rift Valley fever, Flaviviruses, dengue virus
- Filoviruses: Ebola, Marburg

NIAID: category B

- *Burkholderia pseudomallei*

Coxiella burnetii (Q fever)

Brucella species (brucellosis)

Burkholderia mallei (glanders)

Chlamydia psittaci (psittacosis)

Ricin toxin (from *Ricinus communis*)

Epsilon toxin of *Clostridium perfringens*

Staphylococcus enterotoxin B

Typhus fever (*Rickettsia prowazekii*)

Food- and waterborne pathogens

Diarrheagenic *Escherichia coli*

Pathogenic vibrios

Shigella species

Salmonella

Listeria monocytogenes

Campylobacter jejuni

Yersinia enterocolitica

Viruses (Caliciviruses, Hepatitis A)

Protozoa: *Cryptosporidium parvum*, *Cyclospora cayetanensis*, *Giardia lamblia*, *Entamoeba histolytica*, *Toxoplasma*

Fungi

Microsporidia

Additional viral encephalitides: West Nile virus, La Crosse virus, California encephalitis virus, Venezuelan equine encephalitis virus, Eastern equine encephalitis virus, Western equine encephalitis, Japanese encephalitis virus, Kyasanur forest virus

NIAID: category C

Emerging infectious disease threats such as Nipah virus and additional hantaviruses

NIAID priority areas

Tick-borne hemorrhagic fever viruses: Crimean-Congo hemorrhagic fever virus

Tick-borne encephalitis viruses

Yellow fever

Multidrug-resistant tuberculosis

Influenza

Other rickettsias

Rabies

Prions

Chikungunya virus

Severe acute respiratory syndrome–associated coronavirus

Antimicrobial resistance, excluding research on sexually transmitted organisms

Research on mechanisms of antimicrobial resistance

Studies of the emergence and/or spread of antimicrobial resistance genes within pathogen populations

Studies of the emergence and/or spread of antimicrobial-resistant pathogens in human populations

Research on therapeutic approaches that target resistance mechanisms

Modification of existing antimicrobials to overcome emergent resistance

Antimicrobial research, as related to engineered threats and naturally occurring drug-resistant pathogens, focused on the development of broad-spectrum antimicrobials

Innate immunity, defined as the study of nonadaptive immune mechanisms that recognize, and respond to, microorganisms, microbial products, and antigens

Coccidioides immitis

Coccidioides posadasii

methods offers great promise not only in research and development but also in the diagnostic setting (eg, stool samples) (**Table 4**).[11,12] Clearly, metagenomics, in which genetic material is directly retrieved from environmental sources, will play a critical role in the future development of determining infectious agents of the GI tract. The use of high-throughput technology has already produced important findings in relation to the GI tract microflora, including the differences between adults and children, with numerous uncultured organisms being the crux of the normal human adult gut flora which remain stable but other organisms change depending on environmental and genetic factors, whereas in infants there appear to be a constant transformation of organisms over time (**Figs. 3** and **4**).[11] There have been several new detection methods developed, with some of these using nanoscale electrochemical detectors and others using DNA sensors (extrachromosomal DNA).[13] The use of stable-isotope probing is also being investigated, but even this technique has limitations.[14] Although these technologies are increasing the understanding of the gut microflora, there remains large gaps of knowledge regarding the metabolic functions of these organisms and the relationship they have with human GI disease. These will be extremely fruitful areas of research and development in the coming years.

Box 2
Bradford Hill's criteria for causality

Consistency: The association is consistent when results are replicated in studies in different settings using different methods.

Strength: This is defined by the size of the risk as measured by appropriate statistical tests.

Specificity: This is established when a single putative cause produces a specific effect.

Dose-response relationship: An increasing level of exposure (in amount and/or time) increases the risk.

Temporal relationship: Exposure always precedes the outcome.

Biologic plausibility: The association agrees with currently accepted understanding of pathobiologic processes. This criterion should be applied with caution.

Coherence: The association should be compatible with existing theory and knowledge.

Experiment: The condition can be altered by an appropriate experimental regimen. Experiment is possibly the most important support for a causal relationship.

Table 3
Organisms associated with GI tract disease in humans

GI Tract Disease	Bacteria	Virus	Parasite	Fungi
Esophageal Cancer	α-hemolytic streptococcus, β-hemolytic streptococcus, *Bacteroides fragilis*, *Bacteroides melaninogenicus*, *Bacteroides* sp, *Clostridium* sp, coagulase-negative *Staphylococcus*, *Corynebacterium* sp, *Escherichia coli*, *Fusobacteria* sp, *Haemophilus influenzae*, *Lactobacillus* sp, *Neisseria catarrhalis*, nonhemolytic streptococcus, *Peptococcus*, *Pneumococcus*, *Proteus mirabilis*, *Staphylococcus albus*, *Staphylococcus aureus*, *Streptococcus pyogenes*, *Streptococcus viridans*, *Candida albicans* *Mycobacterium avium*, *Mycobacterium tuberculosis*	Cytomegalovirus, Epstein-Barr virus, Herpes simplex virus, Varicella-zoster virus	Cryptosporidium	Histoplasma capsulatum,
Gastric Cancer	*H pylori*	Epstein-Barr virus	—	—
Cholangiocarcinoma	—	Hepatitis C virus, Hepatitis B virus	*Clonorchis sinensis*, *Opistochus vivarini*	—
Gall Bladder Disease	*E coli*, *H pylori*, *Helicobacter* sp, Enterobacteriaceae, Leptospira, *Salmonella enteritidis*, *Salmonella typhi*, *Staphylococcus aureus*, *Micrococcus* sp	Cytomegalovirus, Epstein-Barr virus, Dengue virus	*C sinensis*, *O vivarini*, *Ascaris lumbricoides*, *Dolosigranulum pigrum*	*Actinomyces* sp, *Candida* sp,
Hepatocellular Carcinoma	—	Hepatitis B virus, Hepatitis C virus	—	—

Acute Pancreatitis	*Mycoplasma pneumoniae, S typhi, Leptospira, Yersinia enterocolitica, Yersinia pseudotuberculosis, Campylobacter jejuni, M tuberculosis, M avium, Legionella* sp, *Brucellosis, Actinomyces, Nocardia*	Measles virus, Coxsackie B virus, hepatitis B virus, Cytomegalovirus, herpes simplex virus, varicella virus, human immunodeficiency virus, Epstein-Barr virus, vaccinia, rubella, adenovirus	*A lumbricoides, Echinococcus granulosus*	*Aspergillus* sp, *Cryptococcus neoformans, Coccidioides immitis, Paracoccidioides brasiliensis, Histoplasma capsulatum, Pneumocystis carinii*
Small Intestinal Bacterial Overgrowth	*Streptococcus* sp, *E coli, Staphylococcus* sp, *Micrococcus* sp, *Klebsiella* sp, *Methanobrevibacter smithii, Bacteroides* sp, *Firmicutes* sp	—	—	—
Irritable Bowel Syndrome	*Salmonella* sp, *Campylobacter* sp, *Shigella* sp, Enterobacteriaceae, Clostridia	—	—	—
Inflammatory Bowel Disease	*E coli, M avium, Streptococcus* sp, Clostridia, Actinobacteria, Proteobacteria, *Clostridium leptum, Faecalibacterium prausnitzii, Bacteroides,* Fusobacteria	—	—	—
Appendicitis	*Y enterocolitica, Y pseudotuberculosis, Actinomyces israelii, Mycobacterium, C jejuni, Clostridium difficile, Salmonella* sp, *B fragilis*	Adenovirus, cytomegalovirus, measles virus (rubeola virus)	*A lumbricoides, Enterobius vermicularis, Strongyloides stercoralis, Schistosomiasis haematobium, Entamoeba histolytica, Trichuris* sp	Mucormycosis, histoplasma capsulatum
Colorectal Cancer	*Helicobacter hepaticus, Enterococcus faecalis, Streptococcus bovis, H pylori, Clostridium septicum, E coli, Streptococcus sanguis, Streptococcus salivarius*	Human papillomavirus, JC virus, Epstein-Barr virus, cytomegalovirus	—	—

Table 4
Automatic nucleic acid extraction methods from bacteria

Instrument	Method	Number of Samples	Time Required
ABI PRISM 6100 nucleic acid PrepStation (Applied Biosystems)	Silica membrane bind/elute protocols with vacuum processing (RNA and DNA)	Up to 96	30 min
ABI PRISM 6700 automated nucleic acid workstation (Applied Biosystems)	Silica membrane bind/elute protocols with vacuum processing (RNA and DNA)	Up to 96	90 min
BioRobot EZ1 workstation (QIAGEN)	Silica membrane bind/elute protocols using magnetic-particle handling (RNA and DNA)	1–6	15–20 min
iPrep Purification Instrument (Invitrogen)	Based on a unique, ionizable nucleic acid-binding ligand whose charge can be switched based on the pH of the surrounding medium (DNA)	Up to 12	18 min
KingFisher ML/96 (Thermo Scientific)	Silica membrane bind/elute protocols using magnetic-particle handling (RNA and DNA)	1–96	20–30 min
MagNA pure compact/LC (Roche Applied Science)	Silica membrane bind/elute protocols using magnetic-particle handling (RNA and DNA)	1–32	15–40 min
Maxwell 16 Instrument (Promega)	Silica membrane bind/elute protocols using magnetic-particle handling (RNA and DNA)	Up to 16	30 min
NucliSens miniMAG (BioMérieux)	Silica membrane bind/elute protocols using magnetic-particle handling (RNA and DNA)	Up to 12	45 min
QIAcube (QIAGEN)	Silica membrane bind/elute protocols with built in centrifuge (RNA and DNA)	Up to 12	60 min, user-developed protocols
X-Tractor Gene RNA/DNA Extraction System (Corbett Life Science)	Silica membrane bind/elute protocols with vacuum processing (RNA and DNA)	8–96	1 h

Data from Barken KB, Haagensen JA, Tolker-Nielsen T. Advances in nucleic acid-based diagnostics of bacterial infections. Clin Chim Acta 2007;384:1–11.

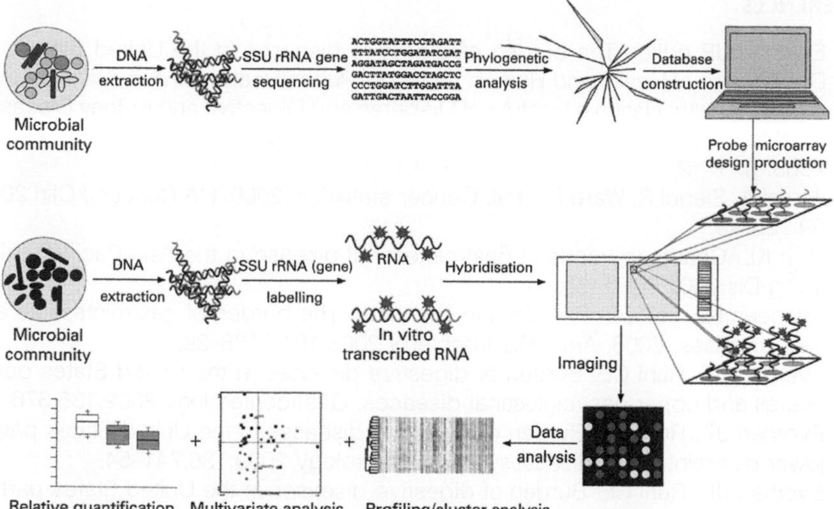

Fig. 3. High-throughput analysis of human GI tract microbiota via brute force sequencing and phylogenetic microarray analysis. SSU rRNA, small subunit ribosomal RNA. (*From* Zoetendal EG, Rajilic-Stojanovic M, de Vos WM. High-throughput diversity and functionality analysis of the gastrointestinal tract microbiota. Gut 2008;57:1605–15; with permission.)

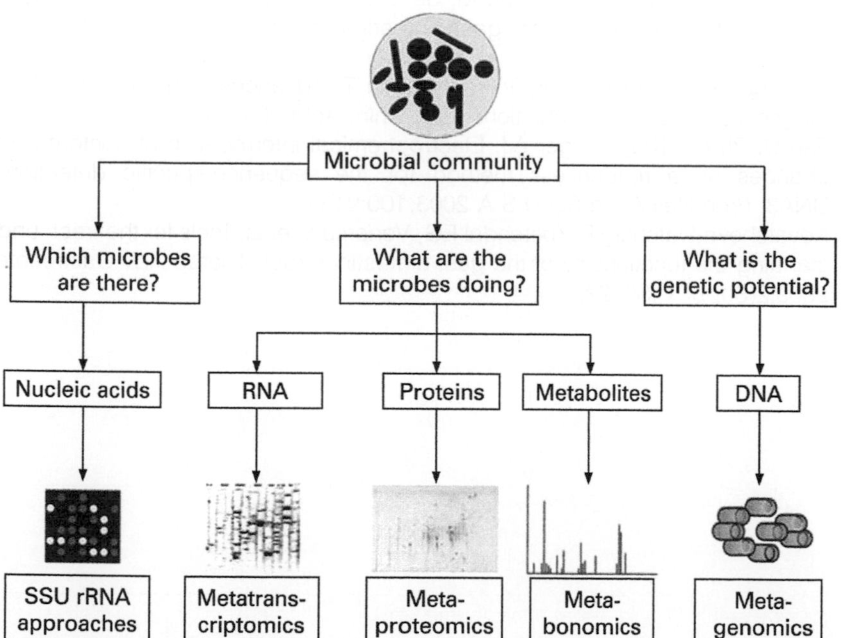

Fig. 4. Metagenomics and other community-based "omics" approaches. SSU rRNA, small subunit ribosomal RNA. (*From* Zoetendal EG, Rajilic-Stojanovic M, de Vos WM, High-throughput diversity and functionality analysis of the gastrointestinal tract microbiota. Gut 2008;57:1605–15, with permission.)

REFERENCES

1. Everhart JE editor. The burden of digestive diseases in the United States. US Department of Health and Human Services, Public Health Service, National Institutes of Health, National Institute of Diabetes and Digestive and Kidney Diseases. Washington, DC: US Government Printing Office. NIH Publication No. 09–6443; 2008. p. 1–12
2. Jemal A, Siegel R, Ward E, et al. Cancer statistics, 2009. CA Cancer J Clin 2009; 59:225–49.
3. Goh KL. Changing trends in gastrointestinal disease in the Asia-Pacific region. J Dig Dis 2007;8:179–85.
4. Shaheen NJ, Hansen RA, Morgan DR, et al. The burden of gastrointestinal and liver diseases, 2006. Am J Gastroenterol 2006;101:2128–38.
5. Everhart JE, Ruhl CE. Burden of digestive diseases in the United States part I: overall and upper gastrointestinal diseases. Gastroenterology 2009;136:376–86.
6. Everhart JE, Ruhl CE. Burden of digestive diseases in the United States part II: lower gastrointestinal diseases. Gastroenterology 2009;136:741–54.
7. Everhart JE, Ruhl CE. Burden of digestive diseases in the United States part III: liver, biliary tract, and pancreas. Gastroenterology 2009;136:1134–44.
8. Hellier MD, Williams JG. The burden of gastrointestinal disease: implications for the provision of care in the UK. Gut 2007;56:165–6.
9. Schlenker C, Surawicz C. Emerging infections of the gastrointestinal tract. Best Pract Res Clin Gastroenterol 2009;23:89–99.
10. Hill AB. The environment and disease: association or causation? Proc R Soc Med 1965;58:295–300.
11. Zoetendal EG, Rajilic-Stojanovic M, de Vos WM. High-throughput diversity and functionality analysis of the gastrointestinal tract microbiota. Gut 2008;57: 1605–15.
12. Barken KB, Haagensen JA, Tolker-Nielsen T. Advances in nucleic acid-based diagnostics of bacterial infections. Clin Chim Acta 2007;384:1–11.
13. Fan C, Plaxco KW, Heeger AJ. Electrochemical interrogation of conformational changes as a reagentless method for the sequence-specific detection of DNA3. Proc Natl Acad Sci U S A 2003;100:9134–7.
14. Kovatcheva-Datchary P, Zoetendal EG, Venema V, et al. Tools for the tract: understanding the functionality of the gastrointestinal tract. Therap Adv Gastroenterol 2009;2(Suppl 1):S9–22.

Index

Note: Page numbers of article titles are in **boldface** type.

Infect Dis Clin N Am 24 (2010) 1059–1066
doi:10.1016/S0891-5520(10)00082-6

D

J

L

M

N

O

P

R

S

T

V

Y

United States Postal Service

Statement of Ownership, Management, and Circulation
(All Periodicals Publications Except Requestor Publications)

1. Publication Title	2. Publication Number	3. Filing Date
Infectious Disease Clinics of North America	0 0 1 - 5 5 6	9/15/10
4. Issue Frequency: Mar, Jun, Sep, Dec	5. Number of Issues Published Annually: 4	6. Annual Subscription Price: $235.00

7. Complete Mailing Address of Known Office of Publication (*Not printer*) (*Street, city, county, state, and ZIP+4®*)

Elsevier Inc.
360 Park Avenue South
New York, NY 10010-1710

Contact Person: Stephen Bushing
Telephone (Include area code): 215-239-3688

8. Complete Mailing Address of Headquarters or General Business Office of Publisher (*Not printer*)

Elsevier Inc., 360 Park Avenue South, New York, NY 10010-1710

9. Full Names and Complete Mailing Addresses of Publisher, Editor, and Managing Editor (*Do not leave blank*)

Publisher (*Name and complete mailing address*)

Kim Murphy, Elsevier, Inc., 1600 John F. Kennedy Blvd. Suite 1800, Philadelphia, PA 19103-2899

Editor (*Name and complete mailing address*)

Barbara Cohen-Kligerman, Elsevier, Inc., 1600 John F. Kennedy Blvd. Suite 1800, Philadelphia, PA 19103-2899

Managing Editor (*Name and complete mailing address*)

Catherine Bewick, Elsevier, Inc., 1600 John F. Kennedy Blvd. Suite 1800, Philadelphia, PA 19103-2899

10. Owner (*Do not leave blank. If the publication is owned by a corporation, give the name and address of the corporation immediately followed by the names and addresses of all stockholders owning or holding 1 percent or more of the total amount of stock. If not owned by a corporation, give the names and addresses of the individual owners. If owned by a partnership or other unincorporated firm, give its name and address as well as those of each individual owner. If the publication is published by a nonprofit organization, give its name and address.*)

Full Name	Complete Mailing Address
Wholly owned subsidiary of	4520 East-West Highway
Reed/Elsevier, US holdings	Bethesda, MD 20814

11. Known Bondholders, Mortgagees, and Other Security Holders Owning or Holding 1 Percent or More of Total Amount of Bonds, Mortgages, or Other Securities. If none, check box → ☐ None

Full Name	Complete Mailing Address
N/A	

12. Tax Status (*For completion by nonprofit organizations authorized to mail at nonprofit rates*) (*Check one*)
The purpose, function, and nonprofit status of this organization and the exempt status for federal income tax purposes:
☐ Has Not Changed During Preceding 12 Months
☐ Has Changed During Preceding 12 Months (*Publisher must submit explanation of change with this statement*)

PS Form 3526, September 2007 (Page 1 of 3 (Instructions Page 3)) PSN 7530-01-000-9931 **PRIVACY NOTICE:** See our Privacy policy in www.usps.com

13. Publication Title: Infectious Disease Clinics of North America

14. Issue Date for Circulation Data Below: September 2010

15. Extent and Nature of Circulation		Average No. Copies Each Issue During Preceding 12 Months	No. Copies of Single Issue Published Nearest to Filing Date
a. Total Number of Copies (*Net press run*)		1621	1524
b. Paid Circulation (By Mail and Outside the Mail)	(1) Mailed Outside-County Paid Subscriptions Stated on PS Form 3541. (*Include paid distribution above nominal rate, advertiser's proof copies, and exchange copies*)	882	807
	(2) Mailed In-County Paid Subscriptions Stated on PS Form 3541 (*Include paid distribution above nominal rate, advertiser's proof copies, and exchange copies*)		
	(3) Paid Distribution Outside the Mails Including Sales Through Dealers and Carriers, Street Vendors, Counter Sales, and Other Paid Distribution Outside USPS®	261	258
	(4) Paid Distribution by Other Classes Mailed Through the USPS (e.g. First-Class Mail®)		
c. Total Paid Distribution (*Sum of 15b (1), (2), (3), and (4)*) ►		1143	1065
d. Free or Nominal Rate Distribution (By Mail and Outside the Mail)	(1) Free or Nominal Rate Outside-County Copies Included on PS Form 3541	70	69
	(2) Free or Nominal Rate In-County Copies Included on PS Form 3541		
	(3) Free or Nominal Rate Copies Mailed at Other Classes Through the USPS (e.g. First-Class Mail)		
	(4) Free or Nominal Rate Distribution Outside the Mail (Carriers or other means)		
e. Total Free or Nominal Rate Distribution (Sum of 15d (1), (2), (3) and (4))		70	69
f. Total Distribution (Sum of 15c and 15e) ►		1213	1134
g. Copies not Distributed (See instructions to publishers #4 (page #3)) ►		408	390
h. Total (Sum of 15f and g)		1621	1524
i. Percent Paid (15c divided by 15f times 100) ►		94.23%	93.92%

16. Publication of Statement of Ownership

If the publication is a general publication, publication of this statement is required. Will be printed in the **December 2010** issue of this publication. | Publication not required

17. Signature and Title of Editor, Publisher, Business Manager, or Owner

Stephen R. Bushing – Fulfillment/Inventory Specialist — Date: September 15, 2010

I certify that all information furnished on this form is true and complete. I understand that anyone who furnishes false or misleading information on this form or who omits material or information requested on the form may be subject to criminal sanctions (including fines and imprisonment) and/or civil sanctions (including civil penalties).

PS Form 3526, September 2007 (Page 2 of 3)

Moving?

Make sure your subscription moves with you!

To notify us of your new address, find your **Clinics Account Number** (located on your mailing label above your name), and contact customer service at:

Email: journalscustomerservice-usa@elsevier.com

800-654-2452 **(subscribers in the U.S. & Canada)**
314-447-8871 **(subscribers outside of the U.S. & Canada)**

Fax number: 314-447-8029

Elsevier Health Sciences Division
Subscription Customer Service
3251 Riverport Lane
Maryland Heights, MO 63043

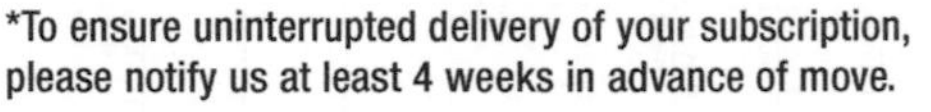

*To ensure uninterrupted delivery of your subscription, please notify us at least 4 weeks in advance of move.

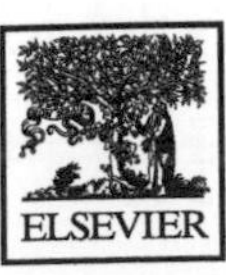

Printed and bound by CPI Group (UK) Ltd, Croydon, CR0 4YY
23/10/2024
01778007-0001